Synthesis Lectures on Biomedical Engineering

This series consists of concise books on advanced and state-of-the-art topics that span the field of biomedical engineering. Each Lecture covers the fundamental principles in a unified manner, develops underlying concepts needed for sequential material, and progresses to more advanced topics and design. The authors selected to write the Lectures are leading experts on the subject who have extensive background in theory, application, and design. The series is designed to meet the demands of the 21st century technology and the rapid advancements in the all-encompassing field of biomedical engineering.

Vytautas Ostasevicius · Vytautas Jurenas ·
Mantas Venslauskas · Laura Kizauskiene

Noninvasive Therapeutic Technologies

Stimulation of Physiological Processes

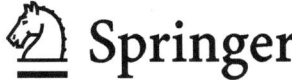

Vytautas Ostasevicius
Institute of Mechatronics
Kaunas University of Technology
Kaunas, Lithuania

Mantas Venslauskas
Institute of Mechatronics
Kaunas University of Technology
Kaunas, Lithuania

Vytautas Jurenas
Institute of Mechatronics
Kaunas University of Technology
Kaunas, Lithuania

Laura Kizauskiene
Faculty of Informatics
Kaunas University of Technology
Kaunas, Lithuania

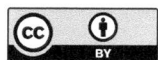

ISSN 1930-0328   ISSN 1930-0336 (electronic)
Synthesis Lectures on Biomedical Engineering
ISBN 978-3-031-79024-9   ISBN 978-3-031-79025-6 (eBook)
https://doi.org/10.1007/978-3-031-79025-6

This work was supported by Kauno Technologijos Universitetas.

This Springer imprint is published by the registered company Springer Nature Switzerland AG
The registered company address is: Gewerbestrasse 11, 6330 Cham, Switzerland

If disposing of this product, please recycle the paper.

Preface

According to the World Health Organization, the number of people over the age of 65 in Europe will increase to 70% by 2050, and the number of people over the age of 80–170%. In addition to the benefits of drug-based treatment methods, the medical community and people with disabilities need noninvasive smart technologies and tools that can be applied to be applied to improve health outcomes. Since human organ systems work according to the laws of physiology, dynamic activation of these processes increases the therapeutic effect. This book is a comprehensive work that uses digital twins and artificial intelligence to focus on the development of noninvasive technologies that improve blood circulation. It presents the authors' solutions published in the scientific press and protected by patents. Methods of hemodynamic activation and blood bioparticle separation are proposed. The revealed characteristics of the therapeutic effect allow to choose the most appropriate modes of vibration, ultrasound, electromagnetic, or other effects for effective therapy. The focus is on low-cost, portable therapy equipment adapted to the clinical and patient home environment. The developed equipment protects against mechanical or thermal damage to biological tissues. After obtaining ethical clearances, the advantages of the equipment have been demonstrated in ex vivo and in vivo applications.

This research was funded by special program "Information technologies for the development of science and knowledge society" grant (P-ITP-24-3) from the Research Council of Lithuania.

Kaunas, Lithuania
November 2024

Vytautas Ostasevicius
Vytautas Jurenas
Mantas Venslauskas
Laura Kizauskiene

Contents

A Narrative Review of Noninvasive Therapy

1.1   Introduction

This chapter discusses the current theoretical and practical applications of ultrasound-assisted or vibratory blood flow activation and bioparticle separation technologies. The disadvantages of high megahertz ultrasound, which is widely used in medical practice for diagnostic and sometimes therapeutic purposes, are related to the limited penetration depth of the acoustic signal, the scattered effect on biological tissues and the overheating. Emphasis is placed on the use of ultrasound to activate the delivery of drugs to the target by disrupting the biofilm covering the bacteria and, at the same time, to activate the effect of antibiotics in the treatment of inflammatory processes. The effect of ultrasound on cardiac valve vascular plaques and wound healing is analyzed. Efforts to mitigate the effects of COVID-19 are becoming increasingly important in the management of pulmonary hypertension. The application of artificial intelligence is accelerating the diagnosis of ailments and the effectiveness of treatment at the origin of the disease. While many studies have looked at the effects of whole-body vibration, the treatment of diabetes and arthritis also requires the use of specific body part therapies. This is particularly important for wheelchair users or people with other mobility problems, as they are unable to stimulate the blood circulation naturally. Ultrasonic excitation in micro-channels for single bioparticles or centrifugation to extract more of them from the blood involves stationary equipment that is not suitable for use in emergency situations.

© The Author(s) 2025   1
V. Ostasevicius et al., *Noninvasive Therapeutic Technologies*, Synthesis Lectures on
Biomedical Engineering, https://doi.org/10.1007/978-3-031-79025-6_1

1.2   Therapeutic Applications of Ultrasound

The primary function of the blood is to deliver oxygen and nutrients to the body cells, and to remove waste from them. Specific functions of the blood also include defense, and maintain homeostasis, such as distributing heat where it is needed. The benefits of ultrasound for the blood have not yet been fully disclosed. Medical ultrasound can be classified into diagnostic ultrasound and therapeutic ultrasound. Diagnostic ultrasound is used to assess health conditions, while therapeutic ultrasound is used to treat health problems. The safety of ultrasound exposure is crucial to the patient's well-being. According to the standard of the World Federation of Ultrasound in Medicine and Biology, and the Food and Drug Administration (USA), the acoustic intensity emitted by medical ultrasound diagnostic equipment must not exceed 720 mW/cm^2 in the frequency range of 1–10 MHz [1]. Experiments on the effect of ultrasound on fat lipolysis have shown that an acoustic intensity of 800–1000 mW/cm^2 and an ultrasound frequency of 1 MHz, the effective depth, or living body fat lipolysis, is 0.9 cm for muscle and 1.7 cm for fat [2], while for biological tissue, the penetration depth of ultrasound at this frequency is 3–5 cm, which increases with decreasing ultrasound frequency. The acoustic intensity of ultrasound decreases exponentially as it penetrates deeper into biological tissue. The attenuation coefficient of biological tissues is proportional to the frequency of ultrasound applied to the human body. It means that low-frequency (20–100 kHz) ultrasound would be suitable to therapeutically affect deeper internal organs.

The results of the study of the effect of high-frequency (3 MHz) continuous ultrasound on blood cells of rats are presented in paper [3]. The analysis revealed that platelets, hematocrit, and hemoglobin levels were significantly different between the experimental and sham groups and indicated that high-frequency ultrasound could reduce hematocrit and hemoglobin levels. The findings of this study, presenting the harmful hematological effects of continuous high-frequency ultrasound, may change our attitude towards the frequent careless diagnostic use of ultrasound in clinics. On the other hand, new aspects of the therapeutic use of ultrasound are suggested for consideration.

Vascular endothelial dysfunction is a pathological condition characterized mainly by an imbalance between vasodilators and vasoconstrictors and is thought to play an important role in the development of atherosclerotic cardiovascular disease. A study [4] showed that pulsed and continuous wave high-frequency ultrasound improved endothelium-dependent vasodilation in patients with Type 2 diabetes mellitus. Further studies should investigate the effect of therapeutic ultrasound on local vascular complications in patients with diabetes. This therapeutic resource is a non-pharmacological, non-invasive, inexpensive, and easy-to-use tool to improve endothelial function in Type 2 diabetes mellitus patients. The article [5] reviews the status of high and low focused ultrasound in the treatment of atherosclerosis. It summarises the findings of studies in animal models and in humans concerning the effects of ultrasound on arterial plaques and arterial wall thrombolysis in carotid, coronary and peripheral arteries. The potential advantages of focused ultrasound, including its noninvasiveness, precise targeting, and real-time monitoring capabilities, are highlighted as an attractive modality for the treatment of atherosclerosis.

A study [6] has shown that low-intensity focused ultrasound stimulation of the vagus nerve can modulate blood pressure. Compared with baseline and control groups, a sustained significant decrease in the ratio of blood pressure, pulse rate, respiratory rate, normalised low-frequency heart rate variability power and low-to-high-frequency heart rate variability power was found, indicating suppression of sympathetic nervous system activity.

Red blood cells (RBCs) or erythrocytes are innate carriers that can also be engineered to improve the pharmacokinetics and pharmacodynamics of many drugs, especially biotherapeutics. It has been shown that many drugs can be successfully loaded both inside and on the outer surface of erythrocytes (RBCs), including anti-inflammatory, antimicrobial and antithrombotic drugs. The article [7] shows that low-frequency ultrasound (20–100 kHz) improves the transdermal transport of various drugs by increasing the permeability of the skin for a variety of low molecular weight drugs as well as for high molecular weight drugs. Onychomycosis (fungal infection of the nail plate) and psoriasis are the two most common nail diseases. Onychomycosis is usually treated with oral antifungal drugs, while psoriasis requires repeated monthly corticosteroid injections into the nail folds, which are limited by the very poor permeability of the drug to the nail plate. Work [8] shows increased drug permeability to the nail through ultrasound-treated bovine hoof membranes, while the work [9] discusses the possibilities of improving drug delivery to the anterior and posterior segments of the eye and shows that ultrasound-induced biological effects reduce the barriers to drug delivery to the eye.

The COVID-19 pandemic has intensified the use of antibiotics and accelerated the development of pathogen resistance, posing a serious threat to global public health. A promising synergistic bactericidal effect of low frequency ultrasound with antibiotics against both planktonic and biofilm bacteria is reported in article [10]. It can also facilitate the release of antibiotics from medical implants. As a non-invasive and targeted therapy, low-frequency ultrasound has great potential in the treatment of bacterial infections. Ultrasound has been shown to reduce inflammation by decreasing the amount of fibrinogen in the blood in animal studies (rats) [11]. The effects of COVID-19 are creating a need for variety of pulmonary therapy devices. The aim of the study [12] was to evaluate whether low-frequency ultrasound can be used for the detection of air trapping in chronic obstructive pulmonary disease. In addition, the ability of low-frequency ultrasound to detect the effects of short-acting bronchodilators was evaluated. Ultrasound at a frequency of 20–40 kHz was transmitted to the sternum and received at the back during inspiration and expiration. The inspiratory and expiratory signals and their difference were used to determine the high pass rate. A significant difference between subjects with chronic obstructive pulmonary disease and healthy subjects was found in the inspiratory and expiratory signals. It was concluded that low-frequency ultrasound is cost-effective, easy to perform, and suitable for detecting air trapping.

Platelets perform many functions in the human body. They maintain hemostasis by adhering to the vascular endothelium, aggregating with other platelets, and initiating the coagulation cascade that leads to the formation of a fibrin meshwork that effectively prevents major blood loss. Platelets are also critical to inflammation, tissue growth, and the immune response. As noted in [13], low-intensity ultrasound combined with a dose of synthetic particles accelerated clot density and stiffness. This suggests that this treatment may lead to better healing of fractures and injuries. Both histology and immunohistochemistry were used to assess the extent of damage to the atherosclerotic tissue and the presence of platelets on the endothelial surface. The aim of the study in [14] was the development of a new ultrasound method based on the simultaneous observation of the change in ultrasound velocity and the frequency spectrum of the signal propagating in coagulating blood and its application to the automatic estimation of blood coagulation parameters. The results have shown that the ultrasound velocity and the frequency spectrum of the ultrasound signal should be used simultaneously during blood clotting to determine the onset and duration of clot retraction. The results confirmed that clot retraction is influenced by fibrinogen concentration and platelet receptor activity. These are determined by the carrier genotype.

Calcific aortic stenosis is the most common heart valve disorder in developed countries. It is characterized by progressive fibrocalcific remodeling and thickening of the aortic valve leaflets, which restricts the amount of blood flowing through the valve. Calcific aortic stenosis is usually treated with surgical or transcatheter aortic valve replacement. However, many patients are not considered suitable candidates for these interventions due to severe comorbidities and limited life expectancy. Thus, non-invasive treatment may offer alternative treatment options for these patients. The study [15] aims to evaluate the safety and ability of non-invasive ultrasound therapy to improve valve function by softening calcified valve tissue. The paper [16] demonstrates the in vivo feasibility and safety of transthoracic noninvasive ultrasound therapy on aortic valves in a porcine model without serious adverse events. The article [17] proposes a non-invasive therapeutic approach based on the use of pulsed cavitation ultrasound to improve the degenerative calcified function of bioprosthetic valves, as most implanted heart valve prostheses are tissue valves that can calcify over time and eventually fail, and surgical or percutaneous redo valve replacement is associated with a higher complication rate.

Machine learning is a field of study and application within the broader domain of Artificial Intelligence that focuses on developing algorithms and techniques that enable computers or machines to learn from data and make predictions. Paper [18] reviews machine learning methods in medical ultrasound diagnostic research. Challenges are associated with limited possibility of image quality control due to the volume of calculations and gradual miniaturization of ultrasound diagnostic devices. Work [19] presents studies of platelet activation and cell surface dynamics. Machine learning made it possible to predict changes in the shape of platelets under the influence of ultrasound. Appropriate parameters such as area or perimeter were used as input for platelet characterization.

1.3 Vibrational Blood Flow Activation

Cardiovascular diseases are an important public health problem, causing about 45% of deaths worldwide. Its management includes medication, lifestyle changes, and exercise, with whole-body vibration exercises being a promising source of treatment. The effects of whole-body vibration, alone or in combination with other types of exercise, in the treatment of cardiovascular disease are investigated in this paper [20]. The effects of whole-body vibration on hemodynamics, cardiovascular, vascular/arterial and muscle parameters were analyzed. The whole-body vibration pulsatility index decreased in the popliteal artery after maximal exercise and was effective in increasing performance in subsequent exercise tests [21]. The effect of whole-body vibration on leg blood flow was investigated in young adult males. Subjects performed a series of random vibration and non-vibration exercise trials while squatting on a vibrating plate. Common femoral artery blood pressure and blood cell velocity were measured in a standing or resting position before, during and after each bout. This study [22] shows that leg blood flow increases systematically during vibration exercise. The study on twenty healthy adults [23] was performed on the vibration platform, which imitates mechanical vibrations of 26 Hz. The mean blood flow velocity in the popliteal artery increased from 6.5 to 13.0 cm $\times$ s^{-1}. In study [24] of patients with type II diabetes mellitus who performed vibration exercise suggested that vibration exercise may be an effective and time-saving tool for improving glycaemic control. The studies [25] showed a significant increase in skin blood flow after five minutes of vibration at 30 or 50 Hz. In patients with pulmonary arterial hypertension, supportive therapy has been used in addition to targeted medical therapy [26]. The effectiveness and safety of oscillatory whole-body vibration was evaluated in patients on stable therapy for pulmonary arterial hypertension. Whole-body vibration significantly improved exercise capacity. This method can be used in a structured training programme and may be feasible for continuous long-term physical exercise in these patients. The study [27] showed the increased skin blood flow after whole body vibration exercise at post-intervention time intervals, which is suitable for diabetes mellitus with poor circulation.

The highest concentration of capillaries can be found in the skin and muscles. Naturally, blood flow through capillaries is mainly regulated by vasomotor nerve fibres and local chemical conditions. There are two possible routes of blood flow through capillaries. When the pre-capillary sphincters are open, blood flows through the true capillaries. When the pre-capillary sphincters are closed, blood flows through a shunt, bypassing the tissue cells without exchanging nutrients. This is how capillary flow is described in cardiovascular theory. However, in some cases there may be other causes of dysfunction. Katsuzo Nishi [28] suggested that human organs are duplicated, and capillaries can be considered as a second heart that can be dynamically activated while lying on the back by shaking the raised arms and legs to promote blood flow. RBCs can be significantly affected by genetic or some pathological conditions. Healthy erythrocytes are disc-shaped with a diameter of 8 μm and have a flexible membrane. The high surface-to-volume ratio facilitates reversible elastic deformation, which is essential for continuous passage through the 6 μm diameter capillaries, transporting nutrients and oxygen. Pathological conditions can significantly affect the shape or membrane properties of the disc-shaped RBC. The erythrocytes of a patient with diabetes mellitus become stiffer and therefore get stuck in smaller diameter capillaries, causing blood flow to be obstructed. This can lead to necrosis and organ damage [29].

The wound healing process depends on the blood supply to the skin. Sufficient blood flow ensures delivery of oxygen and nutrients that are crucial to the healing process. The results of the diabetic mice study show that low-intensity vibration training may be a novel therapeutic method for healing diabetic wounds [30]. People who are confined to wheelchairs or have other mobility problems cannot stimulate their blood circulation naturally. Insufficient blood volume can lead to problems such as cold feet, numbness, ulcers or even amputation. Electrical muscle stimulators could be used to increase circulation in the legs. Electrical impulses delivered through electrodes cause muscles to contract, increasing blood flow. However, this method is controversial and long-term studies are needed. In most cases, physiotherapists recommend imitating natural movements rather than using electrical muscle stimulation.

In recent decades, however, evidence has accumulated that RBCs have the ability to sense low oxygen tensions in hypoxic tissues and subsequently release signalling molecules that influence the distribution of blood flow [31]. The emergence of the integration of physical and molecular processes in fields such as mechanobiology is thus providing new and invaluable insights, even in areas such as erythrocyte physiology that were previously thought to be well understood.

Multivariate regression analysis showed that under resting conditions there was no correlation between rheological parameters and erythrocyte velocity in capillaries. Blood flow regulation appeared to be so effective that pathological changes in blood fluidity had no effect on the velocity of an erythrocyte passing through the capillaries [32]. During vasoparalysis in the early phase of post-ischemic hyperemia, a very clear correlation between plasma viscosity and maximum post-ischemic erythrocyte velocity in ipsilateral skin capillaries was observed after 3 min of stasis in the vasculature distal to a pressure cuff applied to the upper arm ($p < 0.0001$). None of the other rheological parameters seemed to play a role. Oxygen transport between blood and tissue is limited by the capillary transit time of the blood, understood as the time available for diffusional exchange before the blood returns to the heart. If all capillaries always contribute equally to tissue oxygenation, this physical limitation will render vasodilation and increased blood flow insufficient to meet the increased metabolic demands of the heart, muscle and other organs. The review [33] describes how natural changes in capillary transit-time heterogeneity and capillary hematocrit across open capillaries during blood flow augmentation can provide a match between oxygen availability and metabolic demands in normal tissue.

In addition to blood flow activation, blood flow restriction [34] is also applied, enhancing the muscle's ability to achieve similar increases in strength and hypertrophy at lower loads, which is particularly beneficial in populations that cannot tolerate heavy-load resistance training, such as patients and athletes recovering from surgery or injury, or those suffering from frailty.

1.4 Separation of Biological Microparticles

The separation of micro-sized bioparticles is an important issue for identification and analysis in industrial, biochemical, and clinical applications. To achieve this goal, microfluidics has been actively adapted because of its ability to precisely manipulate microparticles. Microfluidic bioparticle separation techniques have been divided into two categories: active and passive methods. Active methods use external forces such as electric or magnetic fields, acoustic waves and optical interactions by exploiting the dielectric, magnetic or optical properties of particles. Passive methods use distinctive physical properties of the particles, such as size, density and deformability of the cells. However, passive methods tend to suffer from lower selectivity than active methods. The intensification of life and the development of technologies increasingly require the treatment of larger volumes of bioparticles. There is an obvious need for low-cost and energy-efficient bioparticles separation/purification devices that are easy to transport and quick to prepare for work under extreme conditions. The research and development of such measures is intended for this work.

The separation of microparticles is important in modern biomedical technologies. Currently available erythrocytes separation techniques based on centrifugal sedimentation, magnetic, plasmapheresis or dialysis phenomena require expensive medical equipment and have limitations related to particle quantity requirements. In addition to the widely used centrifugal sedimentation of microparticles, the method of magnetic separation in a microchannel is spreading [35]. Magnetic particles are transported by ratcheting through a wheel using magnetically soft micro-pillars in combination with a directionally cycled rotating magnetic field to dynamically modify the potential energy landscape. The separation of micro-scale particles is an important issue in industrial, biochemical and clinical applications for the identification and analysis of specific particles. Circulating tumour cells are likely to be derived from clones of the primary tumour, so it can be argued that they can be used for all biological studies that apply to the primary cells. Screen Cell devices are disposable and inexpensive innovative devices that use a filter to isolate and sort tumour cells by size [36].

The preparation of monodisperse emulsions is one of the most important methods used in the field of precision chemical or pharmaceutical engineering, where the same physical properties are required for precise control of chemical reactions or physical interaction with external substrates. The report [37] presents a microfluidic system for continuous and droplet separation using microscale hydrodynamics. The paper [38] provides lateral driven continuous dielectrophoresis micro separators for red and white blood cells suspended in a highly conductive, dilute whole blood. Continuous micro-separators allow blood cells to be separated by the lateral dielectrophoretic force generated by a planar array of interdigitated electrodes arranged at an angle to the direction of flow. A simplified linear charge model that is developed for theoretical analysis was verified by comparing it with simulated and measured results. It is shown that the design of a lateral-driven continuous dielectrophoresis micro-separator is practical for the permanent separation of blood cells without the need to control the conductivity of the suspension medium by overcoming the critical deficiencies of the dielectrophoresis micro separators. For the separation of microparticles at the lower (sonic) frequencies, several scenarios have been examined, and the first investigations were related to the collection of microparticles in fluids around resonant plaques. In [39] it was shown that the particle clumping in the vibrating capillary tube is the same as that of macroscopic patterns in sand ripples.

The acoustic radiation force based on the compressibility installation described in [40] for better particle separation efficiency, is defined as the fraction of the particles collected in the centre outlet. The technology presented in this paper allows solving the problem of embolization with the possibility of separating red blood cells or erythrocytes from lipid particles. Since the particles are red blood cells and lipid droplets in plasma, the erythrocytes gather in the pressure node (in the centre of the channel), and the lipid particles gather in the pressure anti-node (near the side walls).

The erythrocyte sedimentation rate is one of the oldest medical diagnostic tools. However, there is currently some debate about the structure formed by the cells during the sedimentation process. In the article [41] a direct probe of the structures formed by erythrocytes in the blood during sedimentation is achieved. It was proved that erythrocyte sedimentation occurs as a dynamic compression of a colloidal gel with plasma channels. Blood cells are suspended in a yellowish substance called plasma. Plasma consists of water and various dissolved molecules. Together, the components of blood plasma account for its large volume in the blood ($\pm55\%$). Blood separation by plasmapheresis can be used to replace unhealthy plasma in patients with healthy plasma from a donor [42]. Removal of erythrocytes from whole blood is an essential step in sample preparations intended for biomedical analysis and clinical diagnosis. To address the limitations of current methods, such as centrifugation and chemical lysis, a novel microfluidic device for high-efficiency erythrocyte removal and leukocyte separation from bulk flows of highly concentrated erythrocytes using a viscoelastic non-Newtonian fluid is proposed in [43]. Erythrocytes are abundant endogenous cells in the blood and are continuously renewed, with a long-life span of 100–120 days. Hence, loading nanoparticles onto the surface of erythrocytes to protect the nanoparticles could be highly effective in prolonging their in vivo circulation time. The review [44] describes various methods for attaching nanoparticles and drugs to the erythrocyte surface and discusses the key factors that influence the stability and circulation properties of the erythrocytes-based delivery system in vivo. The paper [45] presents protocols for blood collection, separation of leukocytes from whole blood by erythrocyte lysis, isolation of mononuclear cells by density gradient separation and various non-flow sorting methods, such as magnetic bead separation, for enrichment of specific cell populations, including monocytes, T lymphocytes, B lymphocytes, neutrophils and platelets, prior to flow cytometric analysis. A protocol for cryopreservation of cells is also provided, as clinical research often involves retrospective flow cytometric analysis of samples stored over a period of months or years. Sensor-loaded erythrocytes, called erythrosensors, could be reinfused into the bloodstream, stimulated non-invasively through the skin and used to measure analyte levels in the bloodstream. There are several techniques for loading erythrocytes to produce carrier erythrocytes. However, their cellular properties remain largely unstudied. Changes in cellular characteristics lead to removal from the bloodstream. The authors of the paper [46] hypothesize that erythrocyte carriers must retain the characteristics of native erythrocytes to serve as a long-term sensing platform and investigate two loading techniques and the characteristics of the resulting erythrocyte carriers. In [47], a comprehensive review from fabrication to applications of erythrocyte-inspired functional materials is given. After summarizing the biomaterials that mimic the biological functions of erythrocytes, the synthesis strategies of particles with erythrocyte-inspired morphologies are presented. The focus is on the practical biomedical applications of these bioinspired functional materials. The prospects of advanced erythrocyte-inspired biomaterials will also be discussed. It is hoped that the summary of existing studies will inspire researchers to develop novel biomaterials, thus accelerating the progress of these biomaterials towards clinical biomedical applications.

Erythrocytes play an important role in the immune system [48]. Erythrocytes recognise and adhere to antigens and promote phagocytosis. The abnormal morphology and function of erythrocytes are also involved in the pathological processes of some diseases. Due to the large number and immune properties of erythrocytes, their immune functions should not be ignored. Based on the characteristics of erythrocyte immunity, various drug delivery systems have been developed for the treatment of diseases and are now a hotspot of research. In medical science, the examination of blood smears for erythrocyte abnormalities leads to the crucial determination of several diseases. The research study [49] has proposed an image analysis perspective to characterise the erythrocytes based on their morphological changes.

References

1. Moyano DB, Paraiso DA, Gonzales-Lezcano RA (2022) Possible effects on health of ultrasound exposure, risk factors in the work environment and occupational safety review. Healthcare (Basel) 10(3):423
2. Lioce EEAN, Novello M, Guiot C (2017) Therapeutic ultrasound: physical basis and clinical assessment. Clin Phys Ther 213–220

3. Mehrpour M, Shakeri-Zadeh A, Basir P, Jamei B, Ghaheri H, Shiran MB (2016) Effects of low-intensity continuous ultrasound on hematological parameters of rats. J Biomed Phys Eng 6(3):195–200

4. Signori LU, Neto LJR, Jaenisch RB, Puntel CO, Nunes GS, Paulitsh FS, Hauck M, da Silva AMV (2023) Effects of therapeutic ultrasound on the endothelial function of patients with type 2 diabetes mellitus. Braz J Med Biol Res 56

5. Imtiaz C, Farooqi M-A, Bhatti T, Lee J, Moin R, Kang C, Farooqi H (2023) Focused ultrasound, an emerging tool for atherosclerosis treatment: a comprehensive review. Life (Basel) 13(8):1783

6. Ji N, Li J, Wei J, Chen F, Xu L, Li G, Lin W-H (2022) Autonomic modulation by low-intensity focused ultrasound stimulation of the vagus nerve. J. Neural Eng 19:066036

7. Cui J, Wei Y, Wang H (2017) The study of low-frequency ultrasound to enhance transdermal drug delivery. In: IEE/ICME international conference on complex medical engineering

8. Torkar A, Krist J, Murdan S (2007) Low-frequency ultrasound to enhance topical drug delivery to the nail. In: AAPS annual meeting expo

9. Duncan B, Al-Kassas R, Zhang G, Hughes D, Qui Y (2023) Ultrasound-mediated ocular drug delivery: from physics and instrumentation to future directions. Micromachines (Basel) 14(8):1575

10. Cai Y, Wang J, Liu X, Wang R, Xia L (2017) A review of the combination therapy of low frequency ultrasound with antibiotics. BioMed Res Int 2317846:14

11. Signori LU, Teixeira AO, da Silva AMV, da Costa ST (2014) Effects of therapeutic ultrasound on hematological dynamics and fibrinogen during the inflammatory phase after muscle injury in rats. Acta Scient Health Sci 36(1):25–31

12. Morenz K, Biller H, Wolfram F, Leonhardt S, Rutter D, Glaab T, Uhlig S, Hohlfeld JM (2012) Detection of air trapping in chronic obstructive pulmonary disease by low frequency ultrasound. BMC Pulm Med 112(1):8

13. Nandi S, Mohanty K, Nellenbach K, Erb M (2020) Ultrasound enhanced synthetic platelet therapy for augmented wound repair. ACS Biomater Sci Eng 6(5):3026–3036

14. Tatarunas V, Voleisis A, Sliteris R, Kazys R, Mazeika L, Lesauskaite V (2018) A novel ultrasonic method for evaluation of blood clotting parameters. J Med Ultrason 45:545–553

15. Messas E, Ijsselmuiden A, Trifunovic-Zamaklar D, Cholley B, Puymirat E, Halim J, Karan R, van Gameren M, Terezic D, Milisevic V, Tanter M, Pernot M, Goudot G (2023) Treatment of severe symptomatic aortic valve stenosis using non-invasive ultrasound therapy: a cohort study. Lancet 402(10419):2317–2325

16. Messas E, Rémond MC, Goudot G, Zarka S, Penot R, Mateo P, Kwiecinski W, Escudero DE, Bel A, Radio NI (2020) Feasibility and safety of non-invasive ultrasound therapy (NIUT) on an porcine aortic valve. Phys Med Biol 65:215004

17. Villemain O, Robina J, Belc A, Kwiecinskia W, Brunevald P, Arnala B, Rémonde M, Tantera M, Messas E, Pernot M (2017) Pulsed cavitational ultrasound softening: a new non-invasive therapeutic approach of calcified bioprosthetic valve stenosis. JACC Basic Transl Sci 2(4):372–383

18. Brattain LJ, Telfer BA, Dhyani M, Grajo JR, Samir AE (2018) Machine learning for medical ultrasound: status, methods, and future opportunities. Abdom Radiol 43:786–799

19. Neeb H, Grieger S, Luxem K, Strasser EF, Kraus M-J (2014) Active or not—machine-learning based prediction of platelet activation. In: Proceedings of the world congress on engineering and computer science, vol I, pp 22–24

20. Gonzales AI, Do Nasimento GB, Da Silva A, Bernardo-Filho M, De Sa-Caputo DC, Sanza A (2023) Whole-body vibration exercise in the management of cardiovascular diseases: a systematic review. J Bodyw Mov Ther 36:20–29

21. Otsuki T, Takanami Y, Aoi W, Kawai Y, Ichikawa H, Yoshikawa T (2008) Arterial stiffness acutely decreases after whole-body vibration in humans. Acta Physiol 194:189–194

22. Lythgoe N, Eser P, de Groot P, Galea M (2008) Whole-body vibration dosage alters leg blood flow. Scand Soc Clin Physiol Nucl Med 29(1):53–59
23. Kerschan-Schindl K, Grampp S, Henk C, Resch H, Preisinger E, Fialka-Moser V, Imhof H (2001) Whole-body vibration exercise leads to alterations in muscle blood volume. Clin Phys 21(3):377–382
24. Baum K, Votteler T, Schiab J (2007) Efficiency of vibration exercise for glycemic control in type 2 diabetes patients. Int J Med Sci 31; 4(3):159–163
25. Maloney-Hinds C, Petrofsky JS, Zimmerman G (2008) The effect of 30 Hz vs. 50 Hz passive vibration and duration of vibration on skin blood flow in the arm. Med Sci Monit 14(3):112–116
26. Gerhardt F, Dumitrescu D, Gartner C, Beccard R, Viethen T, Kramar T, Baldus S, Hellmich M, Schonau E, Rosenkranz S (2017) Oscillatory whole-body vibration improves exercise capacity and physical performance in pulmonary arterial hypertension: a randomised clinical study. Heart 103(8):592–598
27. Lohman EB, Petrofsky JS, Maloney-Hinds C, Betts-Schwab H, Thorpe D (2007) The effect of whole-body vibration on lower extremity skin blood flow in normal subjects. Med Sci Monit 13(2):71–76
28. Wikipedia. Katsuzo Nishi (2013) [Online] http://en.wikipedia.org/wiki/Katsuzō_Nishi
29. Diez-Silva M, Dao M, Han J, Lim C-T, Suresh S (2010) Shape and biomechanical characteristics of human red blood cells in health and disease. MRS Bull 35(5):382–388
30. Weinheimer-Haus EM, Judex S, Ennis WJ, Koh TJ (2014) Low-intensity vibration improves angiogenesis and wound healing in diabetic mice. PLoS One 9(3):e91355
31. Richardson KJ, Kuck L, Simmonds MJ (2020) Beyond oxygen transport: active role of erythrocytes in the regulation of blood flow. Am J Physiol Heart Circ Physiol 3196(4):H866–H872
32. Jung F, Mrowiets C, Hiebl B, Franke RP, Pindur G, Sternitzky R (2011) Influence of rheological parameters on the velocity of erythrocytes passing nailfold capillaries in humans. Clin Hemorheol Microcirc 48(1):129–139
33. Østergaard L (2020) Blood flow, capillary transit times, and tissue oxygenation: the centennial of capillary recruitment. J Appl Physiol 129(6):1413–1421
34. Whipple M, Terese MD, Rachel ADO, Donnenwerth JJ, Andrew RMD (2021) Blood flow restriction in exercise and rehabilitation. ACSM's Health Fitness J 25(5):6–9
35. Murray C, Pao E, Tseng P, Aftab S, Kulkarni R, Rettig M, Di Carlo D (2016) Quantitative magnetic separation of particles and cells using gradient magnetic ratcheting small. 12(14):1891–1899
36. Desitter I, Guerrouahen BS, Benali-Foret N, WechslerJ JPA, KuangY YM, Wang L, Berkowitz JA, Distel RJ, Cayre YE (2011) A new device for rapid isolation by size and characterization of rare circulating tumor cells. Anticancer Res 31(2):427–441
37. Maenaka H, Yamada M, Yasuda M, Seki M (2008) Continuous and size-dependent sorting of emulsion droplets using hydrodynamics in pinched microchannels. Langmuir 24(8):4405–4410
38. Han K-H, Frazier AB (2008) Lateral-driven continuous dielectrophoretic microseparators for blood cells suspended in a highly conductive medium. J Lab Chip 8(7):1079–1086
39. Zoueshtiagh F, Thomas PJ, Thomy V, Merlen A (2008) Micrometric granular ripple patterns in a capillary tube. Phys Rev Lett 100:054501
40. Peterson F, Nilsson A, Holm C, Jonsson H, Laurell T (2005) Continuous separation of lipid particles from erythrocytes by means of laminar flow and acoustic standing wave forces. Lab Chip 5(1):20–22
41. Darras A, Breunig HG, John T, Zhao R, Koch J, Kummerow C, König K, Wagner C, Kaestner K (2022) Imaging erythrocyte sedimentation in whole blood. Front Physiol 12:729191
42. Castel L (2023) The most effective blood separation methods. Med Life Sci

43. Nam J, Yoon J, Kim J, Jang WS, Lim CS (2019) Continuous erythrocyte removal and leuko-cyte separation from whole blood based on viscoelastic cell focusing and the margination phenomenon. J Chrom 21(1595):230–239

44. Zhang S-q, Fu Q, Zhang Y-j, Pan J-x, Zhang L, Zhang Z-r, Liu Z-m (2021) Surface loading of nanoparticles on engineered or natural erythrocytes for prolonged circulation time: strategies and applications. Act Pharm Sini 42:1040–1054

45. Pradeep K, Dugur J. McCoy P (2015) Collection, storage, and preparation of human blood cells. Curr Protoc Cytom 73:5.1.1–5.1.16

46. Lopez SCB, Meissner KE (2017) Characterization of carrier erythrocytes for biosensing appli-cations. J Biomed Opt 22(9):091510

47. Luo Z, Sun L, Bian F, Wang Y, Yu Y, Gu Z, Zhao Y (2022) Erythrocyte-inspired functional materials for biomedical applications. Adv Sci 10(6):2206150

48. Ren Y, Yan C, Yang H (2023) Erythrocytes: member of the immune system that should not be ignored. Crit Rev Oncol/Hemat 187:104039

49. Kumar P, Babulal KS (2023) Hematological image analysis for segmentation and characteriza-tion of erythrocytes using FC-TriSDR. Track 2 Med Appl Multimed 82:7861–7886

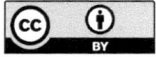

Acoustic Activation of Human Circulatory Parameters

2

2.1 Introduction

To ensure the patient's well-being, safe ultrasound therapy technologies are necessary. According to the standard, the sound intensity level of medical ultrasound diagnostic equipment must not exceed 1000 mW/cm^2 in the high frequency range from 1 to 10 MHz, which ensures an acoustic signal penetration of up to 1.7 cm. The acoustic intensity decreases exponentially in proportion to the depth of biological tissue exposure and the frequency-dependent attenuation coefficient of acoustic energy. For the first time in medical practice, the effects of low-frequency ultrasound on the blood were revealed, where the acoustic waves transmitted through the blood separated individual erythrocytes from their aggregates. To this end, a low-frequency ultrasound actuator, utilizing digital twin technology, was developed and patented to deliver focused acoustic waves deeper into the tissue. An artificial intelligence technique has been demonstrated to predict the consequences of ultrasound treatment of blood samples. In animal experiments, low-frequency ultrasound has been shown to significantly reduce blood pressure and pulse rate and improve blood gas exchange, without the use of drugs, which is applicable to the treatment of pulmonary hypertension.

2.2 Prediction of Changes in Blood Parameters Induced by Low-Frequency Ultrasound

2.2.1 Sonication of Blood Samples

In search of opportunities to improve blood circulation and speed up the analysis and interpretation of blood indicators by non-invasive means, ultrasound technology was used.

© The Author(s) 2025

V. Ostasevicius et al., *Noninvasive Therapeutic Technologies*, Synthesis Lectures on Biomedical Engineering, https://doi.org/10.1007/978-3-031-79025-6_2

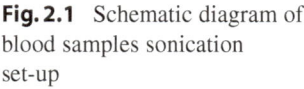

Fig. 2.1 Schematic diagram of blood samples sonication set-up

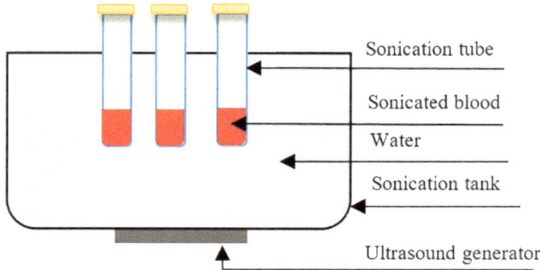

Blood sonication was performed using water bath sonication technology with ultrasonic cleaner CT-400 (Wah Loen Electronic Co., Ltd), which operates at a frequency of 46 ± 2 kHz with different intensities and durations of ultrasound. To ensure the ultrasound frequency, measure the ultrasonic intensity and maintain constant parameters during each stage of the experiment, the tests were carried out using a hydrophone HCT-0320 connected to an acoustic cavitation meter MCT-2000 (Ondo Corp., USA). Since ultrasound with electric power leads to higher temperatures that might degrade the blood samples, the temperature was strictly monitored and controlled in the range of 20–28 °C. The sonication platform is shown in Fig. 2.1. The water temperature in the ultrasonic bath varied from 20 °C (room temperature) to 28 °C. Water temperature fluctuations were caused by the periodic operation of the ultrasonic bath. The study measured the highest rise in water temperature within the bath over a continuous period of 180 s. while generating ultrasound at an intensity of 100–150 mW/cm^2. Following each ultrasound bath operation, a pause was implemented until the water temperature within the bath returned to a range of 21–23 °C.

After sonication, the blood was analyzed using Swelab Alfa system [1], which is an automated hematology analyzer for in vitro diagnostics under laboratory conditions. A complete blood count with 20 different components was performed on all blood samples. Blood was collected from 42 lung disease patients by certified nurses into Vacuette tube 3 ml K2E K2EDTA 13×75 lavender cap-black ring. One person's blood from one Vacuette tube was divided into seven samples. One sample was control, this blood was not affected by ultrasound, and measurement was performed two times (at the beginning of the experiment and at the end), remaining samples were sonicated at three different intensities and two different times. So, each person's blood was tested for all six variables of ultrasound intensity and time as well as without affecting it with ultrasound. All experiments with the blood were performed during the first hours after collecting it. Only prior to affecting the blood with the ultrasound, it was divided into seven samples and transferred from the K2EDTA Vacuette tube to the smaller Eppendorf tube. All the divided blood was tested for complete blood count within a few minutes after affecting it with ultrasound.

Table 2.1 Characteristics of low-frequency ultrasound acting on blood samples

Intensity and duration of ultrasound exposure
K, D, E, F—A control blood sample was not exposed to ultrasound
A and 5—Exposure 90 s, US intensity ~100–150 mW/cm^2 at 48 kHz; high power ultrasound
B—Exposure 180 s, US intensity ~100–150 mW/cm^2 at 48 kHz high power ultrasound
C and 1—Exposure 90 s, US intensity ~50–70 mW/cm^2 at 44 kHz medium power ultrasound
D and 2—Exposure 180 s, US intensity ~50–70 mW/cm^2 at 44 kHz medium power ultrasound
E—Exposure 90 s, US intensity ~5–12 mW/cm^2 at 44 kHz low power ultrasound
F—Exposure 180 s, US intensity ~5–12 mW/cm^2 at 44 kHz low power ultrasound
3—Exposure 270 s, US intensity ~50–70 mW/cm^2 at 44 kHz medium power ultrasound
4—Exposure 360 s, US intensity ~50–70 mW/cm^2 at 44 kHz medium power ultrasound
4a—Exposure 270 s, US intensity ~5–12 mW/cm^2 at 44 kHz low power ultrasound
5a—Exposure 360 s, US intensity ~5–12 mW/cm^2 at 44 kHz low power ultrasound
6—Water

The characteristics of low-frequency ultrasound acting on blood samples are presented in Table 2.1. Blood sample analysis was performed with Swe lab Alfa hematology analyzer.

Hematological analysis is an important test for the detection of disease and for monitoring the health of humans and animals. Automated hematology analyzers have been routinely used as a rapid, accurate and simple diagnostic method. The automated hematology analyzer has replaced the traditional manual assay methods and eye counting when determining hematological parameters. Recently, they have been widely used in laboratories and hospitals for counting blood cells necessary for diagnosis and for monitoring treatment of various disorders.

2.2.2 Changes in Blood Parameters Affected by Ultrasound

Certified nurses collected blood from lung disease patients into a 3 ml Vacuette K2E K2EDTA 13 × 75 tube with a lavender cap-black ring and it was equally divided into 7 samples, so each part of ~0.43 ml was exposed to ultrasound. The Swelab Alfa analyzer was used for enumeration of red blood cells (RBC); mean cell volume of red cells (MCV); red cell distribution relative and absolute volumes (RDW%, RDWa); hematocrit (HTC); platelet count (PLT); mean platelet volume (MPV); platelet distribution width (PDW); plateletcrit (PCT); platelet large cell ratio (LPCR); white blood cells (WBC); hemoglobin (HGB); mean corpuscular hemoglobin (MCH); mean corpuscular hemoglobin concentration (MCHC); lymphocytes (LYM); granulocytes (GRAN); minimum inhibitory dilution (MID); lymphocytes percentage (LYM%); granulocyte percentage (GRA%); mid-sized white cells percentage (MID%). All experiments with patient blood were carried out within the first hour after blood collection. The characteristics of low-frequency ultrasound acting on blood samples are presented in Table 2.1.

The automated hematology analyzer is not used to make diagnoses on patients. It is designed to collect data reflecting the patient's hematological status. This data, in conjunction with other diagnostic information and the evaluation of the patient's condition, can be used by a trained clinician to establish the patient's diagnosis and to define clinical treatment. The changes in the parameters of the blood affected by these low-frequency ultrasound modes are presented in Fig. 2.2.

Since hemoglobin is the carrier of oxygen from the lungs, the effect of ultrasound on changes in mean corpuscular hemoglobin concentration (MCHC) and mean corpuscular hemoglobin (MCH) was subjected to assessment using a blood analyzer (Fig. 2.2m, n). These parameters indicate the amount of hemoglobin per cell and the amount of hemoglobin per unit volume, respectively. The difference between MCH and MCHC is that MCHC considers the volume or size of red blood cells, while MCH does not. The role of hemoglobin in conveying oxygen from the pulmonary alveoli to the somatic cells is paramount. Hematological parameters reflect the current state of health of the body. The range of MCH is 27–33 pg/cell, and the range of MCHC is 33–36 g/dL of red blood cells. It has been observed that when exposed to low-frequency ultrasound, as shown in Fig. 2.3, the MCH and MCHC values tend to exceed the permissible ranges. This could potentially be related to an increase in blood oxygen saturation.

Repeated measures ANOVA was performed to compare the effect of different ultrasound exposures on different blood parameters. 42 participants were tested for 20 blood parameters in 6 different ultrasound combinations (Table 2.1). The ANOVA results revealed that there was a statistically significant (p-value is <0.05) difference in 15 blood parameters between at least two groups. MATLAB R2018a was used to perform statistical analysis for these 15 parameters (Table 2.2). The F-statistic is the ratio of the mean squared errors, where d_1 is equal to 40 (for the numerator) and $d_2 = 6$ (for the denominator).

Multiple tests found that the mean value of 49 ultrasound conditions was significantly different from control group. Mainly high-power ultrasound influenced test parameters (Table 2.3).

There was no statistically significant difference between 5 groups, $p > 0.05$ (Table 2.4).

2.2.3 Nonparametric Kruskal–Walli's Test for Blood Analysis

The Kruskal–Walli's test is a popular non-parametric statistical test used in medicine to compare the distribution of a continuous variable among multiple groups or treatments [2–4]. It is often used when the assumptions of parametric tests cannot be met, in such cases

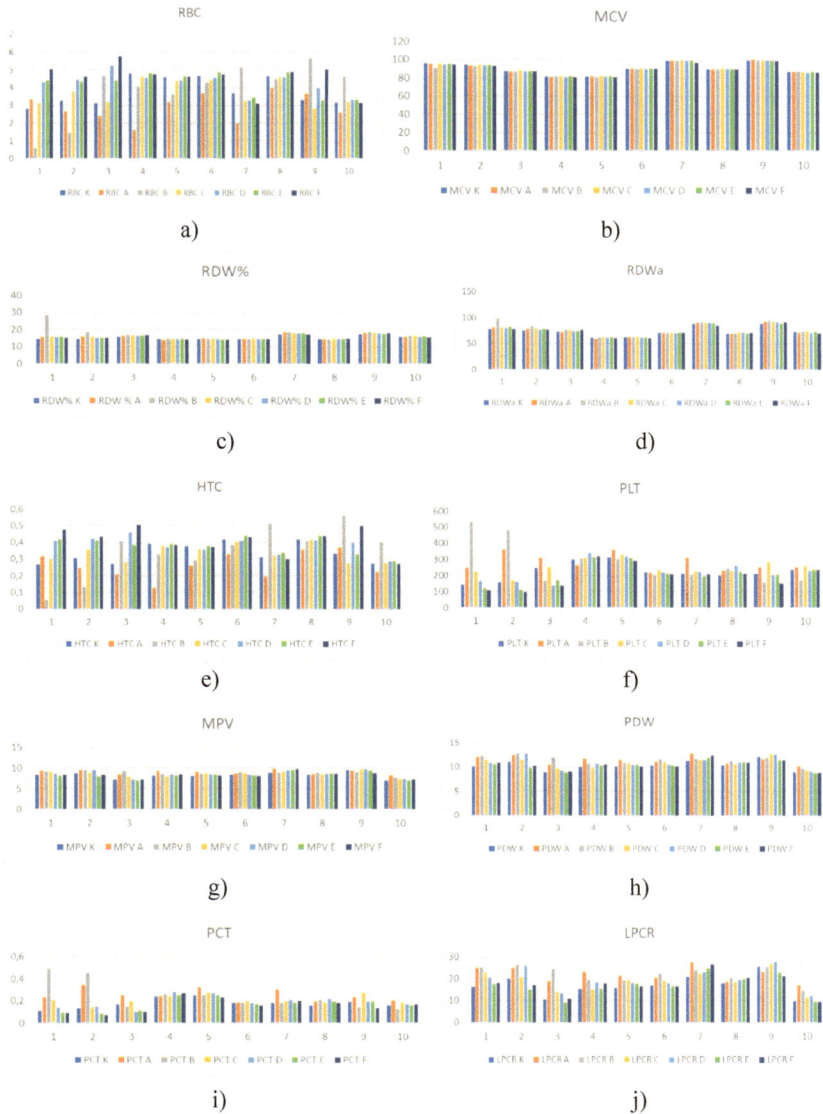

Fig. 2.2 Parameters of blood samples exposed to low-frequency ultrasound: **a** RBC—red blood cell; **b** MCV—mean corpuscular volume; **c** RDW%—red cell distribution with; **d** RDWa—red cell distribution volume; **e** HTC—hematocrit; **f** PLT—platelet count; **g** MPV—mean platelet volume; **h** PDW—platelet distribution width; **i** PCT—plateletcrit; **j** LPCR—platelet large cell ratio; **k** WBC—white blood cell count; **l** HGB—hemoglobin; **m** MCH—mean corpuscular hemoglobin; **n** MCHC—mean corpuscular hemoglobin concentration; **o** LYM—lymphocytes; **p** GRAN—granulocytes; **r** MID—minimum inhibitory dilution; **s** LYM%—lymphocytes percent; **t** GRA%—granulocyte percent; **u** MID%—minimum inhibitory dilution percent

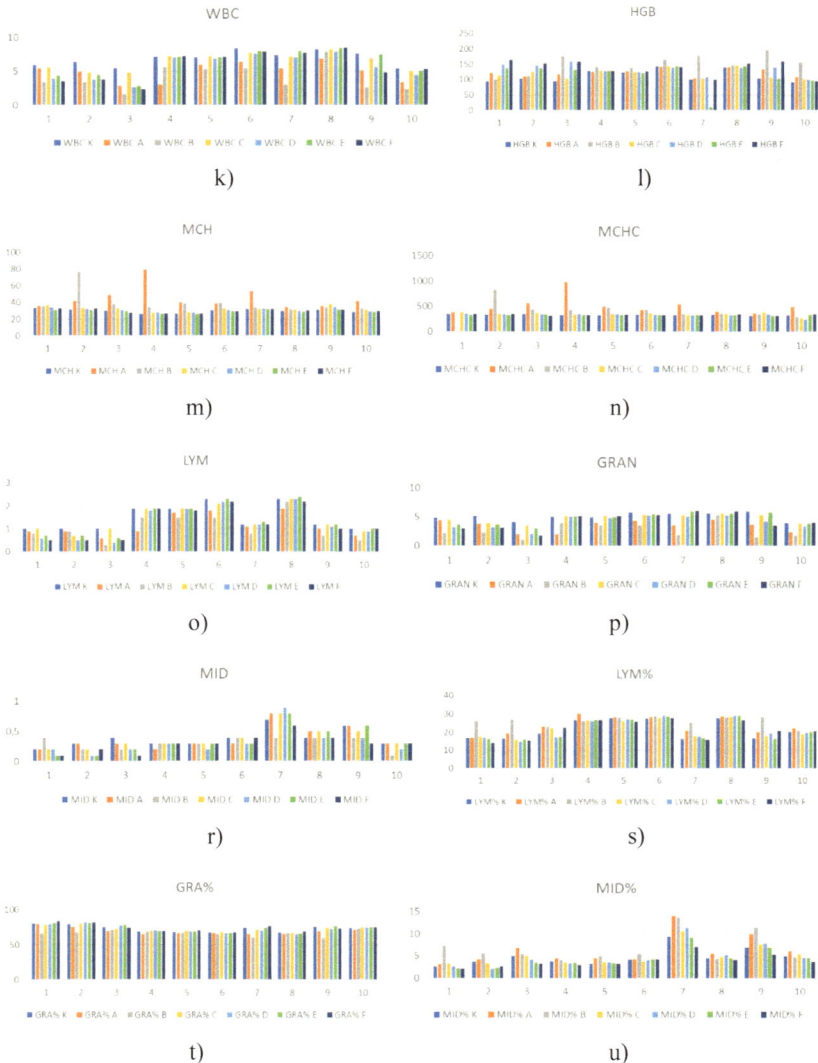

Fig. 2.2 (continued)

when the data is not normally distributed, or the variances are not equal. The Kruskal–Walli's test compares the sums of the ranks among the groups. If the sums of the ranks differ significantly among the groups, then it can be concluded that at least one group is different from the others [5]. When the null hypothesis of the test is rejected at the user-defined significance level α, it indicates that at least one of the groups being compared

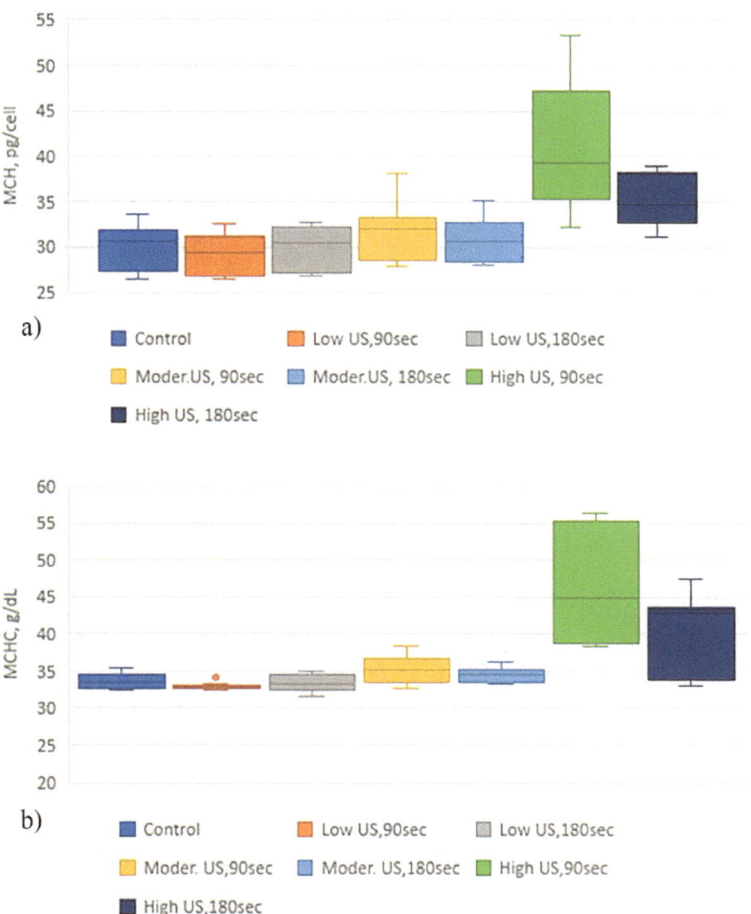

Fig. 2.3 The MCH (**a**) and MCHC (**b**) changes under the influence of various intensities and durations of ultrasound exposure, where in blue—a control blood sample not exposed to ultrasound; the blood samples of other colors are exposed to ultrasound: exposures are 90 and 180 s, low acoustic intensity—5–12 mW/cm^2, moderate acoustic intensity—40–80 mW/cm^2 and high intensity 100–150 mW/cm^2 at frequency of 44–48 kHz. The error bars are dispersion of the measured MCH and MCHC values. The low-, medium-, or high-intensities ultrasound settings in this figure have been selected according to the specifications of the developed transducer. The ultrasound intensity was 10–150 mW/cm^2, and the electric power consumption of the ultrasound bath was 10–60 W

exhibits a statistically significant difference from the others concerning the dependent variable under investigation. Multiple comparison procedures can be used to identify where the differences lie among the populations. Pairwise multiple comparisons compare each pair of groups to determine which groups are significantly different, while the stepwise stepdown procedure is a sequential testing procedure that adjusts the multiple comparisons to reduce the probability of a type I error. The Kruskal–Walli's method is usually

Table 2.2 Repeated measures ANOVA results

Parameter	$F_{40,6}$	p-value
RBC	13.8	<0.01
MCV	12.507	<0.01
HCT	12.612	<0.01
MPV	14.576	<0.01
PDW	15.202	<0.01
LPCR	15.308	<0.01
WBC	29.435	<0.01
HGB	2.254	0.039
MCH	17.344	<0.01
MCHC	2.527	0.021
LYM	16.982	<0.01
GRAN	32.881	<0.01
LYM%	13.522	<0.01
GRA%	7.287	<0.01
MID%	23.488	<0.01

applied to three or more independent groups, but can also be applied to two groups, with a sample size of at least 5 instances in each group. The ranks of the data are used to calculate the test statistic H, which is as follows:

$$H = \frac{12}{N(N+1)} \sum_{i\check{z}1}^{k} \frac{R_i^2}{n_i} - 3(N+1), \tag{2.1}$$

where N is the total number of sample size, k is the number of groups, R_i^2 is the sum of ranks for group i, and n_i is the sample size of group i.

This study uses Dunn's test, which performs pairwise comparisons between each independent group and indicates which groups are statistically significantly different at a given confidence level α. A significance level of 0.05 ($\alpha = 0.05$) is the threshold for rejecting the null hypothesis and confirming the alternative hypothesis. The test uses the average ranks of each group's scores from the Kruskal–Walli's test as an approximate exact statistic for the rank sum test. The test statistic is calculated based on the differences between the mean ranks of the groups and the conclusion is drawn from these differences. When multiple comparisons are made at the same time, it is important to control the (Type I) error rate. One way to do this is to adjust the p-values obtained from multiple comparisons. A common approach is the Bonferroni adjustment, also used in our study.

Blood samples from 10 (of 42) patients were exposed to 6 different low-frequency ultrasound modes (Table 2.3) and changes in 20 blood parameters were identified. The

Table 2.3 Multiple comparisons test results

Parameter	Ultrasound condition	p-value	Lower	Upper
RBC	90 s High power	7.7407e-05	0.24091	0.90982
	180 s High power	0.044232	0.0083252	1.0327
	90 s Medium power	0.01738	0.015071	0.24005
MCV	180 s High power	0.0020901	0.14987	0.14987
	180 s Medium power	0.034435	0.012938	0.54316
	90 s Low power	0.003893	0.068213	0.51228
	180 s Low power	2.1648e-05	0.24868	0.83425
HCT	90 s High power	7.5145e-05	0.021017	0.079129
	90 s Medium power	0.040439	0.00029169	0.021123
MPV	90 s High power	3.9101e-06	−0.55772	−0.18862
	180 s High power	4.1826e-08	−0.55121	−0.25366
	90 s Medium power	0.00068375	−0.37446	−0.074321
	180 s Medium power	6.0592e-07	−0.45315	−0.17124
PDW	90 s High power	1.0374e-05	−0.83408	−0.26348
	180 s High power	1.1562e-06	−0.85447	−0.31139
	90 s Medium power	0.0039076	−0.48651	−0.064706
	180 s Medium power	5.9255e-05	−0.60206	−0.1638
LPCR	90 s High power	1.8239e-05	−4.064	−1.2287
	180 s High power	4.1615e-08	−4.0771	−1.879
	90 s Medium power	0.002002	−2.4268	−0.3878
	180 s Medium power	1.3404e-07	−3.157	−1.2967
WBC	90 s High power	2.0324e-07	0.85458	2.1308
	180 s High power	3.5534e-07	1.0971	2.82
	90 s Medium power	1.2307e-07	0.22664	0.54897

(continued)

Table 2.3 (continued)

Parameter	Ultrasound condition	p-value	Lower	Upper
	180 s Medium power	1.3434e-05	0.31494	1.0168
HGB	90 s Medium power	0.049301	−5.8834	−0.02976
MCH	90 s High power	0.00030284	−14.117	−3.1883
	180 s High power	0.00057798	−15.648	−3.207
	90 s Medium power	0.0022027	−2.6109	−0.40914
	180 s Medium power	0.0001132	−2.7524	−0.70262
MCHC	90 s High power	2.0957e-06	−120.72	−42.679
	180 s High power	0.0008265	−178.16	−34.342
	90 s Medium power	0.0029628	−30.701	−4.4493
LYM	90 s High power	2.9031e-06	0.1163	0.33735
	180 s High power	2.5463e-05	0.12192	0.41466
GRAN	90 s High power	3.7899e-07	0.68411	1.7647
	180 s High power	1.7658e-07	1.0223	2.5289
	90 s Medium power	1.7658e-07	0.22266	0.50905
	180 s Medium power	2.2056e-06	0.34071	0.97149
LYM%	90 s High power	0.00024894	−1.8705	−0.43199
	180 s High power	0.00056303	−3.6677	−0.75182
	90 s Medium power	0.036038	−1.6292	−0.03425
	180 s Medium power	0.00099011	−1.3988	−0.25973
GRA%	90 s High power	0.00054481	0.62761	3.0456
	180 s High power	5.0931e-06	2.3153	6.9676
	180 s Medium power	0.0025352	0.42076	2.7939
MID%	180 s High power	0.016738	−1.3377	−0.086654

(continued)

Table 2.3 (continued)

Parameter	Ultrasound condition	p-value	Lower	Upper
	180 s High power	4.0561e-05	−3.8352	−1.0819
	180 s Medium power	0.042034	−1.5917	−0.018056

Table 2.4 Multiple comparisons test results with no statistically significant difference

Parameter	$F_{40,6}$	p-value
RDW%	1.293	0.26
RDWa	0.317	0.927
PLT	1.266	0.273
PCT	1.696	0.123
MID	2.097	0.055

blood of each patient was sonicated under six different ultrasound intensity and time variables (A, B, C, D, E, F), as well as without any ultrasound exposure (K). To ensure the statistical validity of our analyses, we assessed the normality of the data using the Kolmogorov–Smirnov test. In cases where significant deviations from normality were detected, suitable transformations were applied to address this issue. Subsequently, paired sample t-tests were conducted to compare means between groups, and if significant differences were observed, an ANOVA was performed to evaluate overall significance. These steps were taken to meet the assumptions of the statistical tests and ensure the reliability of our data analysis. A repeated measures ANOVA was performed to compare the effect of different ultrasound exposure (Table 2.2) on different blood parameters. The ANOVA results revealed that there was a statistically significant (p-value is <0.05) difference in 15 blood parameters between at least two groups. MATLAB R2018a was used to perform statistical analysis for these 15 parameters. The F-statistic is the ratio of the mean squared errors, where $d_1 = 40$ (for the numerator) and $d_2 = 6$ (for the denominator).

A multiple comparisons test showed that the mean value of 49 ultrasound conditions was significantly different from the control group. Mainly higher-power ultrasound had the greatest effect on test parameters. We used the Kruskal–Walli's test with Dunn's post-hoc test to determine whether there is a significant difference in the effect of ultrasound (in terms of different intensities and durations) on different blood parameters. In the table below each row represents the null hypothesis that the distribution of the two samples is the same. When there is no evidence to reject the null hypothesis, then there is no significant difference, meaning that ultrasound has no effect (or very small effect) on a particular blood parameter. Otherwise, if the null hypothesis is rejected, this indicates that there is a significant difference between the values of the blood parameters affected by the ultrasound signals. Table 2.5 shows that for 11 out of 20 parameters, the impact of the ultrasound signals (6 different ultrasound influences) is statistically significant (p-value is <0.05).

The diagrams presented in Fig. 2.4 show the results of the Kruskal–Walli's test for different blood parameters with p-value>0.05 (null hypothesis is retained), starting from the baseline value and affected by ultrasound signals that vary in strength (high—H, medium—M, low—W) and duration (90 and 180 s). The changes in RDW values after exposure to ultrasound in the blood are very minor, with a slightly larger increase observed when exposed to the highest ultrasound signal for 180 s (180H). By exposing the blood with a high ultrasound signal for 180 s, we can see that the set of recorded RDW results in values that are outside the normal range. However, the median line between all sets except 180H is almost straight. As we can see, the MCV values are almost non-sensitive

Table 2.5   Kruskal–Wallis null hypothesis test results

No.	Null hypothesis: the distribution of X parameter is the same across categories of ultrasound signals	p-value	Kruskal–Wallis test
1	Parameter X = RDW	0.990	Retain the null hypothesis
2	Parameter X = RBC	**<0.001**	Reject the null hypothesis
3	Parameter X = MCV	0.842	Retain the null hypothesis
4	Parameter X = RDWa	0.977	Retain the null hypothesis
5	Parameter X = HTC	**<0.001**	Reject the null hypothesis
6	Parameter X = PLT	0.885	Retain the null hypothesis
7	Parameter X = MPV	**0.037**	Reject the null hypothesis
8	Parameter X = PDW	**0.044**	Reject the null hypothesis
9	Parameter X = PCT	0.808	Retain the null hypothesis
10	Parameter X = LPCR	**0.015**	Reject the null hypothesis
11	Parameter X = WBC	**0.010**	Reject the null hypothesis
12	Parameter X = HGB	0.584	Retain the null hypothesis
13	Parameter X = MCH	**<0.001**	Reject the null hypothesis
14	Parameter X = MCHC	**<0.001**	Reject the null hypothesis
15	Parameter X = LYM	0.166	Retain the null hypothesis
16	Parameter X = GRAN	**0.002**	Reject the null hypothesis
17	Parameter X = MID	0.467	Retain the null hypothesis
18	Parameter X = LYM (%)	0.157	Retain the null hypothesis
19	Parameter X = GRA (%)	**0.006**	Reject the null hypothesis
20	Parameter X = MID (%)	**<0.001**	Reject the null hypothesis

to the ultrasound signal and all values in this blood set are within the normal range [75–100]. A similar situation can be observed with such parameters as HGB and LYM, where only the 180H has an ultrasound signal. A similar situation applies to parameters such as HGB and PDW, where only the highest ultrasound signal of 90 s (90H) and 180 s (180H) duration influences the values of parameters. A review of all the blood parameters for which the null hypothesis is retained reveals that the parameter values at 90H and 180H slightly increase or decrease.

The boxplot diagrams in Fig. 2.5 show the results of the Kruskal–Walli's test for different blood parameters for which the p-value is very low <0.001 (null hypothesis is rejected), and the effect of ultrasound on these parameters is therefore most significant. In a set of 20 blood parameters, 5 of them respond quite severely to ultrasound high intensity signal. Analyzing the RBC values, we can see that a strong ultrasound signal causes a sharp decrease in values, a medium intensity signal has almost no effect, and a weak one has a slight increase in values. Similar situation can be observed with HTC parameter. From the results with MCH and MCHC parameters we can see that, in contrast to RBC and HTC, a strong ultrasound signal leads to an increase in parameter values outside the normal range, including extreme values. In the case of the MID (%) parameter, there is

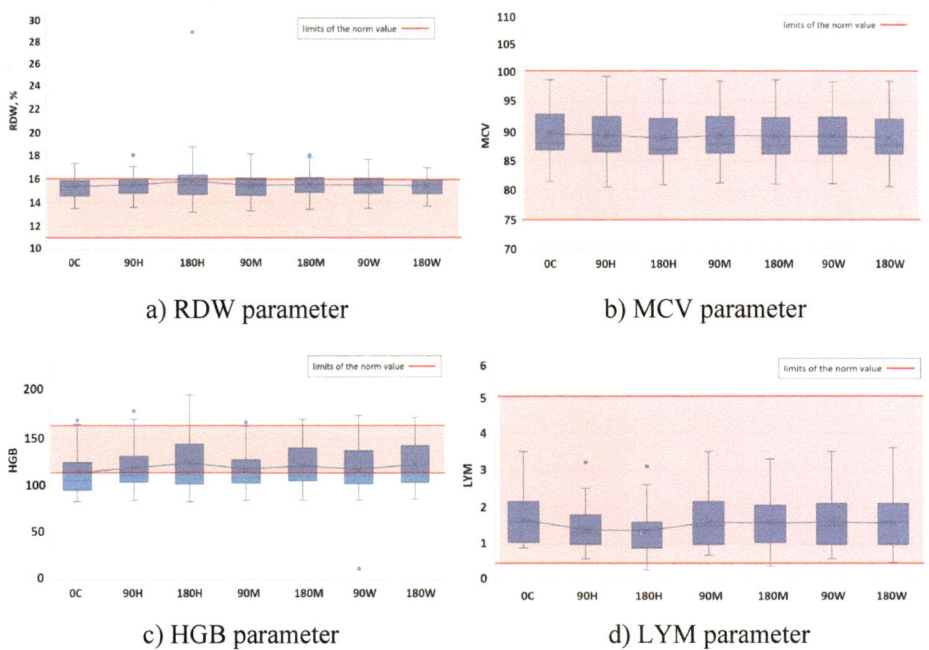

Fig. 2.4 Independent-Samples Kruskal–Walli's test results for four different blood parameters with an p-value >0.05 (null hypothesis is retained). Red line—the limits of the norm for a particular parameter, the norm area, which defines normal range for the denoted blood parameter

also an increase in values when exposed to a strong ultrasound signal for both 90 and 180 s.

The research method of Pairwise Comparison of ultrasound signal values for the five most responsive blood parameters (RBC, HTC, MCH, MCHC, MID (%)) was applied and is denoted in (Fig. 2.6). With all other blood parameters, the same heptagon pattern was obtained—with all red linear connections.

The heptagon vertices depicted in Fig. 2.6 correspond to the following ultrasonic exposure values: initial status (0H); 1 (180H); 2 (180M); 3 (90W); 4 (90H); 5 (90M); 6

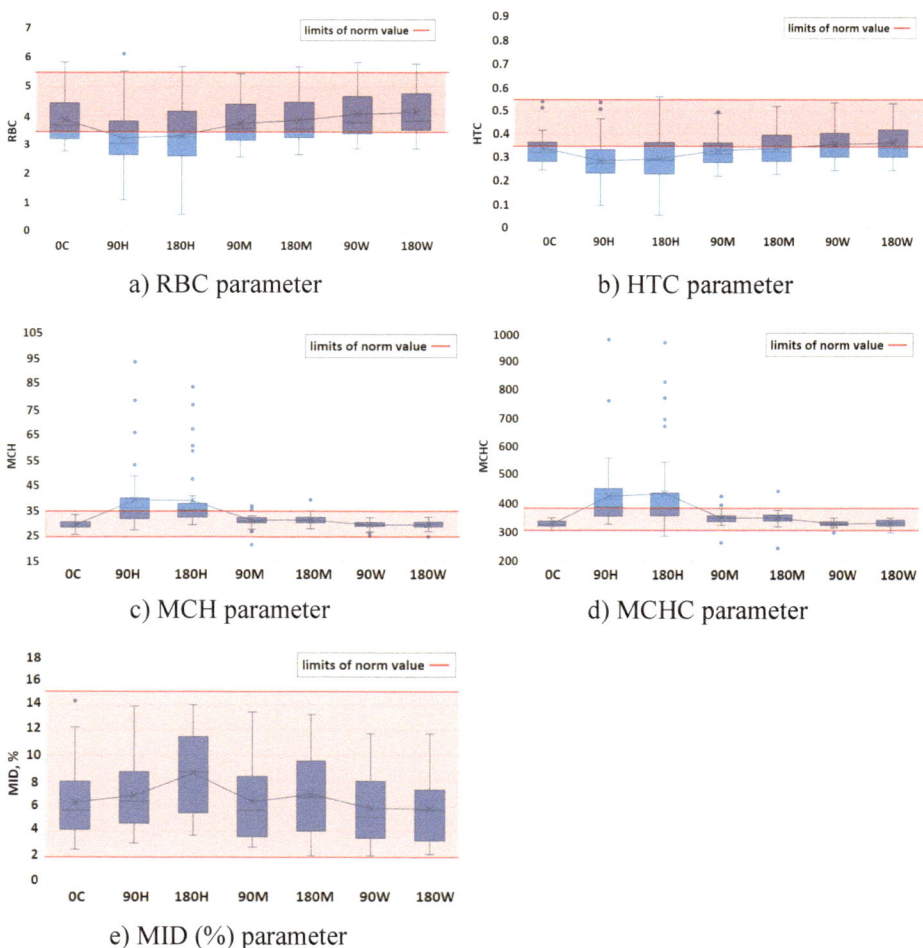

a) RBC parameter

b) HTC parameter

c) MCH parameter

d) MCHC parameter

e) MID (%) parameter

Fig. 2.5 Independent-Samples Kruskal–Walli's Test results on different blood parameters with a very low p-value < 0.001. The red line—shows the limits of the norm for a particular parameter, the norm area, which defines the normal range for the denoted blood parameter

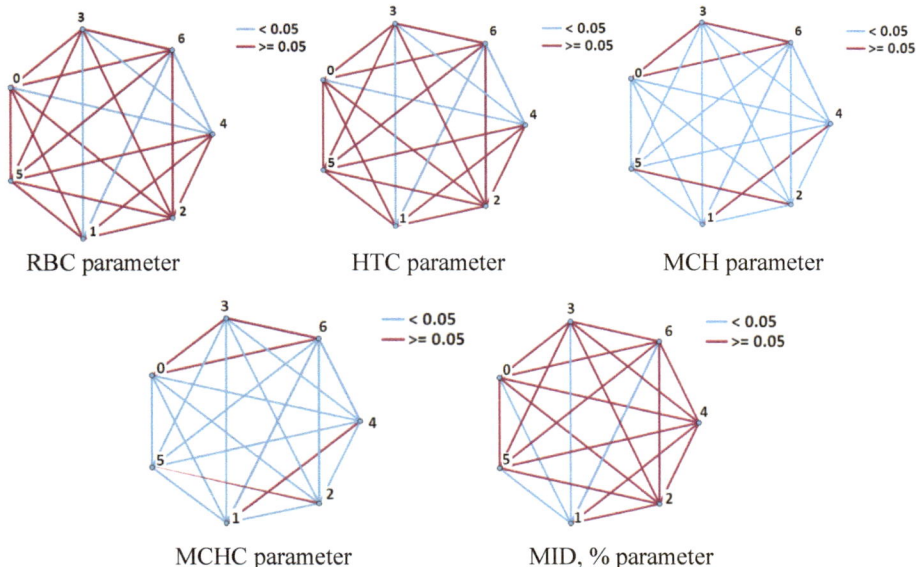

Fig. 2.6 Pairwise comparison of each parameter (V1) where each node shows the sample average rank of V1. Vertices of the hexagon correspond to the following values of ultrasonic exposure: 0 (0C); 1 (180H); 2 (180M); 3 (90W); 4 (90H); 5 (90M); 6 (180W)

(180W). Different colors of the junctions between the peaks indicate different p-values between the pairs (the values of the corresponding blood parameter affected by the different ultrasound signals). If the line is blue, the p-value is <0.05; otherwise, the line is red. Nevertheless, our primary focus lies in the pairs featuring a zero-heptagon vertex, which refers to the initial values of the blood parameter. When considering a zero vertex, blue connections are frequently observed with vertices 4 (90H) and 1 (180H), which serve as indications of a high-intensity ultrasound signal lasting for 90 and 180 s, respectively. Furthermore, there exists a more pronounced interdependence among vertices 1, 3, and 6. More details are provided in Table 2.6, which shows the specific p-values adjusted for Bonferroni connection between blood parameter initial value and those exposed to different ultrasound signals. The table reveals a significant impact of the 90H ultrasound signal on denoted blood parameter values. In contrast, medium ultrasound signals (90M and 180M) exhibit a considerably lower effect, and weak signals do not appear to have a significant influence on any of the five blood parameters.

The graphs in Fig. 2.7 show the results of the Kruskal–Walli's test for blood parameters with a significance level >0.05. It is evident that exposure to high intensity 180H and 90H ultrasound signals can lead to both an increase and a decrease in parameter values.

Upon analyzing the overall significant impact of ultrasound on all blood parameters at their initial state (0C), it becomes evident that most blood parameters are influenced by

Table 2.6 Dunn test results for the blood parameters most affected by the ultrasound signal

Blood parameter	p-Values adjusted by the Bonferroni correction					
	0C-180W	0C-90M	0C-180H	0C-90H	0C-90W	0C-180M
RBC	1.000	1.000	0.469	0.037	1.000	1.000
HTC	1.000	1.000	0.324	0.047	1.000	1.000
MCH	1.000	0.008	0.000	0.000	1.000	0.03
MCHC	1.000	0.000	0.000	0.000	1.000	0.000
MID, %	1.000	1.000	0.028	1.000	1.000	1.000

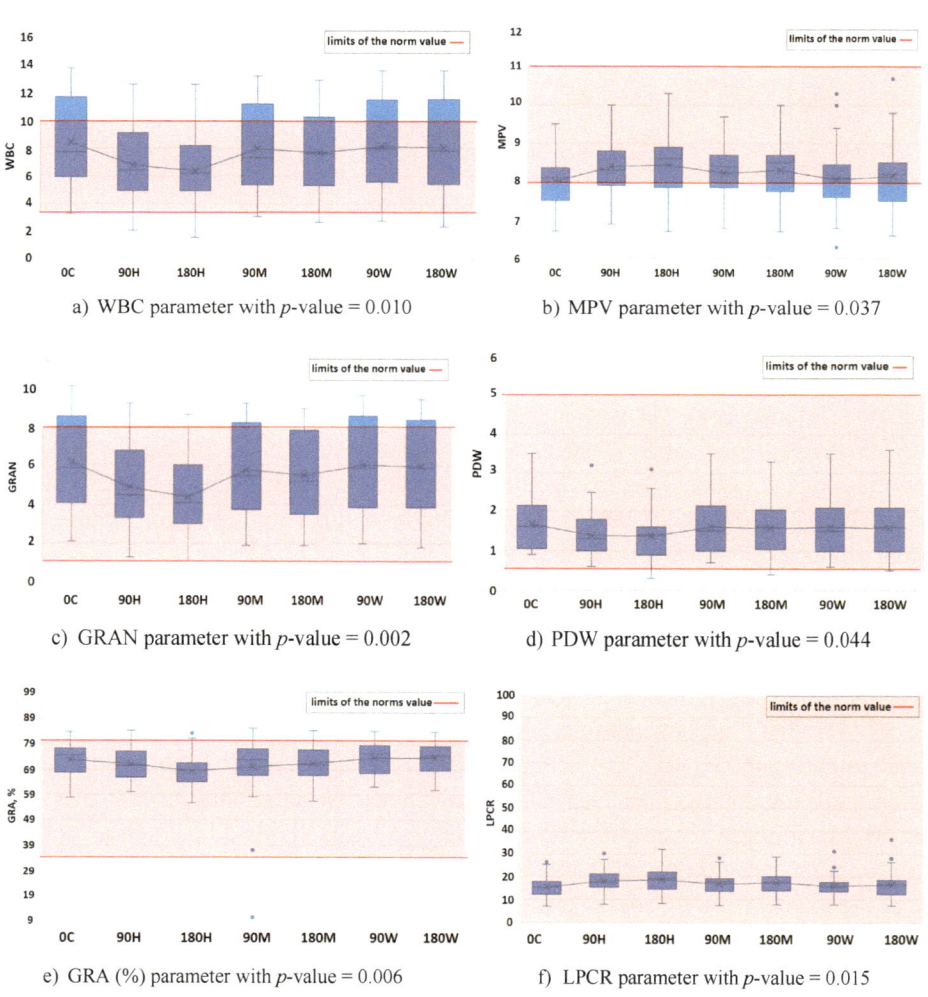

a) WBC parameter with p-value = 0.010

b) MPV parameter with p-value = 0.037

c) GRAN parameter with p-value = 0.002

d) PDW parameter with p-value = 0.044

e) GRA (%) parameter with p-value = 0.006

f) LPCR parameter with p-value = 0.015

Fig. 2.7 Independent-samples Kruskal–Walli's test results on different blood parameters with an p-value <0.05. The red line shows the limits of the norm for a particular parameter, the norm area

Fig. 2.8 Frequencies of significant ultrasound exposure among all blood parameters

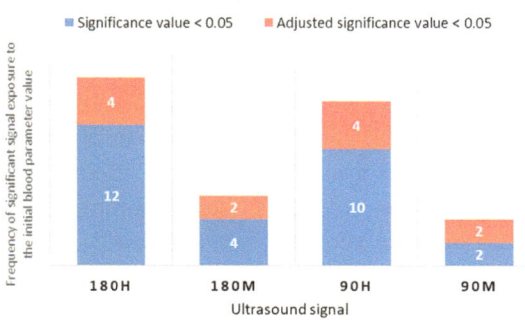

the 180H signal. Specifically, 12 out of 20 parameters exhibit a p-value < 0.05, while 4 out of 20 parameters demonstrate an adjusted p-value < 0.05. In terms of these two significance indicators, the 90H effect ranks second, with 10 out of 20 parameters showing a p-value < 0.05 and 4 out of 20 parameters displaying an adjusted p-value < 0.05. A medium signal has a significant effect on 2–3 times fewer blood parameters (p-value < 0.05 only for 2 parameters) than a strong signal, while a weak signal has no significant effect at all (Fig. 2.8).

2.2.4   Investigation of Platelet Aggregation Using Artificial Intelligence Algorithms

To demonstrate that the selected frequency and intensity of ultrasound induces platelet activation in a dose-dependent manner, a single individual's blood was analyzed utilizing a platelet aggregometer. Two blood samples were collected for testing purposes. One sample served as the control, without any ultrasound exposure and instead treated with epinephrine (adrenaline) to induce platelet aggregation. Another sample was divided into 4 tubes and exposed to ultrasound for varying lengths of time and intensities. It was exposed to ultrasound for 90 s or 180 s time and after exposure it was treated with epinephrine to induce platelet aggregation. The ultrasound tests were carried out at different ultrasound signals, i.e., some samples were tested, at electric power of 35 W (US intensity ~50–70 mW/cm^2), as shown in Table 2.3, and others at 60 W (US intensity ~100–150 mW/cm^2). The time and frequency of 44 kHz were the same to ensure that the ultrasound effect would not be harmful. The platelet aggregation test was conducted at the Laboratory of Molecular Cardiology, Institute of Cardiology, Lithuanian University of Health Sciences, located in Kaunas, Lithuania. The test followed the established classical Born method and utilized a semi-automatic CE IVD certified platelet aggregometer TA-8V from SD Medical (Frouard, France). Platelet aggregation was assessed by comparing the intensity of light transmission between platelet-rich and platelet-poor plasma samples after induction with epinephrine (adrenaline). Transmission of platelet—poor plasma was considered 100%. The final concentration of epinephrine was 10 µM (Chrono-Log,

Havertown, Pennsylvania, USA). Preparation of platelet-rich plasma was carried out by centrifuging of whole blood at $100 \times g$ for 15 min. Platelet-poor plasma was prepared by centrifuging the platelet-rich plasma at $1000 \times g$ for 30 min. AFI LISA 2.5 L refrigerated centrifuge (Château-Goutier, France) was used to prepare blood samples. The aggregation of platelets was measured as % Agr. Different measures of accuracy were calculated from the experiments, i.e. Mean Squared Error (MSE), Root Mean Square Error (RMSE) and Mean Absolute Percentage Error (MAPE) [6]. The MSE is a measure representing the average of the squared difference between actual and predicted values in a dataset. The RMSE is just the square root of the root mean square error, the only difference being that the MSE measures the variance of the residuals, while the RMSE measures the standard deviation of the residuals.

$$RMSE = \sqrt{MSE}, \text{ where } \quad MSE = \frac{1}{n} \sum_{t=1}^{n} |y_t - \hat{y}_t|^2 \qquad (2.2)$$

where n—number of time point, y_t—is the actual value at a given time t, and $\hat{y}_t$—is the predicted value, t observation in a dataset.

MAPE also evaluates the accuracy of the model's predictions, but it measures the average absolute percentage difference between the predicted and actual values:

$$MAPE = \frac{100\%}{n} \sum_{t=1}^{n} \left| \frac{y_t - \hat{y}_t}{y_t} \right|. \qquad (2.3)$$

The results of a blood test with a platelet aggregometer (Fig. 2.9) conducted with epinephrine, which can also show the suppression of other receptors. The study showed that in the absence of ultrasound, the maximum platelet aggregation recorded was 104% (Fig. 2.9a). Conversely, when sonicated with ultrasound, achieving 100% platelet aggregation was not observed (Fig. 2.9b). Instead, a gradual decrease in platelet aggregation was observed as follows: 95% at an ultrasound intensity of 100–150 mW/cm^2 with a duration of 180 s, 92% at an ultrasound intensity of 100–150 mW/cm^2 with a duration of 90 s, 86% at an ultrasound intensity of 50–70 mW/cm^2 with a duration of 180 s, and 80% at an ultrasound intensity of 50–70 mW/cm^2 with a duration of 90 s.

Test results shown in Fig. 2.9 indicate that the process of blood platelet aggregation begins faster with sonicated samples compared to the sample treated only with epinephrine (adrenaline). For the sonicated samples, 10% platelet aggregation was achieved within 1 min and 40%—within 2 min after induction of platelet aggregation with epinephrine. For the blood samples treated only with epinephrine (adrenaline), 5% platelet aggregation was achieved within 1 min and 10%—within 2 min. In vitro [7] it was found that ultrasound produces more stable platelet aggregates than a natural platelet aggregation stimulant. Ultrasound-induced platelet aggregation holds promise as a potential solution for addressing platelet receptor (P2Y$_{12}$ receptor) issues such as defective response to soluble agonists [8] and effectively controlling bleeding.

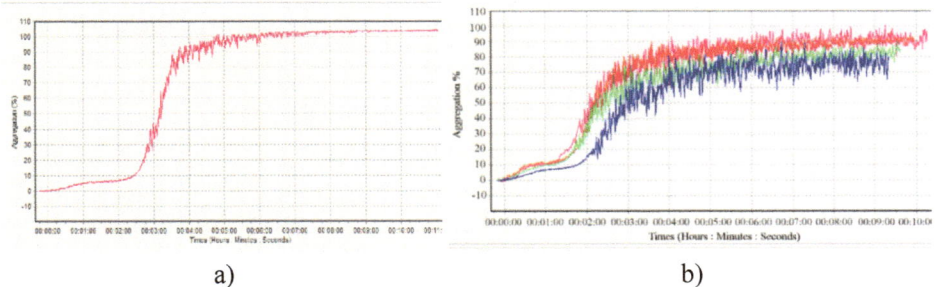

a)   b)

Fig. 2.9 Blood platelet aggregation with epinephrine (**a**) and low-frequency ultrasound (**b**) in vitro. In graphic **b** two samples are sonicated with ultrasound at 60 W electric power (pink, red) and two samples sonicated with ultrasound at 35 W electric power (green, blue)

Ongoing efforts are underway to predict platelet (PLT) values based on the influence of ultrasound signals, their duration, and intensity. Machine learning algorithms are well-suited for PLT value prediction. Among the various algorithms used for regression problems, the study employed the five most popular ones. Based on the experimental results of 10 tests, the support vector regression (SVR) algorithm with a linear kernel was found to be the most accurate algorithm, as determined by the root-mean-square-error (RMSE) metric. Table 2.7 PLT prediction results providing the average RMSE value obtained from 10 tests for five different ML algorithms: Decision Trees (DT), Random Forest (RF), Artificial Neural Network (ANN), Linear Regression (LR), and Support Vector Regression (SVR).

Considering the results of all the Machine learning algorithms, we can see that the highest error values are obtained with the three-layer ANN, with an average RMSE value of 72.47 for all 6 different ultrasound signals (Table 2.7). The largest prediction errors are observed for the high impact signal, i.e., 90H and 180H, while the best prediction results are obtained for the PLT values exposed with medium signal (90M and 180M). The same tendency can be seen with the remaining models. LR model has an average error of 55.50, DT − 47.61, RF − 44.39 and SVR have demonstrated the best prediction accuracy with an average RMSE of 32.06 (MAPE = 10.38%, Fig. 2.10).

Table 2.7 PLT prediction results

ML algorithm	90W	180W	90M	180M	90H	180H
DT	44.156	36.61	41.61	35.8	67.34	60.16
RF	47.822	33.68	34.49	29.75	67.98	52.63
ANN	66.04	51.84	27.04	41.75	154.24	93.96
LR	48.99	42.83	43.54	38.77	76.05	82.83
SVR	23.45	27.73	22.90	27.12	35.41	55.80

Fig. 2.10 Prediction accuracy with an average *RMSE*

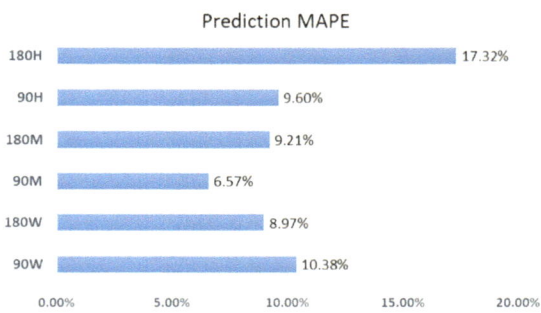

Figure 2.11 shows the results of the SVR model's prediction of the PLT value (in terms of MAPE value) using different ultrasound signals. The best accuracy of 6.57% was obtained when predicting PLT values exposed with the 90M signal, while the worst accuracy of 17.32% was obtained when exposed with the 180H signal. It can be assumed that the effect of a longer and stronger ultrasound signal is slightly more difficult to predict, as extreme values occur. This is also evident from the results (a)–(b) in Fig. 2.11, where the actual PLT values affected by the ultrasound signal are shown as blue dots and the predicted ones as red dots.

To assess the importance of attributes, we used the *F*-test statistical test [9], which is helpful for feature selection when there are numerous potential predictor factors, as we aim to identify a subset of variables that are most strongly associated with a response variable. The feature importance scores are computed as:

$$Fscore = -\log(p), \tag{2.4}$$

where *p* is the probability of *F*-test.

The importance scores of all blood parameters using the *F*-test algorithm for the prediction of the PLT value, including only the longest ultrasound signals of different strengths, i.e., 180W, 180M and 180H, are shown in Table 2.8, with the Top 5 feature importance scores for each signal highlighted in green. These scores rank the attributes in order of importance, with a higher F-score indicating that the relevant predictor is more important.

The results of the experiments showed that the baseline PLT value and the PCT are the blood factors that have the biggest impact on the predictive value of the PLT value (see Table 2.8, all three columns are in green). The GRAN parameter can be ranked as the third most important, but its importance depends on the ultrasound exposure signal, as in the case of LYM or RDW parameters (one or two columns in green). Meanwhile, we can state that MCV has the least impact on the prediction of the PLT value as it shows the lowest value of the *F* score. Table 2.8 Feature importance scores (*F* scores) using *F*-test algorithm for the PLT value prediction including 180W, 180M and 180H signals.

Human blood is a shear-thinning fluid with a complex reaction that relies heavily on the red blood cells (RBC's) ability to form aggregates. The aggregation of human RBC

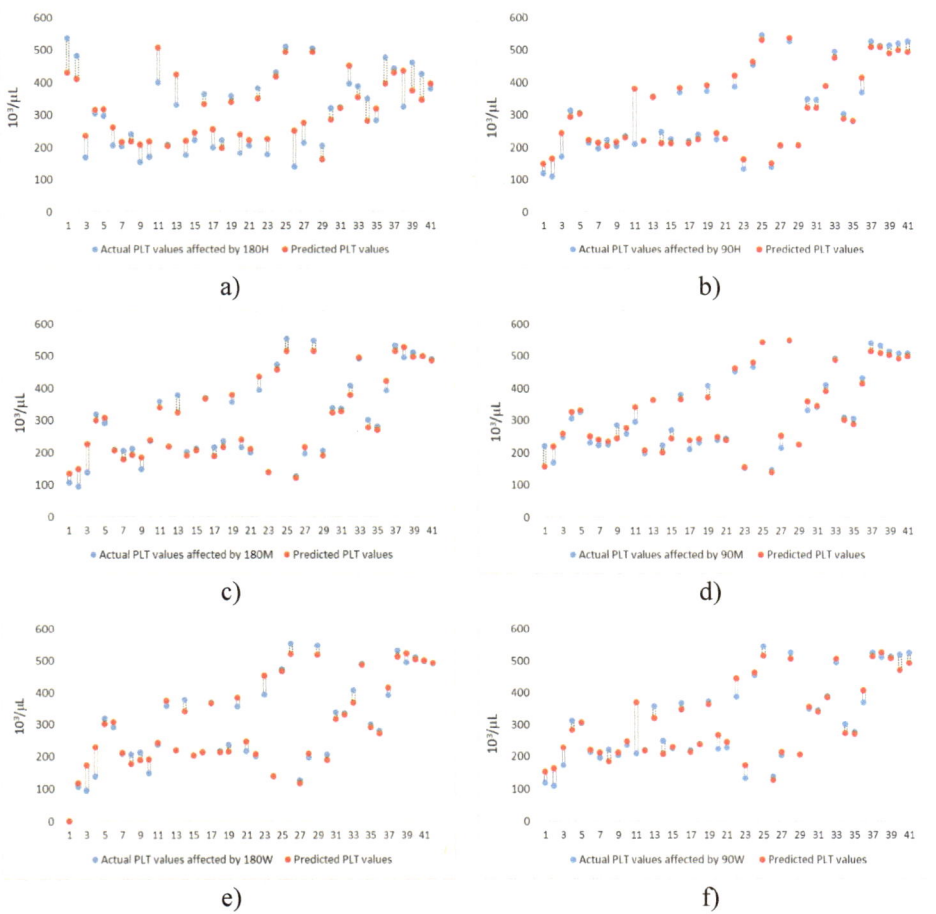

Fig. 2.11 PLT prediction results for the testing data using SVR model

is a major cause of a wide range of pathological conditions, from bacterial infections to cancer. At low shear rates or during hemostasis, RBCs form aggregates that resemble piles of coins, called 'rouleaux'. However, studies have shown that under the influence of low-frequency ultrasound dissociation of RBC aggregates into individual RBC cells occurs. RBC aggregates are separated into single cells, when the shear force is over a certain value caused by ultrasound. Dissociation of RBC aggregates increased with increasing shear rate above a critical value of $\gamma = 5\text{–}10 \text{ s}^{-1}$ [10].

The results of the study show that the observed changes in the parameters provided by the blood analyzer are not only related to the formation of a blood clot, but also to the dissociation of cell aggregates. In addition to this fundamental finding, our research also aimed to propose faster statistical and artificial intelligence methods for processing blood

Table 2.8 Feature importance scores

Parameter	Feature importance scores		
	180W signal	180H signal	180M signal
GRA_	0.3833	6.8175	0.409
GRAN	9.5306	2.7977	10.22
HGB	2.2199	3.4821	3.515
HTC	4.4684	1.6236	6.1263
LYM	2.8005	2.8074	3.634
LYM_	6.4304	1.8829	5.327
LPCR	1.5975	4.2939	2.048
MCH	4.0813	0.6867	4.6901
MCHC	2.9951	0.2831	3.026
MCV	1.2764	0.0996	1.93
MID	1.2299	2.4537	1.62
MID_	1.0965	6.1439	1.573
MPV	1.597	2.5401	1.761
PCT	34.1933	8.0421	40.59
PDW	1.9328	2.9174	2.384
PLT	35.9738	9.1113	35.03
RBC	2.8726	1.3778	2.681
RDW	5.2536	1.6584	4.282
RDW a	2.3421	1.0386	2.011
WBC	2.9999	3.6711	4.152

parameters, avoid the mistakes of inexperienced analysts and confirm the advantages of low-frequency ultrasound. Ultrasound affects the blood by both radiation and flow forces. Shear forces, radiation force and acoustic flow occur together. High-frequency ultrasound induces aggregation of blood particles by exciting standing acoustic waves in the liquid phase of the blood, where aggregated RBCs accumulate in the nodes. In contrast to the standing waves, traveling acoustic waves cause the opposite phenomenon—the mixing of blood aggregates. Therefore, during blood analyzer tests, it was found that the number of single erythrocytes separated from aggregates by low-frequency ultrasound in the volume of a blood analyzer drop is lower than in the same volume of erythrocyte aggregates not affected by ultrasound.

Blood tests revealed several parameters such as mean corpuscular hemoglobin (MCH), mean corpuscular hemoglobin concentration (MCHC) and platelet aggregation (PLT) that showed the greatest changes during exposure to low-frequency ultrasound and exceeded the permissible limits. Parameters such as mean corpuscular hemoglobin (MCH) and mean corpuscular hemoglobin concentration (MCHC) indicate the amount of hemoglobin per cell and, the amount of hemoglobin per unit volume, respectively. Hemoglobin is required to transport oxygen from the lungs to the cells of the body, Ultrasound has an impact on changes in these blood parameters related to erythrocyte function. During this study, venous blood was drawn from a vein near the elbow for laboratory purposes. The venous blood is poor in oxygen. When ultrasound was used on dissociated erythrocytes in an open sample (surrounded by oxygen in Vacuette K2E K2EDTA 13×75 tube) and the shear rate exceeded a critical value, the color of the dissociated erythrocytes changed to a bright red color, as if they had been enriched by oxygen, as in the case of arterial blood. An important property of hemoglobin is that O_2 binding is pH dependent. It has been experimentally observed that CO_2 is released more readily when the pH is acidic, i.e. when there is a lot of CO_2's around. This' is the case for our blood samples before treatment with low-frequency ultrasound. This treatment has potential to render hemoglobin more conductive to binding with CO_2 offering energy for the dispersion of gas bubbles within membranes or the fusion of multiple erythrocytes membranes [11]. The results of these studies are published in the authors' publication [12]. The key finding of this study was to observe changes in gas exchange in the blood under the influence of different intensities of low-frequency ultrasound. This finding holds potential implications for treating pulmonary hypertension using the low-frequency ultrasound transducer. However, paying attention to such blood parameters as platelet count (PLT), plateletcrit (PCT), white blood cells (WBC), lymphocytes (LYM), granulocytes (GRAN), which are also affected by ultrasound, should be mentioned and what ailments it is used for therapy would be useful.

A platelet count (PLT) is a laboratory test that measures the number of platelets in the blood. Platelets are cells that help blood to clot and are essential for the formation of blood clots. A normal platelet count is between 150,000 and 450,000 platelets per microlitre of blood. High or low platelet counts can increase the risk of blood clots or excessive bleeding. Having more than 450,000 platelets is a condition called thrombocytosis; having less than 150,000 is called thrombocytopenia. This condition can be dangerous because it affects the body's ability to form clots, leading to excessive bleeding. Figure 2.2f shows that PLT can be increased under the influence of low frequency ultrasound.

Plateletcrit (PCT) is the calculation of the volume occupied by platelets in the blood, as a calculation of platelet count (PLT) and mean platelet volume (MPV). In general, the number of platelets in the blood is maintained by a constant rate of destruction of old platelets and formation of new platelets. Genetic and environmental factors such as lifestyle and exercise, ethnicity, age, smoking and alcohol consumption can all affect PLT, MPV and PCT levels. In addition, capillary sampling can lower PLT and consequently MPV and PCT, so the venous sampling for PLT biomarkers is recommended. Low platelet counts can lead to excessive blood loss, haemorrhage and internal bleeding, which can be life-threatening. Severe cases of bleeding inside the body and under the skin as a result of not having enough platelets is a bleeding disorder called immune thrombocytopenia. Figure 2.2i shows that PCT can be increased under the influence of low frequency ultrasound.

White blood cells (WBCs), also called leukocytes, are an important part of the body's immune system. These cells help fight infections, heal trauma and recover from illness. A high WBC count can be caused by many conditions, including: autoimmune and inflammatory diseases that cause the immune system to attack healthy tissues; viral or bacterial infections, including rheumatoid arthritis; immunosuppression, an immune disorder; bone marrow disease (myelofibrosis); a reaction to medicines such as adrenaline or corticosteroids; cancers such as leukaemia and Hodgkin's disease; allergic reactions; tissue damage from a burn or surgery. Figure 2.2k shows that WBC can be reduced under the influence of low frequency ultrasound.

Lymphocytes (LYM) are a type of white blood cell that play a vital role in the immune system. They help fight infections, destroy infected or tumour cells and contribute to the immune system's memory. Having high levels of lymphocytes in the blood is called lymphocytosis. Lymphocytosis is an indication that the immune system has been activated in response to a disease or medical condition. Lymphocytosis can lead to lymphadenopathy (swollen lymph nodes) and splenomegaly (enlarged spleen). Splenomegaly can cause a dull pain in the upper right side of the body. Other symptoms may develop depending on the underlying cause. High levels of lymphocytes may indicate, for example, an infection or cancer of the blood or lymphatic system. Figure 2.2o shows that LYM can be reduced under the influence of low frequency ultrasound.

About two-thirds of white blood cells contain granules (small particles). These cells are called granulocytes (GRAN). They're derived from bone marrow and are both short-lived and highly mobile. The most common type of granulocytes are called neutrophils. They are often the first responders to areas of inflammation in the body. They follow chemical signposts to travel through blood vessels to directly fight infection and other causes of inflammation, often within minutes of the initial trauma. If complete blood count (CBC) shows an elevated neutrophil count, this may be due to an infection. Similarly, a low neutrophil count may indicate a weakened immune system. A high number of granulocytes in the blood (granulocytosis) can be a sign that body is fighting off an infection or having an allergic reaction. High levels of granulocytes can also be a sign of a chronic disease or cancer of the blood cells. Figure 2.2p shows that GRAN can be reduced under the influence of low frequency ultrasound.

2.3   Development of a Low-Frequency Piezoelectric Ultrasonic Transducer for Biological Tissue Sonication

The safety of ultrasound exposure is crucial to the patient's well-being. The acoustic intensity level emitted by medical ultrasound diagnostic equipment must not exceed 1000 mW/ cm^2 in the 1–10 MHz frequency range. These frequency waves are significantly absorbed by biological tissue, limiting their therapeutic effect on internal organs. Experiments have shown that, with an acoustic intensity of 800–1000 mW/cm^2, the effective depth of 1 MHz ultrasound is 0.9 cm for muscle and 1.7 cm for fat. The acoustic intensity decreases exponentially and proportionally with biological tissue's attenuation coefficient and depth of action. In addition, this coefficient in the human body is proportional to the frequency of the operating ultrasound. In this ongoing research, low-frequency (20–100 kHz) ultrasound is being studied for its potential to therapeutically affect deeper internal organs. A low-frequency ultrasonic acoustic wave transducer was created, which can excite a higher than the first natural vibration mode. Theoretical studies have confirmed that focused ultrasound signals lead to deeper penetration depth. Unlike flat surface ultrasonic transducers, used so far, that emit a cylinder-shaped, uniformly distributed acoustic signal, a newly created transducer with a cut-out surface emits a ring-shaped acoustic signal that, at a certain distance, interferes and focuses into a narrower beam for deeper tissue penetration. This opens the possibility of using a more targeted and precise ultrasound acoustic wave for treatment, affecting only the treated part of the body, instead of the whole body.

2.3.1 Concept of a Low-Frequency Ultrasound Transducer for Noninvasive Therapy

For blood gas circulation improvement, it is necessary to create dedicated technical means. A low-frequency ultrasonic actuator, which is developed using the principles of digital twins, is the most suitable for that purpose [13]. The term "digital twin" still lacks a common understanding, leading to differences in its technological implementation and objectives. This term covers virtual and physical replicas of a device under development, which are used as a specific testbed for a process or a product, to simulate the changes made before they are implemented in real life, by entitling virtual and physical copies as virtual and physical twins, respectively, and linking them to simulations and experiments resulting in a digital output. Acoustic waves carry energy that can be harnessed to perform useful work. The energy density carried by a plane wave is given by [14]:

$$\varepsilon = p\,v/2c = p^2/2\rho_0 c^2 = \rho\,v^2/\,2 \tag{2.5}$$

where p and v are the acoustic pressure and velocity amplitudes, ρ_0 represents the mass density and c is the sound velocity of the medium.

Another commonly used metric for describing energy propagation in a wave is the wave intensity, which quantifies the rate of energy transfer by the acoustic wave (in units of Wcm^{-2}). The time average intensity for a plane wave in a fluid can be calculated directly from the pressure and fluid properties. The sound intensity I and the sound pressure P are two characteristic parameters describing the acoustic wave propagation and are defined by the following equation [14]:

$$I = p^2/2\rho_0 c = 0.5\,\rho_0 c\omega^2 A^2 \tag{2.6}$$

where ρ_0 represents the mass density and c is the sound velocity of the medium (1 g/cm^3), ω is the angular frequency, and A is the amplitude of the acoustic wave.

An additional important material property for the design of acoustic systems is the material attenuation coefficient. Attenuation describes the loss of acoustic energy irreversibly to heat due to various mechanisms such as viscosity or molecular relaxation [14]. When an acoustic wave propagates in material, the pressure amplitude after a distance L is given by:

$$p = p_0 e^{-\alpha L} \tag{2.7}$$

where p_0 is the initial pressure of the wave and α is the attenuation coefficient in neper per centimeter.

Attenuation is highly frequency-dependent, with higher frequencies being attenuated more strongly than lower ones. Thus, at frequencies below 0.3 MHz, ultrasound has a significantly better effect on deeper biological tissues, and a strong biochemical reaction is more likely to occur. The effects of low-frequency ultrasound on bones, blood vessels and internal organs should therefore be carefully studied. However, cavitation phenomena below 100 kHz can destroy biological tissues and, in some places, raise their temperature above the vital limit. The mechanical index (MI) is an indication of the mechanical damage that may be caused by inertial cavitation:

$$MI = P_{NP}/f_c^{-0.5} \tag{2.8}$$

where peak-negative pressure (P_{NP}) is expressed in MPa, and f_c is expressed in MHz. The value taken for P_{NP} should be the maximum value anywhere in the field, measured in water but reduced by 0.3 dB cm^{-1} MHz^{-1} attenuation.

Furthermore, in this ultrasound frequency range (20–100 kHz), emulsification or dispersion forces acting on blood can easily cause hemolysis. These factors are also frequency and intensity dependent. Therefore, the effects of ultrasound on bones, blood vessels and internal organs must be carefully studied when developing new types of ultrasound emitters operating below 100 kHz.

Three different configurations of Langevin-type ultrasonic transducers were developed. One of them had a cylindrical front mass with a flat ultrasound emitting surface (Fig. 2.12a), and two with different diameters d_1 of 59 mm and of 100 mm, respectively, had a cut-out circular front mass surface (Fig. 2.12b). The design of the latter is based on three concepts: 1—the use of a front mass with a cut-out annular surface produces stronger excitation; 2—the radial mode oscillation of the modified front mass produces a concentrated acoustic field; and 3—more acoustic energy is produced in the higher frequency vibrational mode.

The fabricated transducers were composed of two piezo-ceramic rings (material—PZT-4), a steel cylinder-shaped back mass (St 304), an aluminum cylinder-shaped front mass (Al 7075-T6).

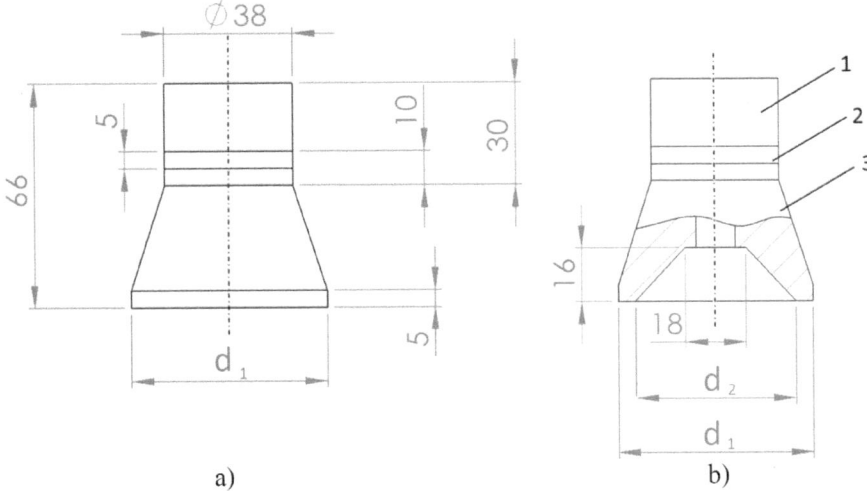

Fig. 2.12 Geometric dimensions of the piezo transducer in mm with flat surface (**a**) and cut-out surface (**b**) of the front mass 3: 1—back mass; 2—two ring-shaped piezoelectric elements

2.3.2 Ultrasonic Transducer Virtual Twin

The FEM models of three Langevin-type ultrasonic transducers with different front mass designs were investigated as virtual twins by comparing two Langevin-type ultrasonic transducers with different diameters of 58 and 100 mm with a cut-out annular surface and one with flat front mass surface. COMSOL Multiphysics 5.6 software was used to create the three-dimensional finite element models (FEM) of the piezo transducers and to perform simulations. This software was used to build a full 3D FEM model and to analyze the transducers to observe its vibration behavior through its simulation by modal analysis and to determine their natural frequencies by harmonic analysis. This was also done to establish the validity of the analytical results. The piezoelectric transducers were modeled using a 3D modeling approach and mesh elements were used for piezoelectric and other components. Modal analysis was used to determine the natural frequencies, mode shapes, and the location of nodal plane. This analysis was performed under resonance conditions with a constant voltage of 50 V applied to the electrical contacts of both ceramic disks. No structural constraint was applied to the modal analysis. This simulates an unconstrained transducer assembly. This state is like the physical test state where the transducer is without any constraints. The transducer properties of the materials used for the simulation are given in Table 2.9.

Muscle material properties (Table 2.10) were selected for the analysis of acoustic wave propagation in human tissue. The attenuation coefficient of a material is frequency dependent. The form $\alpha = \alpha_0 f^b$ s assumed, where α (Np/m) is the absorption coefficient for a

Table 2.9 Properties of the materials used for simulation

Material properties	Piezoceramic PZT-4 [15]	Steel [16]	Aluminum [17]
Young's modulus [N/m^2]		200e+9	71.7e+9
Poison's ratio		0.25	0.33
Density [kg/m^3]	7500	7800	2810
Dielectric permittivity matrix, $\times$ 10^{-7} [F/m]	$\varepsilon_{11} = 11.42$; $\varepsilon_{33} = 8.85$		
Piezoelectric matrix [C/m^2]	$e_{13} = 18.01$; $e_{33} = 29.48$; $e_{52} = 10.34$		
Elasticity matrix, $\times 10^{10}$ [N/m^2]	$c_{11} = 14.68$; $c_{12} = 8.108$; $c_{13} = 8.105$; $c_{33} = 13.17$; $c_{44} = 3.29$; $c_{66} = 3.14$		

Table 2.10 Material properties of muscle [18]

Speed of sound, m/s	1588
Density, kg/m^3	1090
Attenuation coefficient Np/m	0.206 (38 kHz); 0.265 (48 kHz)

given frequency f, α_0 (Np/m/Hz) is a medium constant, and b is also a numerical constant dependent on the tissue type [18].

FEM modeling was used to investigate the vibration modes and sound pressure field in the range 0–100 kHz, including the radiation in the muscle at the two lowest resonant modes of the developed piezoelectric transducer.

2.3.3 Ultrasonic Transducer Physical Twin

Based on the theoretical analysis and simulations, two prototypes of the piezoelectric transducer with different cylindrical front mass designs of diameter 58 mm were made for experimental study to determine the output characteristics of the transducer and to verify the results of the numerical modeling. The dynamics of the transducer has been evaluated by measuring the electrical impedance, resonant frequencies and vibration modes comparing with simulation results. A Polytec Laser Doppler 3D scanning vibrometer PSV-500-3D-HV (Polytech GmbH), linear amplifier P200 (FLC Electronics AB) were used for a high-precision measurement of the three-dimensional vibration distribution on the front surface of the transducer (Fig. 2.13).

The resonant frequencies of the developed piezoelectric transducers were measured using impedance analyzer 6500B (Wayne Kerr Electronics Ltd., UK) presented in Fig. 2.14.

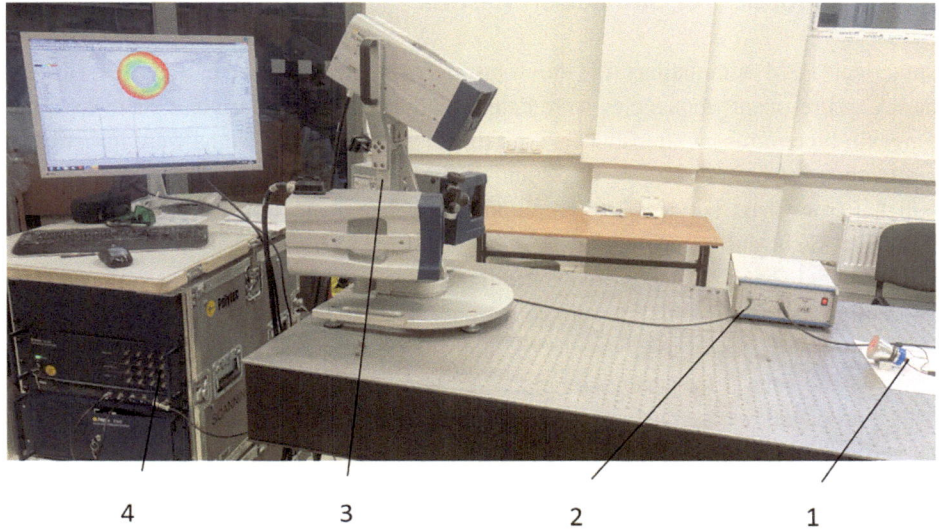

Fig. 2.13 Set-up with Polytec PSV-500-3D scanning laser vibrometer: 1—transducer; 2—linear amplifier; 3—Polytech scanning laser heads; 4—Polytech signal generator/data acquisition system

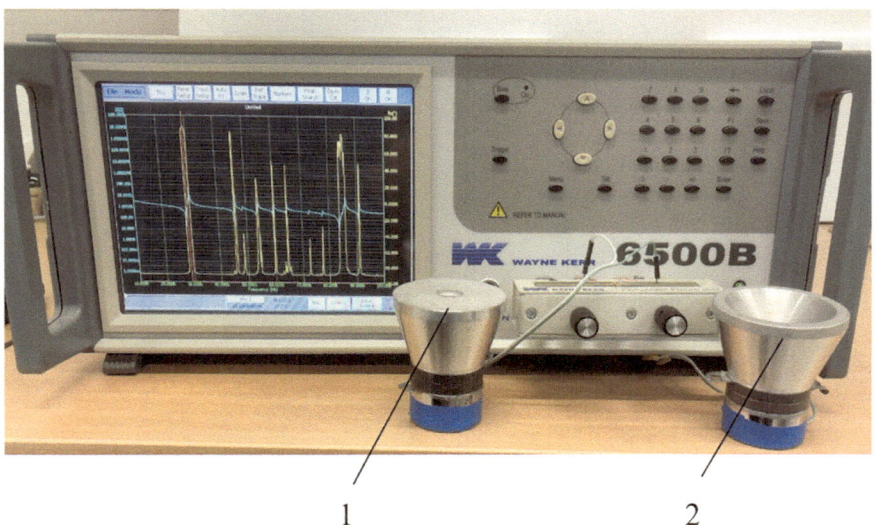

Fig. 2.14 Experimental set-up with impedance analyzer and the two tested transducers: 1—transducer with flat surface; 2—transducer with cut-out surface

2.3.4   Validation of Simulation Results

Numerical FEM simulations of the transducers were performed, and the vibration modes and resonant frequencies were determined using forced harmonic analysis. Three Langevin-type ultrasonic transducers with different front mass designs were investigated: two of them with diameters d_1 of 58 and 100 mm and cut-out annular surface and one with flat front mass surface. The amplitude-frequency characteristics of the transducers with flat and cut-out front mass surfaces are presented in Fig. 2.15 in X, Y, Z axis.

The modal shapes of the piezoelectric transducer with flat and cut-out surfaces at the first natural frequency vibrations are shown in Fig. 2.16.

The modal shapes of the piezoelectric transducers with flat and cut-out front surfaces at the second natural frequency vibrations are presented in Fig. 2.17.

The propagation of acoustic waves excited in muscle by piezoelectric transducers with flat and cut-out surfaces at the first mode are presented in Fig. 2.18.

The propagation of acoustic waves excited in muscle by piezoelectric transducers with flat and cut-out surfaces at the second mode are presented in Fig. 2.19.

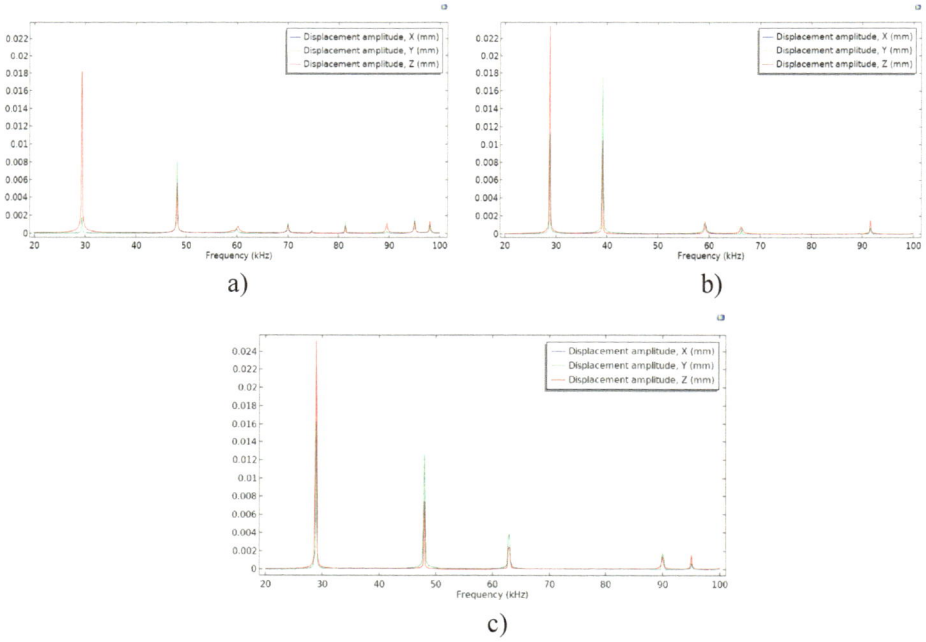

a)

b)

c)

Fig. 2.15 Theoretical amplitude-frequency-characteristics of piezoelectric transducers using COM-SOL Multiphysics: **a**—with flat surface, **b**—with cut-out surface and outer diameter of 59 mm, **c**—with cut-out surface and outer diameter of 100 mm

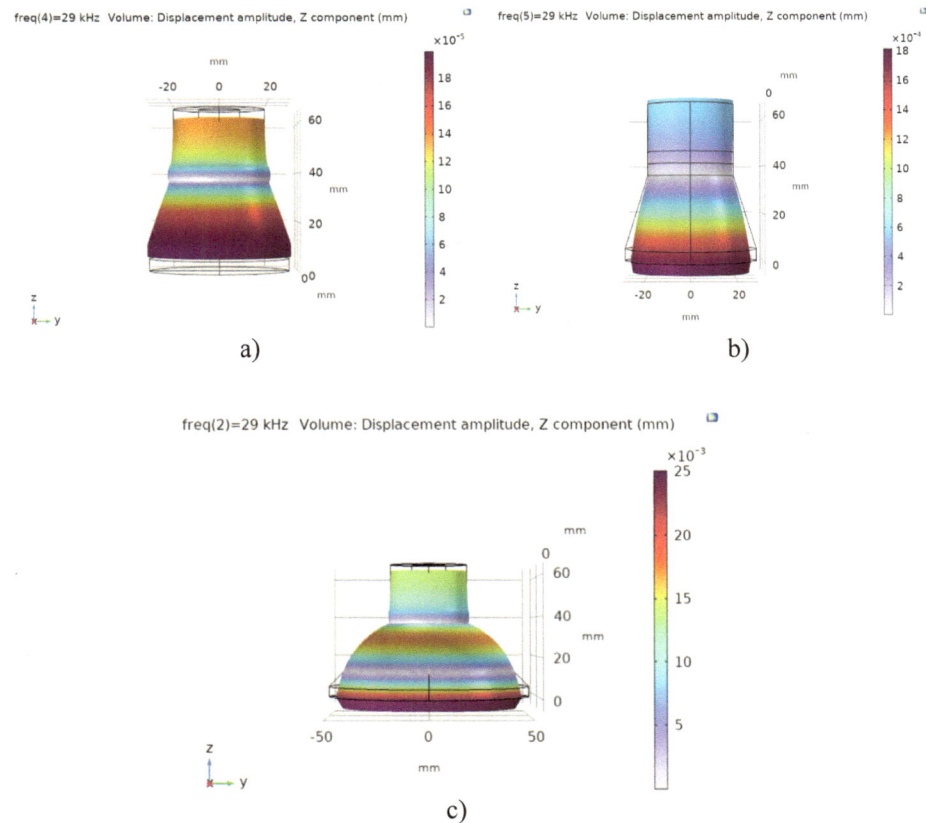

Fig. 2.16 Modal shapes of the piezoelectric transducer at the first natural frequency: **a**—with flat surface, **b**—with 58 mm diameter cut-out surface, **c**—with 100 mm diameter cut-out surface

The boundary condition for zero sound pressure ($p_t = 0$) was selected for the upper surface of muscle medium. It is said to be appropriate for an approximate liquid gas interface. Acoustic analysis requires a mesh that allows to capture the results of wave propagation. The analysis has 5 finite elements for each wavelength of the medium. Distribution of the acoustic pressure level of an ultrasound wave propagating in a muscle tissue, simulated by piezoelectric transducers, in the second natural mode is presented in Fig. 2.20.

The dynamics of the two fabricated transducers with different front mass designs of 58 mm have been evaluated. Using an impedance analyzer 6500B (Wayne Kerr Electronics Ltd., UK) measurement of the electrical impedance, resonant frequencies and vibration modes were performed and validated with simulation results (Fig. 2.21a, b).

A Polytech Laser Doppler 3D scanning vibrometer PSV-500-3D-HV (Polytec GmbH, Germany) was used for high-precision measurement of the three-dimensional vibration

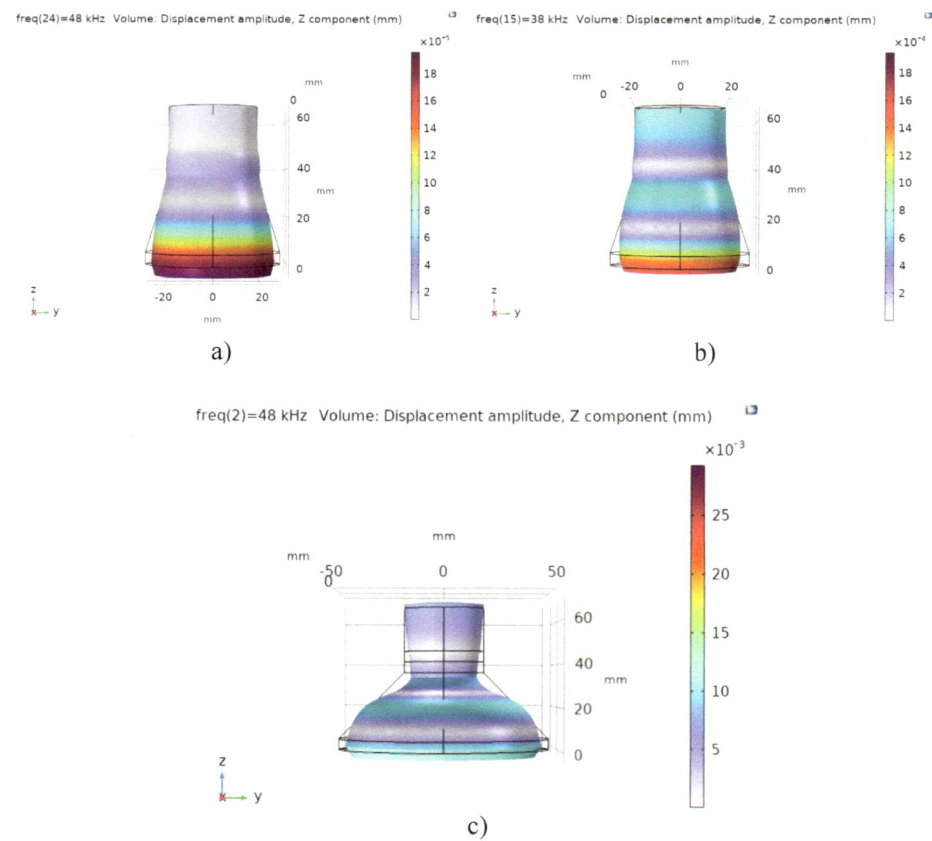

Fig. 2.17 Modal shapes of the piezoelectric transducer at the second natural frequency vibrations: **a**—with flat surface, **b**—with 58 mm diameter cut-out surface, **c**—with 100 mm diameter cut-out surface

distribution of the transducer's front surface (Fig. 2.13). The periodic chirp type driving signal of 50 V was used in the frequency range from 20 to 100 kHz (Fig. 2.22a, b). The longitudinal and radial vibrational modes with the highest velocity amplitudes were measured with Polytech 3D scanning vibrometer at two resonance frequencies respectively: a longitudinal amplitude of 12.8 mm/s at 28.47 kHz and a radial amplitude of 25.5 mm/s at 46.19 kHz for the transducer with a flat surface and a longitudinal amplitude of 9.5 mm/s at 28.13 kHz and a radial amplitude of 42.7 mm/s at 38.04 kHz for the transducer with cut-out surface. Stronger excitation on the second natural frequency was obtained by utilizing a transducer with a cut-out front mass surface.

The Langevin-type ultrasonic wave transducer has been analyzed for its high directivity and long propagation distance properties due to its high frequency (>25 kHz), short wavelength, and has been extensively studied for detection and sensing purposes. Ultrasound

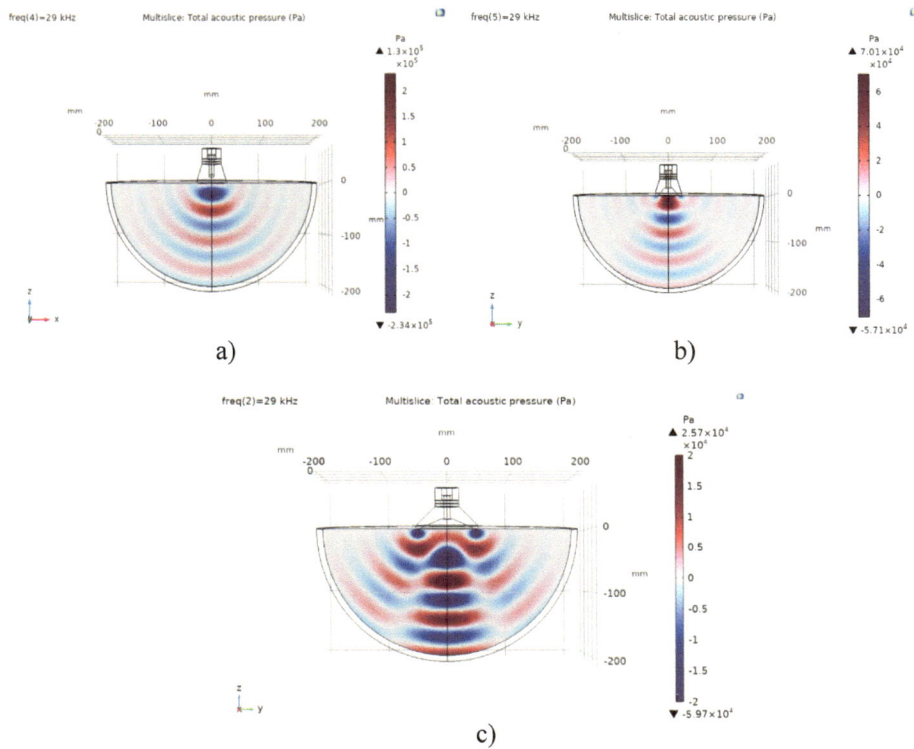

Fig. 2.18 Propagation of acoustic field generated by piezoelectric transducer at the first mode in the muscle: **a**—with flat surface, **b**—with 58 mm diameter cut-out surface, **c**—with 100 mm diameter cut-out surface

sonication is known to have effects on the living body, such as the promotion of enzyme reactions, emulsification, thermogenic effects, expansion of capillary blood vessels, and improving metabolism. Here, "the effective depth of ultrasound exposure is defined as the depth of ultrasound beam close to the body surface of the patient's internal organ, which is effectively treated therapeutically." In this case, the acoustic energy delivered to the organ is proportional to the intensity and duration of the ultrasound. The first five resonant frequencies of the developed 58 mm diameter transducers were modelled, and further analysis showed that the vibrational modes with the largest displacements were found at two resonant frequencies: around 29 and 46 kHz for the flat surface transducer, and around 29 and 40 kHz for the cut-out front mass transducer (Fig. 2.15a, b). The resonant frequencies of the developed 58 mm diameter piezoelectric transducers measured with an impedance analyzer (Fig. 2.21) coincide with frequencies of the first and second resonant modes, measured with Polytech 3D scanning vibrometer (Fig. 2.22) and the resonant frequencies determined using FEM modeling (Fig. 2.15a, b).

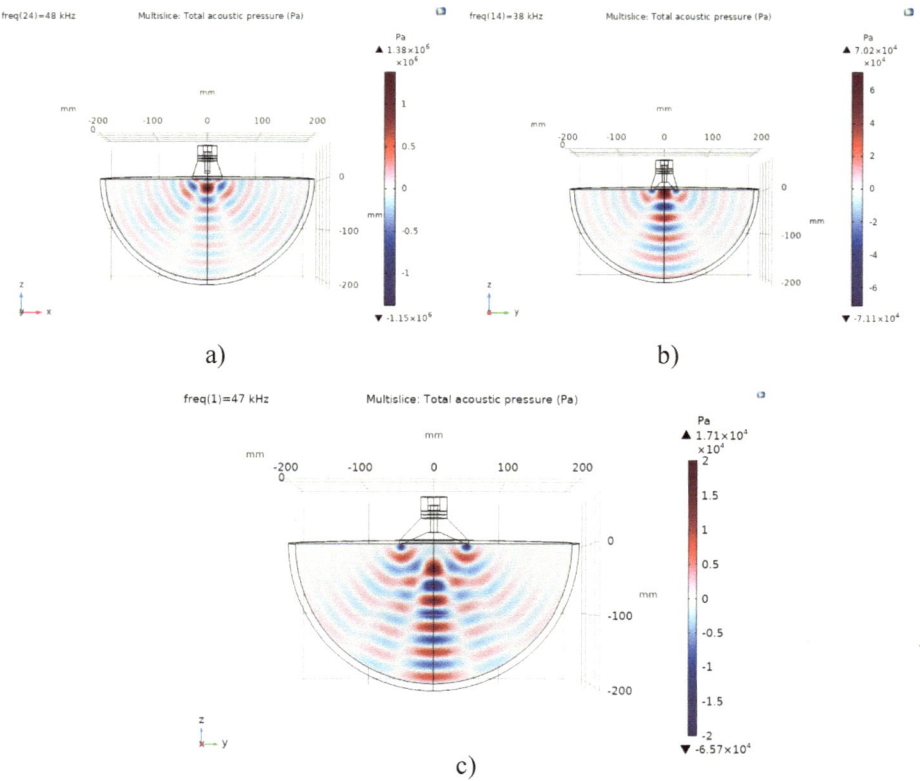

Fig. 2.19 Propagation of acoustic field generated by piezoelectric transducer in muscle tissue at the second mode: **a**—with flat surface, **b**—with cut-out surface of 58 mm diameter, **c**—with cut-out surface of 100 mm diameter

The simulated vibrational modes of the piezo transducer at the first natural frequency indicate that the transducer with flat surface vibrates only in the Z direction of the longitudinal axis, while the cut-out surface transducer is excited by longitudinal and radial vibrations (Fig. 2.17). In the case of a cut-out surface type transducer, since the tip volume is cut out, more deformation is observed in the X and Y-axes. The propagation of acoustic waves excited by flat and cut-out surface piezoelectric transducers in muscle tissue at the second mode show that the radial vibrations are dominating for the transducers with flat and cut-out surfaces, and amplitudes of vibration in X–Y directions are higher for transducers with cut-out surface (Fig. 2.20). The acoustic pressure wave varies above and below the ambient pressure, typically with harmonic (sinusoidal) modulation. Free-field conditions are used for measurements of acoustic pressure. These conditions approximate to those under which the acoustic field consists only of a traveling wave, propagating into

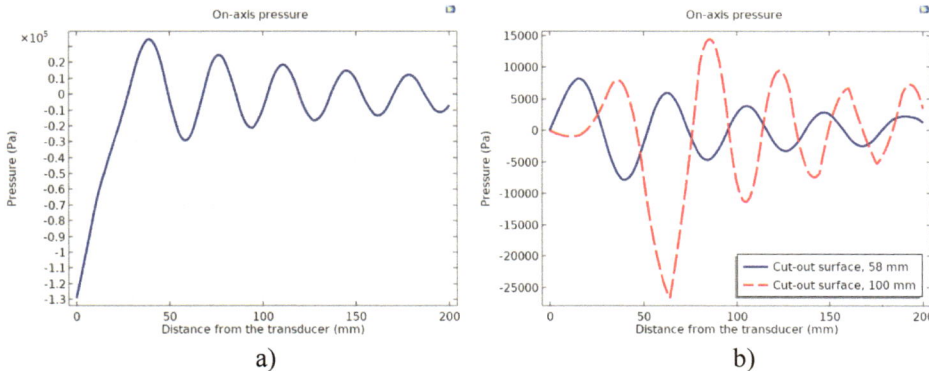

Fig. 2.20 Distribution of the acoustic pressure level of an ultrasound wave propagating in a muscle medium, simulated by piezoelectric transducers, in the second natural mode: **a**—with a flat surface at a resonant frequency of 48 kHz; **b**—with a cut-out surface and the different diameters of: 58 mm at a resonant frequency of 38 kHz (solid line) and with a diameter of 100 mm at resonant frequency of 47 kHz (dashed line)

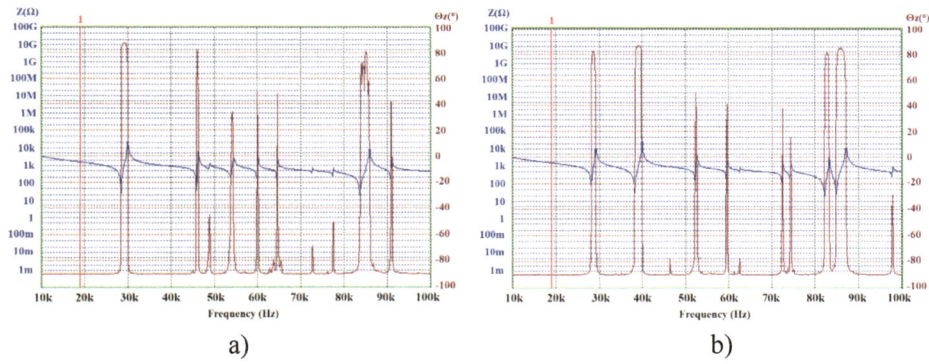

Fig. 2.21 Experimental impedance-phase versus frequency characteristics; **a**—the electric impedance of the transducer with flat surface; **b**—the electric impedance of the transducer with cut-out surface

an infinite medium without boundaries. Due to the relatively thin wall, this type of transducer can generate a more directional and concentrated acoustic wave, as can be seen in Fig. 2.20b. Half of the sphere of 200 mm radius was used for acoustic wave modelling in muscle medium. A perfectly aligned area of 10 mm layers was also used to simulate an open and non-reflecting infinite region to match the model to realistic conditions.

As illustrated by the graphs (Fig. 2.20b), the total acoustic pressure of the cut-out surface transducer type is lower than that of the flat-surface transducer type, but it is more directional, which is very important when trying to use it in a real-world environment.

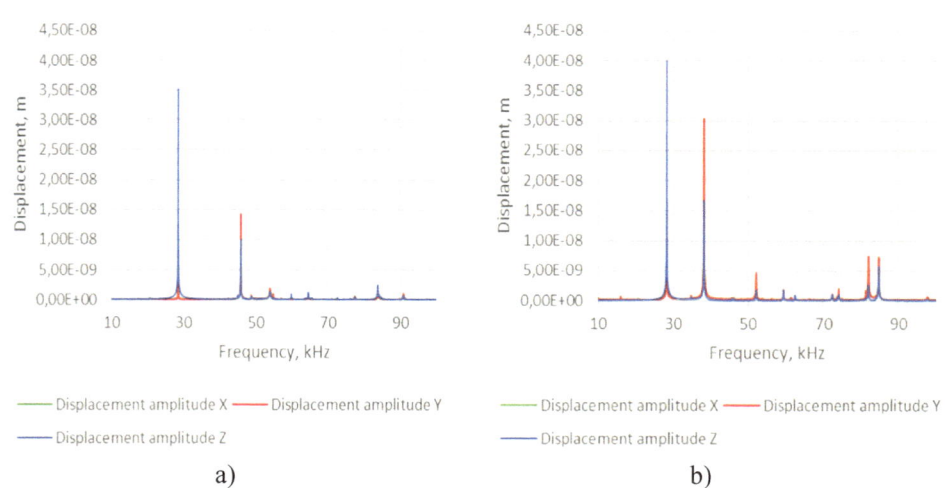

Fig. 2.22 Experimental amplitude-frequency characteristics of the two developed transducers measured with Polytech 3D scanning vibrometer: **a**—with flat surface; **b**—with cut-out surface

However, the same Fig. 2.20b, shows that the acoustic pressure generated by a cut-out transducer of 100 mm diameter at a depth of 6 cm of muscle tissue is almost 5 times higher than the acoustic pressure of a 58 mm diameter cut-out surface transducer. When used to treat the human body, the more directional and precise the wave, the better results can be achieved as only the part of the body being treated is affected, not the whole body. Furthermore, the longitudinal mode is not as suitable for medical applications as the radial mode, because the stronger acoustic signal produced by the second natural frequency mode transducer can be focused on a specific depth of biological tissue. Asymmetry between positive and negative half-cycles can be seen for the simulations of acoustic pressure level distribution in muscle medium and is caused by non-linear propagation of ultrasound wave in an interface layer between transducer and muscle tissue. Under such conditions, the peak rarefaction, p_r, and peak compression, p_c, or peak negative and peak positive pressure, respectively, are separately identified. And only the peak rarefaction is used to estimate the risk of sonicated tissue destruction due to the mechanical cavitation. In this case a Mechanical Index (MI) is used, which is given by the following equation MI $= p_r f^{0.5}$, wherein p_r is the maximum negative peak pressure in units of MPa, and f is the center frequency of the ultrasonic wave in units of kHz. Thus, it is a frequency-weighted acoustic pressure value and indicates the likelihood of cavitation, when MI is higher than 0.6. Therefore, the very high peak negative acoustic pressure generated by the flat surface transducer in an interface layer between the transducer and muscle tissue (Fig. 2.20a) can induce tissue destruction by cavitation.

2.4   Low-Frequency Ultrasound for Pulmonary Hypertension Therapy

Design of the proposed low-frequency ultrasonic acoustic wave Langevin-type [19] piezo-electric transducers with cut-out and flat surfaces of the front mass have been developed and patented [20] to evaluate the therapeutic effects of low frequency sonophoresis on biological tissues (Fig. 2.23).

The transducer consists of two piezoelectric ring-shaped ceramic elements 4 sand-wiched between two metallic masses, called the back mass 5 and the front mass 6. These masses are held in place by a preload bolt 7 which allows the ceramics to be preloaded to avoid undesirable tensile stresses. The back mass and the preload bolt were made of durable high impedance steel SUS 304. The front mass was made of aluminum since it has a lower acoustic impedance than piezoelectric elements and has good acoustic radiation characteristics. Two ring-shaped PZT-4 type piezoelectric ceramic elements 4 were sandwiched between two solid masses 5 and 6, and two 0.5 mm thick copper-nickel electrodes 8 for the input electrical signal connection to the piezoelectric ceramic elements. The ultrasound was transmitted through the sheep's body using two using two different transducers. One transducer had a cut-out front mass surface (Fig. 2.23a-1), and the other had a standard flat front mass surface (Fig. 2.23a-2).

Experimental studies were carried out at the LSMU Veterinary Academy. The sheep were first sedated using Xylazine hydrochloride (1 mg/kg intramuscular (IM), Bela–Pharm GmbH & Co. KG, Germany) as premedication, then transferred to the operating table and injected with Butorphanol (0.2 mg/kg IM, Richter Pharma, Austria). The sheep were

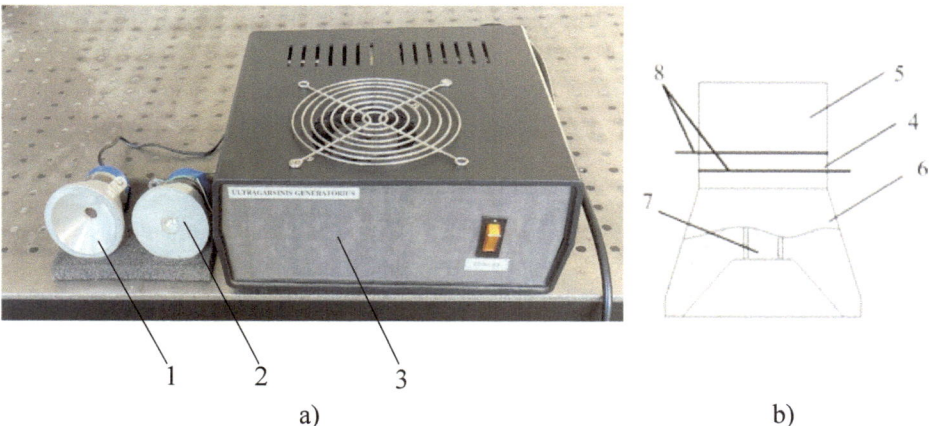

a)   b)

Fig. 2.23 **a**—Ultrasonic transducer with a cut-out (1) and flat (2) surfaces with laboratory-made controller (3); **b**—layout of the ultrasonic transducer with a cut-out surface: 4—ring-shaped piezo-electric element, 5—back mass, 6—front mass, 7—a preload bolt, 8—copper-nickel electrodes

then shaved, hair was removed from both sides of the chest, sternum, jugular vein, and left muzzle. Under sterile conditions, venous catheters (16 G, Provein™, Lars Medicare, India) were inserted into the left jugular vein. Saline solution was injected intravenously at a rate of 5 ml/kg/h. Ketamine (7 mg/kg intravenous (IV)) was used to induce anesthesia and sheep were prepared for intubation. The larynx then was visualized through a laryngoscope and was sprayed with 10% lidocaine spray solution (Egis Pharmaceuticals PLC, Hungary) to avoid respiratory spasm, endotracheal tube (ET, Kruuse, Denmark) was secured, the cuff inflated, and artificial lung ventilation performed using ventilator (model Fabius Tiro, Draeger, Germany). Long-term deep anesthesia was achieved using inhalation gas Sevoflurane 2% (Baxter, Belgium) and maintained with Midazolam (0.1 mg/kg/h, Kalceks, Latvia) and fentanyl (0.05 mg/kg/h, Kalceks, Latvia) using continuous rate infusion. The oxygen level was adjusted by about 21% to keep the animal adequately oxygenated during anesthesia. The sheep were carefully monitored using both manual practices and mechanical tools: eye position, palpebral reflex, mucous membrane color and capillary refill time were checked and recorded at five-minute intervals.

2.4.1 Modal Analysis of the Ultrasonic Transducer

Comparison of the dynamics of conventional and engineered low-frequency ultrasonic acoustic wave transducers. A Polytec laser Doppler 3D-scanning vibrometer PSV-500-3D-HV (Polytec GmbH, Germany) was used for the modal analysis of the transducers with cut-out and flat front surfaces (Fig. 2.13).

When the transducers were excited with 10 V_{P-P} sinusoidal (0–100) kHz frequency signals, their natural oscillation modes were recorded (Fig. 2.24a, b). The transducer with a flat surface has a longitudinal mode at 28.44 kHz frequency and 35.6 nm amplitude. The radial mode is at 45.81 kHz with an amplitude of 14.2 nm. The transducer with a cut-out surface has a longitudinal mode at 28.13 kHz with an amplitude of 39.9 nm and radial mode at frequency of 38.19 kHz and amplitude of 30.1 nm. The measured results show that higher vibration amplitudes are generated by a transducer with a cut-out annular surface of the front mass.

Three-dimensional scanning vibrometer was used to determine the operating deflection shapes and eigenmodes of the developed ultrasound transducer in the frequency range from 0 to 100 kHz. The vibrometer was used to measure the deflection shapes of the transducer's front mass surface at the resonant frequencies of the longitudinal and radial vibration modes and is shown in Fig. 2.25.

The eigenmodes (Fig. 2.25) show that the flat transducer has its largest displacements at 28 and 46 kHz, while the cut-out transducer—at 28 and 38 kHz, respectively. Hence, the efficiency of ultrasonic oscillations for blood micro/macro circulatory structures can be increased by using piezoelectric acoustic transducers with a cut-out surface that can be excited by a higher frequency mode. This cut-out surface transducer has been found

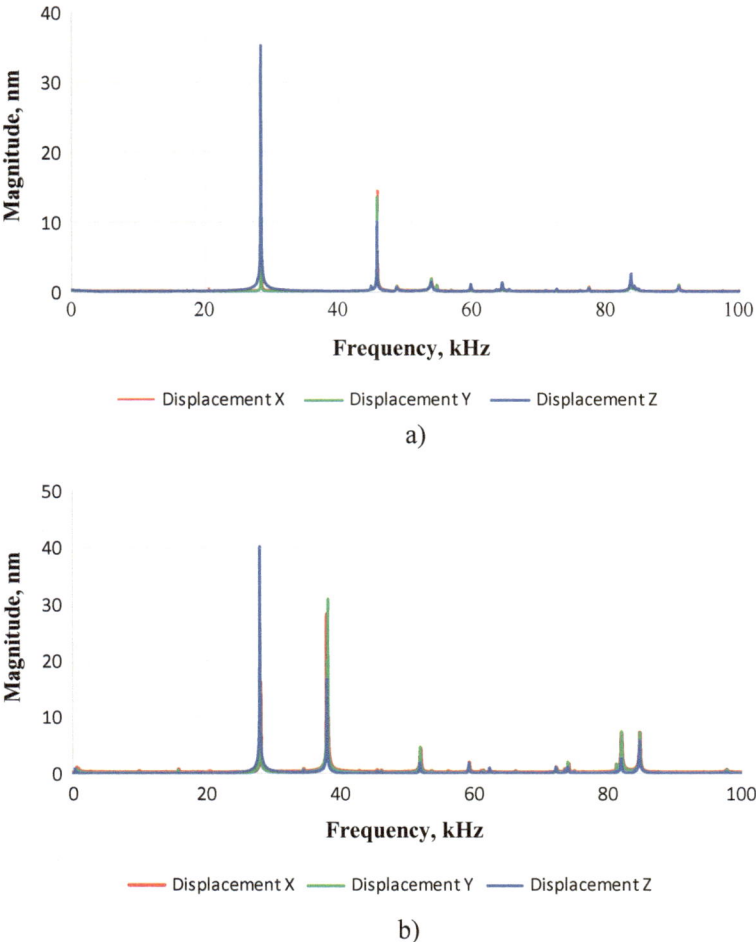

Fig. 2.24 Frequency responses of the two developed transducers: **a**—with flat and **b**—with cut-out surfaces; blue—out-of-plain vibration, red and green—in-plain vibration

to have a more directional overall sound pressure compared to a flat surface, which is very important in real-world applications. The effectiveness of pulmonary hypertension therapy is attributed to its ability to stimulate a directed and deeply penetrating acoustic wave that precisely affects the part of the body to be treated.

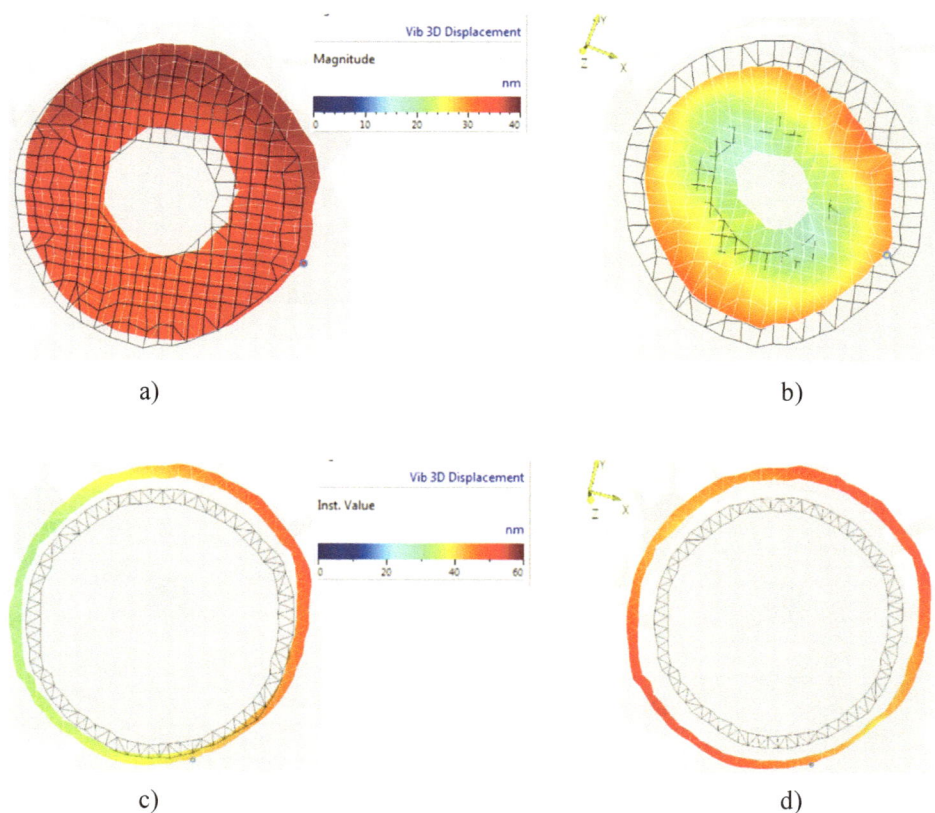

a)　　　　　　　　　　　　　　　　　　　　b)

c)　　　　　　　　　　　　　　　　　　　　d)

Fig. 2.25 The eigenmodes at the resonant frequencies: for transducer with flat surface at frequencies of 28.44 kHz; **b**—transducer with flat surface at frequency of 45.81 kHz; **c**—transducer with cut-out surface at frequency of 28.13 kHz; **d**—transducer with cut-out surface at frequency of 38.19 kHz

2.4.2　Measurement of the Ultrasound Pressure in the Lungs

In experimental studies using ultrasound, a hydrophone was used to measure the acoustic wave pressure and to determine its intensity. Knowing the pressure, velocity, and density of the medium in which this acoustic wave propagates, we can calculate the intensity of the acoustic wave. Before studying ultrasound penetration into biological tissues, it is important to know the intensity of the ultrasonic signal emitted by the transducer. For this purpose, ultrasound level measurement equipment has been developed (Fig. 2.26). This figure presents the setup for measuring the acoustic pressures emitted by transducer 1 immersed in a water bath 3, oscillating at the second vibrational mode of 38 kHz. To suppress the reflected ultrasonic waves from the walls of the bath, an ultrasound-attenuating material 4 was used as a lining. Two different hydrophones were used in the

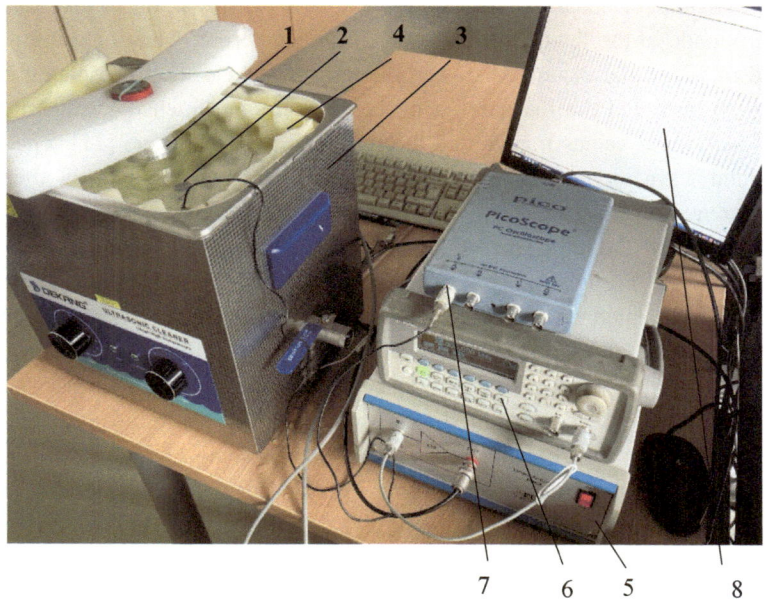

Fig. 2.26 A set up for measurement of the acoustic wave pressure generated by the ultrasonic transducer: 1—ultrasonic transducer; 2—hydrophone; 3—water bath; 4—ultrasound attenuating material; 5—power amplifier P200 (FLC Electronics AB, Sweden); 6—signal generator Agilent 33220A; 7—oscilloscope Pico Scope 3424 (Pico Technology Ltd., UK) 8—PC

experiment. Calibration of a broad-spectrum piezoelectric hydrophone 2 with an active diameter of 15 mm was performed using a hydrophone HCT-0320, coupled with a digital pressure meter MCT-2000 (Onda Corp., USA) in the frequency range of 20–100 kHz. The tests were carried out with transducers excited by a harmonic electrical signal of 50 $V_{P\text{-}P}$.

The waves generated by an acoustic transducer can be used to create an acoustic field, which can be divided into distinct areas called near and far fields. Consequently, within the near field the interference pattern engenders spatial variations in sound pressure levels. As the waves propagate away from the transducer, the sound field gradually equalizes, leading to enhanced predictability and amplification of the emitted waves in the region beyond the near field, often referred to as the "natural focus" [21]. The near-field distance in water of the investigated transducer with a diameter of 40 mm and an operational frequency of 38 kHz is greater than 10 mm. Therefore, the distance between the transducer and the hydrophone was set to more than 10 mm, for the measurements in water and the measured acoustic pressure was determined as the peak output value emitted by the investigated transducer. Characterization of the acoustic fields generated by transducers is necessary for the development of standards that ensure a positive risk–benefit outcome of treatment.

The expression for acoustic intensity given in IEC 61102 assumes that the measurements were made in the far field of the transducer. Therefore, when measurements were performed in water, the distance between the transducer and the hydrophone was set to more than 10 mm, and the measured acoustic pressure and intensity values were determined as peak input values transmitted through the sonicated tissue [21]. The ability of an ultrasound wave to transfer from one type of biological tissue to another depends on the difference in impedance between two different biological tissues and ultrasound attenuation factor. If the impedance is similar, a large part of the incident sound intensity will be transmitted through the boundary interface; if the difference is large, the sound is reflected. As indicated in Table 2.1, bone, soft tissue, and air correspond to the typical ranges of high, medium, and low biological tissue acoustic impedance values. Approximately 1% of the ultrasound intensity is reflected at the fat-muscle interface, with nearly 99% of the intensity being transmitted to deeper biological tissues. Almost 100% of the intensity is reflected at the air-muscle interface. A Transonic G-15 gel (TELIC S.A.U., Spain) placed between the sheep's skin and the transducer is an important part of the standard ultrasound procedure to ensure a good transducer-skin interface by eliminating air that would reflect the ultrasound.

The attenuation coefficient depends on the density and viscosity of the material and the frequency of the ultrasound. The acoustic properties of soft biological tissues, bones and gas inclusions depend on the attenuation coefficient of the acoustic wave passing through these tissues. The attenuation coefficients measured in various biological tissues are reported in the literature [22, 23] (Table 2.11).

The stand shown in Fig. 2.28 was set up for an experimental study of in vivo ultrasound transmission through the body of a sheep. The ultrasonic wave was excited by generator 6 with a sinusoidal signal amplitude of 5 V_{P-P} at the resonance frequency of the investigated transducers and was augmented by a power amplifier 5 with a constant voltage gain of 10. The ultrasound transducer was positioned on the sheep's chest near the lungs at right angles to the ribs and sent ultrasonic waves across a sheep body, which were received by a piezoelectric hydrophone and transmitted to a computer screen through an oscilloscope Pico Scope 3424 (see Figs. 2.27 and 2.28).

2.4.3 Pulmonary Hypertension Study in Vivo

Studies of ultrasound signal transmission through the body of the sheep and its effect on pulmonary hypertension were performed on live sheep (Fig. 2.28). Noradrenaline, or norepinephrine, is important for the body's therapeutic response. As a drug, it produces effects such as increased blood pressure and heart pulse rate, widening pulmonary airways, and constricting blood vessels in nonessential organs. The ultrasound was transmitted through the sheep's body using two different transducers. One transducer had a cut-out front mass surface (Transducer 1), and the other had a standard flat front mass surface (Transducer

Table 2.11 Acoustic parameters of ultrasound in various materials and biological tissues

Tissue	Density, kg/m^3	Longitudinal wave velocity m/s	Acoustic impedance (kg/m^2 s) $\times 10^6$	Attenuation coefficient dB/cm at 1 MHz
Air	1.2	330	0.0004	7.50
Water	1000	1480	1.48	0.0022
Blood	1060	1560	1.62	0.15
Skin	1150	1730	1.99	0.35
Liver	1060	1550	1.64	0.50
Heart	1040	1560	1.62	0.52
Skeletal muscles	1070	1590	1.70	
Parallel fibres				1.40
Perpendicular fibres				0.96
Bone	1380–1810	2700–4100	3.75–7.38	15.0
Lung	400	440–500	0.18–0.20	40.0

2). The test was carried out by exciting the transducers with an electrical signal of 50 V_{P-P}, and the input electrical power used by the transducers was about 20 W. The transducer with a cut-out surface was excited at a frequency of 38 kHz and the transducer with flat surface was excited at 46 kHz. The acoustic pressure transmitted through the body of a sheep was measured with a hydrophone, and the results are presented in Table 2.12.

From Table 2.12, it is evident that the acoustic parameters of the modified transducer with a cut-out surface, such as acoustic pressure through sheep's body is ~1.5 times, acoustic intensity in water ~2.0 times, and acoustic intensity transmitted through sheep's body ~4.0 times higher than the parameters of the transducer with a standard flat surface. The frequencies of the second mode oscillations of the investigated transducers (transducer with a standard flat surface—46 kHz, transducer with a cut-out surface—38 kHz) differ little and the characteristics of the acoustic fields they create can be compared, regardless of the small difference in frequencies. The research results show that the output surface of the modified transducer generates a larger vibration amplitude and due to its circular shape, the acoustic field spreads more directional. The permeability of standard flat and cut-out front mass surface actuators through the sheep's body were compared.

To induce pulmonary hypertension and to measure blood pressure changes in the right ventricle of the sheep's heart under ultrasound, it was necessary to open the thorax after the sheep had been put under general anesthesia. The chest was opened for the sheep, because it was necessary to insert a catheter directly into the pulmonary artery to accurately measure blood pressure changes in the right ventricle of the sheep's heart. During

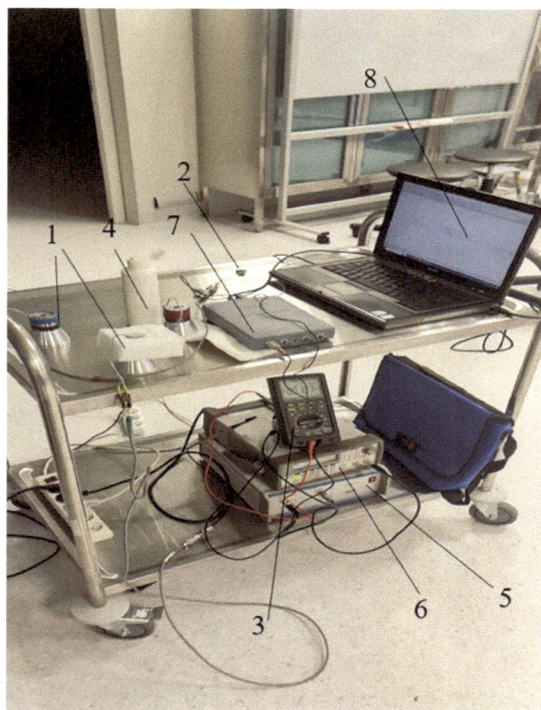

Fig. 2.27 Experimental setup for measurement of the sonication intensity transmitted through tissue by an ultrasonic transducer: 1—ultrasonic transducer; 2—hydrophone; 3—RMS multimeter MS8218 (Mastek Group Ltd.); 4—ultrasonic gel Transonic G-15 (TELIC, S.A.U., Spain); 5—power amplifier P200 (FLC Electronics AB, Sweden); 6—signal generator Agilent 33220A; 7—oscilloscope Pico Scope 3424 (Pico Technology Ltd., UK); 8—PC

tests with 5 sheep, pulmonary hypertension was artificially induced applying vessel ligation and changes in blood oxygen concentration were measured under the influence of low-frequency ultrasound. Measurements of sheep heart pulse rate, pulse oximetry, capnography, IBP and NIBP were performed with a multifunctional monitoring device (Draeger Vista 120, Draeger, Germany). IBP was measured in the left facial artery.

The duration of the process was determined empirically in real-time by determining the effect of ultrasound on the measured physiological parameters of the tested sheep. The testing process lasted for 10 min, and the sonication was stopped after 7 min. The ultrasound effect was determined and then the ultrasound transducer was removed. The dispersion intervals of the values of the measured physiological parameters of the five tested sheep are shown graphically for the individual measurement points. The changes in the oxygen concentration in the lungs of the sheep (Fig. 2.29) show that an increase of the parameter SpO_2 begins after 2 min of sonication. After 7 min of exposure to ultrasound, the oxygen concentration in the blood increases by more than 10%. When the

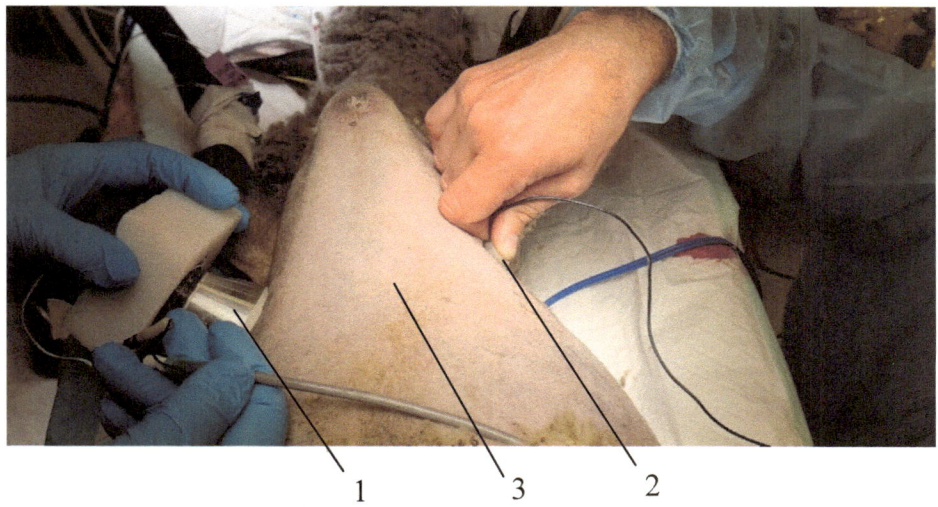

Fig. 2.28 Measurement of the transmitted ultrasound signal through the sheep's body: 1—transducer; 2—hydrophone; 3—a sheep's body

Table 2.12 An approximate acoustic pressure transmitted by the transducer

Transducer type	Acoustic pressure in water kPa	Acoustic pressure through sheep's body kPa	Acoustic intensity in water mW/cm^2	Acoustic intensity transmitted through sheep's body mW/cm^2
Transducer 1	75	1.5	380.07	0.24
Transducer 2	54	0.9	197.03	0.06

ultrasound is stopped, a slight decrease in the oxygen concentration is observed for the next 3 min, until the end of the test.

The exchange of gases in the blood intensifies thanks to the acoustic waves caused by low-frequency ultrasound travelling through the patient's blood vessels, which dissociate erythrocyte aggregates into single erythrocytes. As a result, about 300 million hemoglobin molecules in a single erythrocyte come into contact with oxygen on the entire surface of the erythrocyte, significantly improving lung artery oxygen metabolism. Venous blood flowing to the lungs is saturated with carbon dioxide, which increases the pH of the blood, and this helps to get rid of carbon dioxide in the lungs faster.

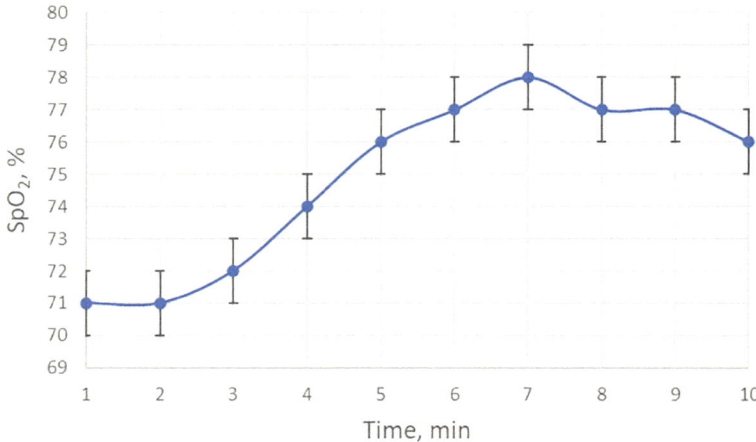

Fig. 2.29 Variation in oxygen concentration in the blood of sheep under the influence of low-frequency ultrasound

During the tests, the sheep's pulse rate was measured (Fig. 2.30). On the time axis the pulse rate is presented from 1 min after the start of sonication. It is evident from this graph that within 7 min of exposure to low-frequency ultrasound, the pulse rate is decreased by approximately 10%. After stopping the ultrasound radiation for the next 3 min, slight fluctuations in sheep pulse rate were observed until the end of the tests.

Blood pressure in the lungs was also measured. It is evident from the graph (Fig. 2.31) that within 7 min of exposure to low-frequency ultrasound, there is a reduction in blood pressure of approximately 13%. After stopping the ultrasound for the next 3 min and

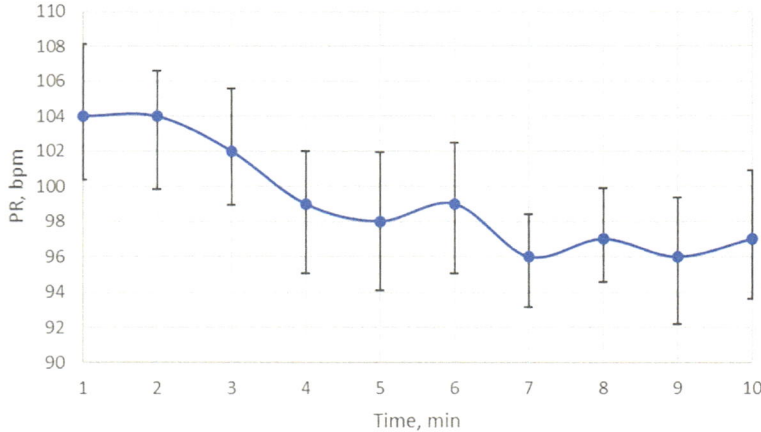

Fig. 2.30 Variation in sheep pulse rate under low-frequency ultrasound

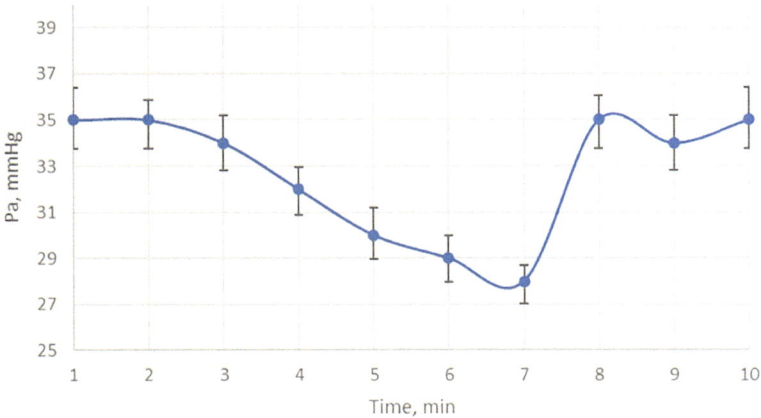

Fig. 2.31 Changes in blood pressure in sheep lungs under low-frequency ultrasound

staying in place with the transducer and hydrophone as shown in Fig. 2.31 until the end of the tests, recovery of blood pressure to the pre-test value was observed.

Blood pressure decreases due to the spaces between the blood cells. The amount of single dissociated erythrocytes number per unit volume becomes smaller than the aggregates of erythrocytes not affected by ultrasound. This significantly reduces blood viscosity. The viscosity of human blood is directly proportional to the hematocrit (the concentration of erythrocytes), which is responsible for the transport of oxygen and carbon dioxide.

Despite modern medical achievements and advanced treatment options, pulmonary arterial hypertension remains an intractable disease with a very high mortality rate. This disease is usually asymptomatic and only becomes apparent when most of the distal pulmonary arteries have become obliterated. Obliteration occurs due to reduced pulmonary arterial compliance and increased deposition of extracellular matrix/collagen in the pulmonary arteries in the presence of hypertension. To date, the quality of life of patients has been improved by prescribing diuretics, anticoagulants, vasodilators, etc. However, dosing, and other problems often arise with these drugs, which are frequently addressed by changing the treatment paradigm for pulmonary hypertension from pharmacological to non-invasive approaches, among which a low-frequency ultrasound transducer for the treatment of artificially induced pulmonary hypertension in sheep has been proposed in this study. When it comes to humans, pulmonary hypertension manifests as chronic pain. Therefore, our proposed low-cost method that does not use drugs that may have side effects on internal organs should reduce pain in this population [24]. As the main function of the lungs is to supply oxygen to the blood, maintaining the level of oxygen concentration in the blood is one of the indicators of the effect of the proposed transducer.

To reduce the risk of mechanical lung injury, efforts were made to shorten the exposure time of low-frequency ultrasound. In this present work, the effect of low-frequency ultrasound on the blood was investigated. Blood is a shear-thinning fluid with a complex reaction that is highly dependent on the ability of red blood cells to form aggregates. The RBC aggregates dissociate into single RBC cells when acoustic signal-induced shear forces exceed $\gamma = 5$–10 s^{-1} [10]. The effect of low-frequency ultrasound on biological cells, occurring at a lower temperature than high-frequency ultrasound, increases oxygen affinity and, consequently, a closer relationship with a higher oxygen saturation.

The presented graph (Fig. 2.29) proves the therapeutic effect of low-frequency ultrasound on the lungs, resulting in an increase in oxygen concentration in pulmonary blood. Oxygen is a pulmonary vasodilator. Although the treatment for pulmonary hypertension focuses on pulmonary vasodilation with oxygen, long-term O_2 therapy is not recommended unless patients develop hypoxemia, which is one of the leading causes of multiple organ injury and death in COVID-19 patients. The evidence presented in [25] suggests that O_2 is a vasodilator in normoxic patients, and that it is not only related to blood-borne (oxyhemoglobin) mechanism, but also to alveoli, and that the therapeutic benefit of O_2 is independent of the arterial oxygen level of 75–100 mm mercury (mmHg). This indicates that O_2 is therapeutically beneficial for pulmonary hypertension patients. The main cause of death from pulmonary hypertension is right ventricular failure [26]. Chronic heart failure develops because of cardiac energy depletion due to oxygen deprivation at the mitochondrial level of cardiomyocytes. Almost 50% of patients with pulmonary hypertension develop iron deficiency [27]. Iron deficiency, due to chronic blood loss or inadequate dietary iron absorption, causes iron deficiency anemia, while inflammation-induced iron retention in innate immune cells and iron uptake blockade cause anemia of chronic disease. Anemia is defined as a decrease in the number of RBCs, or hemoglobin, which carries oxygen in the blood. The amount of hemoglobin, which carries oxygen to the body's cells from the lungs, improves the absorption of iron [28]. Our finding [12] that low-frequency ultrasound 12 dissociates aggregated erythrocytes into single erythrocytes, whose hemoglobin molecules interact with oxygen over the entire erythrocyte surface area than the aggregates of erythrocytes that are not exposed to ultrasound.

According to research in [29], reduced gas transmission in patients with pulmonary hypertension has traditionally been associated with progressive pulmonary arterial attrition and vascular remodeling, which reduces the volume of capillary blood available for gas exchange. Ultrasonic exposure can also be used in clinical applications as focused therapeutic ultrasound with higher acoustic power, using contrast agents, known as microbubbles, for more effective drug absorption. Such improved absorption of drugs into cells is due to the increased permeability of the membrane under the influence of ultrasound [30]. The results of therapeutic drugs delivery using thoracic ultrasound and microbubbles, primarily to damaged areas of the lung, especially to the endothelium, have been described in a study [31]. Using our proposed low-frequency ultrasound transducer, it is possible to select an excitation frequency that coincides with the resonant frequency of the microbubbles, which results in their disruption, thereby accelerating drug delivery. This is also confirmed by the author of [32], who reported that low-frequency 20 kHz ultrasound in vitro (125 mW/cm^2, 100 ms pulses per second) increased the permeability of salicylic acid through human skin by almost 1000 times compared to high-frequency 1 MHz ultrasound (92 W/cm^2). Acoustic cavitation, i.e., the formation and violent collapse of gas microbubbles in a liquid irradiated with low-frequency ultrasound, is a major contributor [33]. Cavitation in the lungs is undesirable because it can destroy the structure of the lung alveoli. In our research the level of cavitation was evaluated by the intensity of the acoustic signal causing cavitation with mechanical index values greater than 0.6. From the equation to calculate mechanical index MI $= P^{r \cdot 3}/\sqrt{f}$ [34] where $P^{r \cdot 3}$ stands for the rarefactional pressure (in unit of MPa) of the ultrasound field with an attenuation coefficient of 0.3 dB (MHz cm^{-1}) and f means the frequency (in unit of MHz) of the ultrasound wave. In the case of sheep, we used low-frequency and low-intensity ultrasound: max acoustic pressure measured was 75 kPa (see Table 2.12), frequency of sonication was 38 kHz and calculated MI $= 0.075/0.195 = 0.385 < \mathbf{0.6}$. The probability of cavitation was therefore very low.

High doses of oxygen cause pulmonary oedema and interstitial fibrosis, whereas continuous exposure to inhaled oxygen does not cause either epithelial damage or alveolar fibrosis [35]. Unlike breathing concentrated oxygen, which produces high levels of oxygen in the blood that can damage and kill cells, mainly in the eyes, the central nervous system and the lungs, the gradual change in blood oxygen levels caused by exposure to low-frequency ultrasound is like human exercise and is beneficial to the body. The research results of the authors of this book show that the effect of low-frequency ultrasound on human pulmonary arteries inhibits their contractions, and that it can be used to treat patients with pulmonary hypertension. Pulmonary vasodilators contain nitric oxide (NO), which is essential for improving oxygen saturation, protecting cells, and preventing inflammation [36]. Inhaled NO is rapidly oxidized to NO_2, which interacts with water to form highly harmful nitric acids that can cause pulmonary oedema and pneumonitis. The positive effects of inhaled NO may give short-term benefits, whereas rapid withdrawal of inhaled NO causes a rebound phenomenon. This is probably due to endogenous NO inhibition, leading to reduced oxygenation and increased pulmonary arterial pressure, so slow and gradual withdrawal of inhaled NO is recommended. Ultrasound-induced release of nitric oxide from tissues in patients with pulmonary hypertension (PH) may be beneficial for oxygenation. Pulmonary vascular remodeling is a major structural change in the vascular wall that is dangerous in pulmonary hypertension. The endothelium is one of the inner layers of the blood vessel wall, lined with endothelial cells. The endothelium is an endocrine organ, that plays a major role in the regulation of angiogenesis, immune responses, and inflammation. A study [37] showed that low-frequency ultrasound increased the expression of vascular endothelial growth factors and influenced the process of neovascularization in a diabetic rat model by promoting the differentiation and proliferation of endothelial fibroblasts. Low-frequency ultrasound has been shown to influence arterial and venous dilation and promote tissue perfusion [38]. In vivo studies in humans have shown that arterial dilation can be observed 1 min. after exposure to ultrasound, partly due to ultrasound-induced release of NO from the tissues, suggesting that ultrasound-mediated vasodilatation in PH patients results in an increase in gas transport.

Sudden cardiac death is the main genesis caused by pulmonary hypertension. Dysfunction of the cardiac autonomic system is assessed by heart rate variability. A low heart rate is favorable in healthy individuals. The changes in pulse rate induced by low-frequency ultrasound are illustrated in Fig. 2.30. Heart rate recovery after exercise is an important indicator of the condition of patients with heart and lung diseases. The study in [39] presents the data on heart rate recovery in pulmonary hypertension patients after a 6-min walk test. The research shows that heart rate recovery is an easily measurable clinical biomarker in the near-term disease space, which allows prediction of worsening clinical survival and hospitalization in patients with PH. The results of our study, which show a marked reduction in pulse rate after 7 min of ultrasound exposure, may provide an alternative for hospitalized patients who cannot walk.

Only a small increase in pulmonary pressure is one of the risk factors predicting the trajectory of clinical outcomes of patients. The presented graph (Fig. 2.31) supports the assumption that low-frequency ultrasound has a therapeutic effect on the lungs, leading to a reduction of pulmonary blood pressure. When exposed to low-frequency ultrasound, the erythrocytes in the aggregates dissociate into single erythrocytes [12] separated by a distance from each other and their number per unit volume of blood is reduced due to the gaps between them compared to the erythrocytes in the aggregates in blood not exposed to ultrasound. Therefore, when ultrasound exposure is discontinued, blood pressure recovers within a minute because the increase in the number of aggregated erythrocytes per unit volume, known as erythrocytosis, is accompanied by an increase in the viscosity of the blood and a recovery of blood pressure to the level it was before the ultrasound exposure. In pulmonary hypertension, the heart pumps blood from the right ventricle to the lungs via blood vessels with increased muscle content in their walls. The small distance of the lungs from the right ventricle results in low blood pressure on this side of the heart and in the artery. The pressure is usually much lower than the systolic or diastolic blood pressure.

The research presented in [40] suggests that in pulmonary arterial hypertension, increased vascular pressure is associated with pulmonary artery vascular remodeling, small-artery obstruction, and increased vascular resistance to pulmonary blood flow. In the long term, high blood pressure can damage the heart and lead to right ventricular failure and, eventually, death. A study in [41] shows that a 10-min treatment with low-frequency ultrasound can reduce the white-coat effect associated with anxiety about healthcare visits and improve clinical hypertension to acceptable blood pressure. The article [42] reported that low-frequency ultrasound induced a significant blood pressure decrease in hypertensive rats. After one week of total ultrasound exposure of 20 min/day, the systolic blood pressure of the rats decreased from 170 ± 4 to 128 ± 4.5 mmHg. Ultrasound stimulation did not cause significant tissue damage, cell apoptosis, or hemorrhage. Functional studies under low-frequency 20 kHz ultrasound were performed on human and rat pulmonary arteries mounted on microvascular myographs [43]. To measure the effect of low-frequency ultrasound on extracellular Ca 2+ entry, preparations were placed in Ca 2+-free solution and, under insonation, the thromboxane agonist U46619 and extracellular calcium were added. In isolated human pulmonary arteries, GYY 4137 induced contractions that were most pronounced in arteries contracted with the thromboxane analog U46619. Transient contractions of GYY4137 were reversed by low-frequency ultrasound, which also induced transient contraction of human pulmonary arteries.

Attempts have been made to use low frequency as a therapeutic modality (e.g. intracoronary ultrasound plaque ablation) [44–46]. By establishing the vasomodulatory effects of ultrasound and mechanical oscillation, the physiological basis for the development of therapeutic and rehabilitation devices that exert therapeutic effects via the aforementioned methods is provided. The aim of the current study was to quantify the vasomodulatory effects of ultrasound and mechanical effects. For this purpose, 2 mm segments of rat (Wistar) superior and small mesenteric arteries were dissected, isolated, transferred to 40 °C physiological saline solution and mounted in myographs (model—420A; DMT, Aarhus, Denmark) for functional studies. The arterial segments were stretched to their appropriate lumen diameter for active tension development. The myograph was used to measure changes in the contractile force of the luminal tissue segments under isometric conditions. Vessels pre-contracted with norepinephrine were subjected to vibrational excitation. Acetylcholine-induced (10 μM ACh) relaxation was used as a control and as evidence of intact endothelial function. Changes in isometric tension were recorded. Vascular relaxation was presented as isometric tension and percentage change in mN from the plateau of vascular contraction with norepinephrine. Data was expressed as median and interquartile range Mdn (IQR). Changes from baseline were evaluated using the Wilcoxon signed ranks test. 12 vessel segments were obtained from 4 male Wistar rats. Polytec laser measurement device + myograph measurement of vessel contraction is shown in Fig. 2.32.

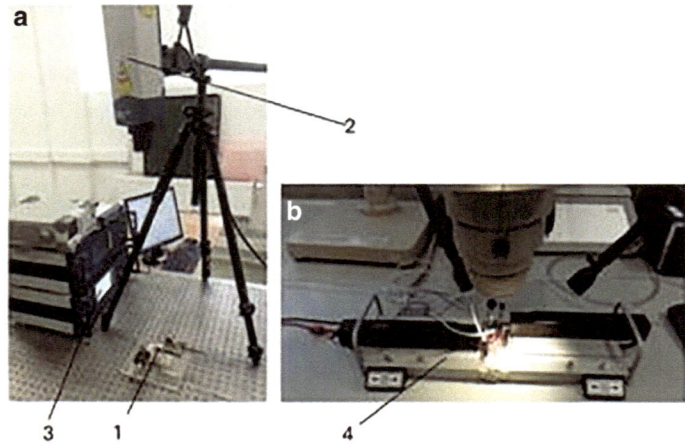

Fig. 2.32 A set-up for the calibration of the mechanical vibration actuator (**a**) and myography system for vessel contraction measurement (**b**): 1—mechanical vibration actuator; 2—laser head Polytec OFV-505; 3—Polytec controller OFV-5000; 4—myograph with an ex vivo mounted vessel

The measurement results are presented in Figs. 2.33 and 2.34. After the blood vessel is constricted and affected by ultrasound (duration—3 s), it causes relaxation of the blood vessel by 5.43%. Gentamicin 10 µM causes no relaxation of blood vessels, and 30 µM causes 20.36% relaxation.

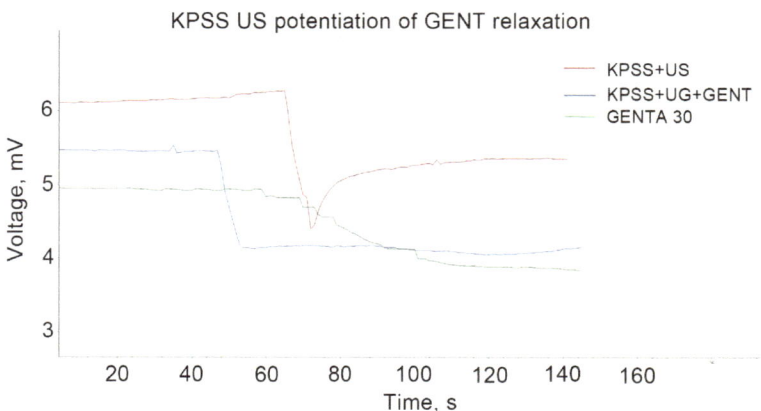

Fig. 2.33 Comparison of medication and vibrational excitation effects on blood vessel relaxation: red—relaxation of the blood vessel by 5.43%, green—gentamicin 10 microMol does not cause relaxation of blood vessels, and 30 microMol—20.36% relaxation and blue-gentamicin 10 microMol and ultrasound relaxation by 22.46%, KPSS-high potassium physiological solution is similar to physiological saline solution but has a greater concentration of potassium

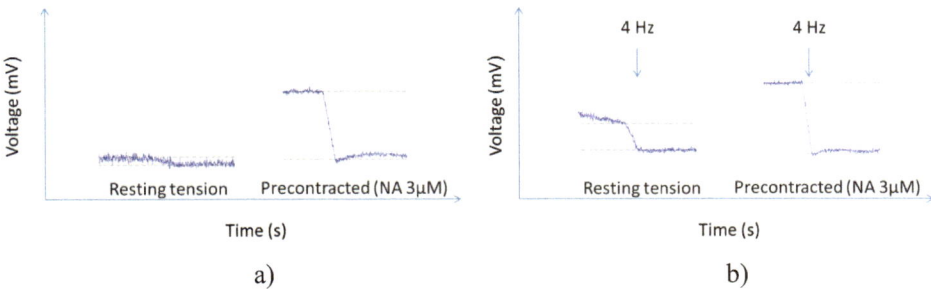

Fig. 2.34 Influence of chemical substance (**a**) and influence vibrational excitation impact (**b**)

10 μM of gentamicin in a 10 mL bath corresponds to 0.06 mcg/mL conc., and 30 μM–0.18 mcg/mL. Meanwhile, the maximum therapeutic concentration in human blood is 3–9 mcg/ml.

Figure 2.34 confirms that the vibrational excitation effect is adequate for drug action and can be used, for example, to prevent a heart attack not only by destabilising atrial fibrillation but also by relaxing blood vessels. Practical advice is to start coughing artificially or beat the chest with your hand when you feel pain in the heart area.

Long-term vasodilator therapy is generally unable to selectively reduce pulmonary vascular resistance and often leads to systemic hypotension, worsening of pulmonary hypertension, exacerbation of right ventricular failure and systemic arterial desaturation [36]. As a result, the average survival rate of patients with pulmonary hypertension remains below three years after diagnosis. Extensive research efforts have led to the emergence of innovative treatments such as stem cell therapy, gene transfer and epigenetic therapy.

Widely used methods of treating pulmonary hypertension, in contrast to our proposed low-frequency ultrasound examination, are invasive and expensive, requiring complex techniques and qualifications. Ultrasound can cause some biophysical effects, including thermal and non-thermal effects on cells, but these effects are significantly less in the case of low-frequency ultrasound than in the case of high-frequency ultrasound. Sonoporation, the most studied non-thermal biological effect of ultrasound, is considered to be the basis for new therapeutic applications. Clinical trials of this innovative low-frequency ultrasound transducer, tested in sheep, will be continued with the aim of obtaining approval for the treatment of pulmonary hypertension in humans. To that end, we offer a skin-friendly version of the low-frequency transducer that is integrated into the cupping lung therapy used in traditional folk medicine (Fig. 2.35).

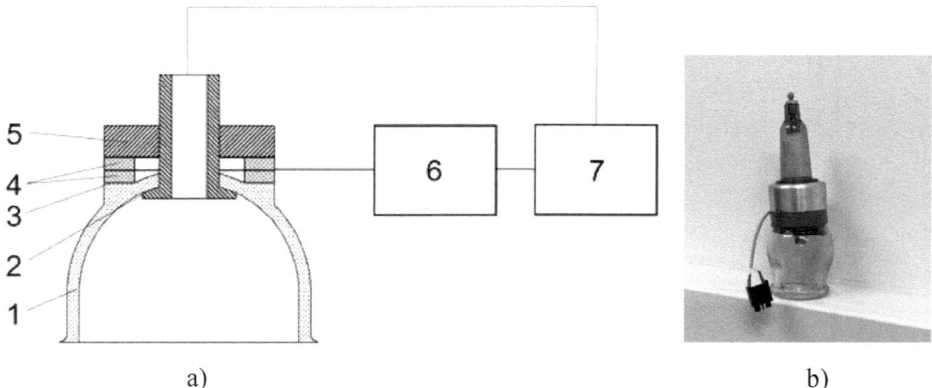

Fig. 2.35 Human-friendly low-frequency ultrasonic actuator control diagram (**a**) and general view (**b**): 1—cup, 2—vacuum supply tube, 3—flat annular surface, 4—piezoceramic rings, 5—sleeve, 6—controller, 7—vacuum pump

Figure 2.35a shows a diagram of a vacuum therapy device with ultrasound stimulation, which includes a vacuum cup 1 with a central hole in which a vacuum supply tube 2 is installed, and a flat annular surface 3 formed around the neck of the vacuum cup 1 at the top, the plane width of which corresponds to the width of the piezoceramic rings 4 pressed from above into the sleeve 5, in which mechanical vibrations are excited by the piezoceramic rings 4 driven by the controller 6, synchronized with the vacuum pump 7. The vacuum pulls the cup towards the body surface, ensuring good contact without the use of ultrasound gel. During the procedure with the device for vacuum therapy with ultrasound stimulation, the vacuum cup 1 is placed on the area of the human body surface prepared for the therapeutic effect, the vacuum pump 7 is switched on, which sucks the air in the vacuum cup 1 through the vacuum supply tube 2 and thus the vacuum cup 1 presses against the surface of the body. At the same time, in the same moment as the start of the vacuum pump, the electric signal from the controller 6 is sent to the piezoceramic rings 4, whose mechanical vibrations spread over the surface of the vacuum cup 1, creating an ultrasonic effect at the point of contact with the body surface, i.e. stimulation. The vacuum pump 7 controlled by the controller 6 in the vacuum cup 1 generates a constant or low-frequency (1–30 Hz) modulated negative pressure, i.e. a pulsating vacuum, which excites low-frequency mechanical vibrations of the part of the body treated by the vacuum cup, thus improving the therapeutic effect. At the same time, the piezoceramic rings 4 are excited by the controller 6 by means of an electrical signal whose frequency coincides with that of the cup-piezoceramic rings-sleeve dynamic system at one of the resonance frequencies in the ultrasonic range from 20 to 100 kHz. During the treatment with a vacuum therapy device, the ultrasound and low-frequency mechanical vibration stimulation can be carried out continuously or at certain intervals by means of the actuator 6. In this way, the low-frequency ultrasound vibrations caused by the radial vibrations of the cup emit a focused acoustic signal into the tissues of the human body, increasing the effectiveness of the therapeutic procedure.

2.4.4 Alternative Therapeutic Applications of Low-Frequency Ultrasound

The applications of the identified hemodynamic features and the developed devices could in the future be linked to the possibility of destroying heart valve plaques by precisely targeting them with a low-frequency acoustic signal. Calcific aortic stenosis is currently the most common heart valve disease. Currently, surgical or transcatheter aortic valve replacement is the only effective treatment. However, 16% of patients with symptomatic severe calcific aortic stenosis are rejected by local heart teams for surgical or transcatheter aortic valve replacement. The use of ultrasound for this purpose relies on the ability to precisely focus the acoustic signal on the area of the heart valve, which could be achieved with our low-frequency ultrasound device.

By using focused acoustic waves, therapeutic ultrasound can induce bioeffects in a precise and targeted manner with minimal or no side effects, making it a promising alternative or complement to traditional therapies. Red blood cells have great potential as a drug delivery system that can lead to unprecedented changes in pharmacokinetics, pharmacodynamics, and immunogenicity. Despite this great potential and nearly 50 years of research, RBC-mediated drug delivery has only recently begun to move out of the academic laboratory and into industrial drug development. Drug loading of RBCs can be accomplished in a variety of ways—by encapsulation within RBCs or surface binding, or ex vivo or in vivo—depending on the intended use. To promote wound healing or to make the healing process more efficient by targeting RBC-encapsulated drugs to a specific organ of the human body, therapeutic agents could be injected to ensure safe drug encapsulation into circulating RBCs without the need for ex vivo modification and RBC infusion. A necessary condition for this is the dissociation of individual erythrocytes from aggregates in the treated body part by irradiation with our invented low frequency ultrasound transducer. Unlike carrier erythrocytes, which are prepared ex vivo by taking a blood sample from the organism of interest and separating the erythrocytes from the plasma by centrifugation, our technique separates erythrocytes in vivo only in the environment of the human organ to be treated. This is achieved by exciting the ultrasound transducer with a higher mode of vibration, which increases the penetration and effect of the acoustic signal on deeper biological tissues and directs the signal precisely to the therapeutically affected area of the body.

Biofilm is a complex structure of microbiome with different bacterial colonies or single type of cells in a group adhering to the surface. These cells are embedded in extracellular polymeric substances, a matrix generally composed of eDNA, proteins and polysaccharides, which shows high resistance to antibiotics. It is one of the major causes of persistence of infection, especially in the nosocomial setting through indwelling devices. Although biofilms are characterized by extremely high resistance to chemical and physical agents, low frequency ultrasound treatment has been suggested as an efficient and safe method for biofilm disruption. Such a technique is particularly useful in cases where biofilms cover internal organ implants, as the penetration of the acoustic signal generated by our device is almost four times greater than that of previously used devices.

The CO_2 is the most potential regulator of cerebral blood flow, and even small fluctuations can cause large changes in cerebral blood flow, as we have revealed a feature of low frequency ultrasound exposure to blood that hemoglobin not only transports more O_2 from the lungs, but also CO_2 from biotissues to the brain can serve to protect a person from dizziness.

2.4.5 Prevention of Limb Amputation in Diabetic Foot Ulcer Patients

The lifetime risk of developing a diabetic foot ulcer in diabetic patients is approximately 25%. Among these individuals, the risk of amputation significantly increases, often leading to worse clinical outcomes. To mitigate the likelihood of lower limb amputation in patients with diabetic foot ulcers, a device utilizing sonic and ultrasonic frequency acoustic stimulation has been developed and patented [47]. The schematic diagram of this device is presented in Fig. 2.36.

The system is most suitable for human lower limbs for several reasons. First, the main blood vessels are positioned shallowly enough and in case of any type of insufficiency of their function, it is not difficult to influence their function, which is not only local, but also systemic, due to the antero-retrograde effect through the vagus-sympathetic system innervating them. Second, there is an important effect on microcirculation, which is realized through the mechanical and partially thermal effects of ultrasound. Third, the effect was determined not only on the functional regulation of blood vessels, but also through the effect on blood-forming elements, i.e. modifying the function of platelets in the desired direction—reducing thrombogenesis as a thromboembolic factor or increasing it in case of a threat of hemorrhages. The system can be used in the presence of pathology of the main vessels of the lower limbs of various origins, especially after reconstructive operations in

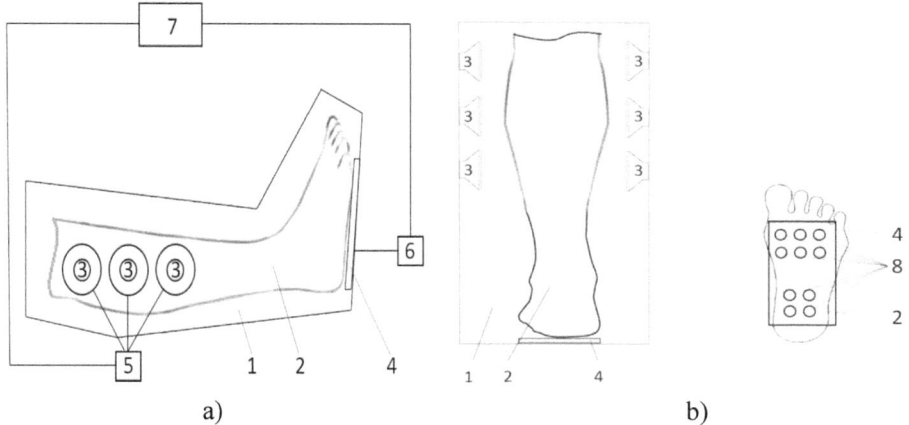

Fig. 2.36 Lower limbs blood flow stimulation system: **a** from the lower leg side with arrayed acoustic speakers and **b** matrix arrangement of bimorph piezoelectric transducers in the plane of the chamber corresponding to the plane of the foot: 1—chamber, 2—feet, 3—speakers, 4—bimorph transducer matrix, 5 and 6—generators, 7—controller, 8—bimorph transducers

the case of diabetic angiopathy and, most importantly, in the case of microcirculatory dysfunction associated with tissue perfusion disorders, characteristic of the highly traumatic "diabetic foot" syndrome, often leading to amputations and irreversible disability. The system uniformly and systematically influences the blood perfusion in the entire human body by affecting the structural elements of the blood: erythrocytes, platelets, leukocytes, etc.

The leg blood flow stimulation system consists of a closed chamber equipped with bimorph-type piezoelectric transducers and in-chamber speakers, which are mounted on the side walls. Both the piezoelectric transducers and speakers are connected to a central controller. The system is designed to accommodate a person's legs up to the knees, which are enclosed within the chamber and secured using a standard elastic splint system. The feet are stimulated by ultrasonic waves generated by the bimorph-type piezoelectric transducers, while the lower legs are affected by acoustic waves emitted from the speakers positioned within the chamber's walls. The controller synchronizes the operation of the piezoelectric transducers and speakers, ensuring that both work in tandem to enhance blood flow activation in the leg tissues, thereby increasing the overall efficiency of blood flow stimulation. A real image of this actuator is provided in Fig. 2.37.

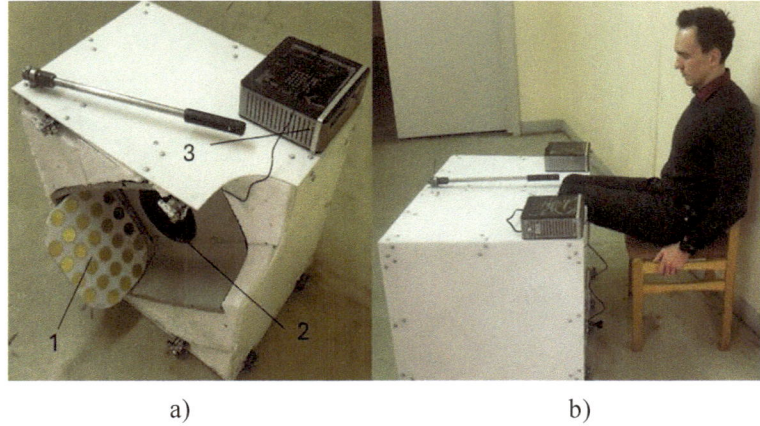

a)   b)

Fig. 2.37 Image of part of the lower limb stimulator (**a**) and patient during therapy (**b**): 1—bimorph-type piezoelectric transducers array; 2—acoustic speaker; 3—controller

References

1. Swelab Alfa PlusUser's Manual (2015)
2. Riffenburgh RH (2012) Statistics in medicine, 3rd edn. Academic Press, p 690
3. Sherwani RAK, Shakeel H, Awan WB, Faheem M, Aslam M (2021) Analysis of COVID-19 data using neutrosophic Kruskal Wallis H test. BMC Med Res Methedol 21(1):215
4. Bayram M, Bayraktar G, Akyol H, Can B (2017) Comparing some blood parameters of ski racers and long-distance athletes. Turk J Sport Exerc 19(3):331–336
5. Knapp H (2017) Intermediate statistics using SPSS, 1st edn. SAGE Publications, p 480
6. Botchkarev A (2019) Performance metrics (error measures) in machine learning regression, forecasting and prognostics: properties and typology. Int J Inf Knowl Manag 14:45–79
7. Otto C, Baumann M, Schreiner T, Bartsch G, Borberg H, Schmid-Schonbein P (2001) Standardized ultrasound as a new method to induce platelet aggregation: evaluation, influence of lipoproteins and of glycoprotein IIb/IIIa antagonist tirofiban. Eur J Ultrasound 14(2–3):157–166
8. Palma-Barqueros V, Revilla N, Sánchez A, Zamora Cánovas A, Rodriguez-Alén A, Marín-Quílez A, González-Porras JR, Vicente V, Lozano ML, Bastida JM, Rivera J (2021) Inherited platelet disorders: an updated overview. Int J Mol Sci 22(9):4521
9. Mahbobi M, Tiemann TK (2015) Introductory business statistics with interactive spreadsheets, 1st Canadian edn, p 102
10. Yeom E, Nam KH, Paeng SJ (2014) Effects of red blood cell aggregates dissociation on the estimation of ultrasound speckle image velocimetry. Ultrasonics 54(6):1480–1487
11. Vidallon MLP, Tabor RF, Bishop AI, Teo BM (2021) Ultrasound-assisted fabrication of acoustically active, erythrocyte membrane "bubbles." Ultrason Sonochem 72:105429
12. Ostasevicius V, Paulauskaite-Taraseviciene A, Lesauskaite V, Jurenas V, Tatarunas V, Stankevicius E, Tunaityte A, Venslauskas M, Kizauskiene L (2023) Prediction of changes in blood parameters induced by low-frequency ultrasound. Appl Syst Innov 6(6):99

13. Ostasevicius V, Jurenas V, Mikuckyte S, Vezys J, Stankevicius E, Bubulis A, Venslauskas M, Kizauskiene L (2023) Development of a low frequency piezoelectric ultrasonic transducer for biological tissue sonication. Sensors 23(7):1–16

14. Kinsler LE, Frey AR, Coppens AB, Sanders JV (2000) Fundamentals of acoustics. Wiley, New York, 99–111; 141–161; 463

15. Berlincourt D, Krueger HHA Properties of Morgan Matroc piezoelectric ceramics, TP-226. Morgan Matroc Inc, 12

16. Steels, General Properties (2023) https://www.matweb.com/search/datasheet.aspx?bassnum=MS0001&ckck=1

17. ASM Aerospace Specification Metals Inc. Aluminum 7075-T6; 7075-T651 (2023) https://asm.matweb.com/search/SpecificMaterial.asp?bassnum=ma7075t6

18. Hasgall PA, Di Gennaro F, Baumgartner C, Neufeld E, Lloyd B, Gosselin MC, Payne D, Klingenböck A, Kuster N (2023) IT'IS database for thermal and electromagnetic parameters of biological tissues. https://itis.swiss/virtual-population/tissue-properties/overview/

19. Ostasevicius V, Jurenas V, Venslauskas M, Kizauskiene L, Zigmantaite V, Stankevicius E, Bubulis A, Vezys J, Mikuckyte S (2024) Low-frequency ultrasound for pulmonary hypertension therapy. Respir Res 70(25):1–12

20. Ostasevicius V, Jurenas V, Bubulis A, Venslauskas M, Vezys J, Stankevicius E, Abramavičius S (2024) Vacuum therapy apparatus with ultrasonic stimulation, EP4374840

21. Jensen JA, Svendsen NB (1992) Calculation of pressure fields from arbitrarily shaped, apodized, and excited ultrasound transducers. IEEE Trans Ultrason Ferroelectr Freq Control 39:262–267

22. Wells PNT (1975) Absorption and dispersion of ultrasound in biological tissue. Ultrasound Med Biol 1:369–376

23. Mast TD (2000) Empirical relationships between acoustic parameters in human soft tissues. Acoust Res Lett 1:37

24. Morris JR, Harrison SL, Robinson J, Martin D, Avery L (2023) Non-pharmacological and non-invasive interventions for chronic pain in people with chronic obstructive pulmonary disease: a systematic review without meta-analysis. Respir Med 211:107191

25. Green S, Stuart D (2021) Oxygen and pulmonary arterial hypertension: effects, mechanisms, and therapeutic benefits. Eur J Prev Cardiol 28(1):127–136

26. Balestra GM, Mik EG, Specht PAC, van der Laarse WJ, Zuurbier CJ, Eerbeek O (2015) Increased in vivo mitochondrial oxygenation with right ventricular failure induced by pulmonary arterial hypertension: mitochondrial inhibition as driver of cardiac failure? Respir Res 16(1):6

27. Xanthouli P, Theobald V, Benjamin N, Marra AM, D'Agostino A, Egenlauf B, Shaukat M, Ding C, Cittadini A, Bossone E, Kögler M, Grünig E, Muckenthaler MU, Eichstaedt CA (2021) Prognostic impact of hypochromic erythrocytes in patients with pulmonary arterial hypertension. Respir Res 22:288

28. Wallace DF (2016) The regulation of iron absorption and homeostasis. Clin Biochem Rev 37(2):51–62

29. Farha S, Laskowski D, Deepa G, Park MM, Tang WHW, Dweik RA, Erzurum SC (2013) Loss of alveolar membrane diffusing capacity and pulmonary capillary blood volume in pulmonary arterial hypertension. Respir Res 14(1):6

30. Kooiman K, Roovers S, Langeveld SAG, Kleven RT, Dewitte H, O'Reilly MA, Escoffre J-M, Bouakaz A, Verweij MD, Hynynen K, Lentacker I, Stride E, Holland CK (2020) Ultrasound-responsive cavitation nuclei for therapy and drug delivery. Ultrasound Med Biol 46(6):1296–1325

31. Sanwal R, Joshi K, Ditmans M, Tsai SSH, Lee WL (2021) Ultrasound and microbubbles for targeted drug delivery to the lung endothelium in ARDS: cellular mechanisms and therapeutic opportunities. Biomedicines 9(7):803

32. Mitragotri S (1996) Transdermal drug delivery using low-frequency sonophoresis. Pharm Res 13(3):411–420

33. Tezel A, Mitragotri S (2003) Interactions of inertial cavitation bubbles with stratum corneum lipid bilayers during low frequency sonophoresis. Biophys J 85:3502–3512

34. Shankar H, Pagel PS, Warner DS (2011) Potential adverse ultrasound-related biological effects: a critical review. Anaesthesiologists 115:1109–1124

35. Aoki T, Yamasawa F, Kawashiro T, Shibata T, Ishizaka A, Urano T, Okada Y (2008) Effects of long-term low-dose oxygen supplementation on the epithelial function, collagen metabolism and interstitial fibrogenesis in the guinea pig lung. Respir Res 9:37

36. Liu K, Wang H, Yu S, Tu G, Luo Z (2021) Inhaled pulmonary vasodilators: a narrative review. Ann Transl Med 9(7):597

37. Chen L, Zheng Q, Chen X, Wang J, Wang L (2019) Low-frequency ultrasound enhances vascular endothelial growth factor expression, thereby promoting the wound healing in diabetic rats. Exp Ther Med 18(5):4040–4048

38. Siegal RJ (2011) Low frequency therapeutic ultrasound causes vasodilation and enhanced tissue perfusion. J Acoust Soc Am 130:2501

39. Minai OA, Nguyen Q, Mummadi S, Walker E, McCarthy K, Dweik RA (2015) Heart rate recovery is an important predictor of outcomes in patients with connective tissue disease-associated pulmonary hypertension. Pulm Circ 5(3):565–576

40. Bisserier M, Pradhan N, Adri L (2020) Current and emerging therapeutic approaches to pulmonary hypertension. Rev Cardiovasc Med 21(2):163–179

41. Nonogaki K, Murakami M, Yamazaki T, Nonogaki N (2018) Low-frequency and low-intensity ultrasound increases cardiac parasympathetic neural activity and decreases clinic hypertension in elderly hypertensive subjects with type 2 diabetes. IJC Heart Vasc 19:34–36

42. Li D, Cui Z, Xu S, Xu T, Wu S, Bouakaz A, Wan M, Zhang S (2020) Low-intensity focused ultrasound stimulation treatment decreases blood pressure in spontaneously hypertensive rats. IEEE Trans Biomed Eng 67(11):3048–3056

43. Tunaitytė A, Abramavicius S, Volkeviciute A, Venslauskas M, Bubulis A, Bajoriunas V, Simonson U, Ostasevicius V, Jurenas V, Briedis K, Stankevicius E (2024) Contractions induced in human pulmonary arteries by a H_2S donor, GYY 4137, are inhibited by low-frequency (20 kHz) ultrasound. Biomolecules 14(3):257

44. Abramavicius S, Ostasevicius V, Jurenas V, Stankevicius E (2018) Ultrasound and mechanical shock induced vascular relaxation. Rehabilitation Yesterday–Today–Tomorrow Dep Clin Rehab Olsztyn 43

45. Abramavicius S, Ostasevicius V, Jurenas V, Stankevicius E (2017) Ultrasound and mechanical shock induced vascular relaxation. In: 75th conference of the University of Latvia, vol 3, p 121

46. Radzeviciene A, Abramavicius S, Zemaityte V, Ostasevicius V, Jurenas V, Stankevicius E (2017) Ultrasound and antibiotic induced vascular relaxation. In: Intrinsic activity: 2nd international conference in pharmacology: from cellular processes to drug targets: Rīga, Latvia, vol 5, suppl 2, pp A2.39–A2.39

47. Ostasevicius V, Jurenas V, Bubulis A, Venslauskas M, Vezys J, Veikutis V, Velicka L (2024) Leg blood flow stimulation system and method for combining low and high-frequency acoustic vibration, LT 7109 B

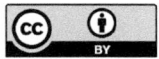

Vibrational Activation of Blood Flow

3

3.1 Introduction

Capillaries connect the flow of arteries and veins, forming a closed blood circuit around the body's cells and tissues to supply and absorb oxygen, nutrients and other substances. The physiological parameters of these flows, such as blood velocity and blood pressure, are highly dependent on capillary blood flow. Given that the diameter of the capillary is smaller than that of the disc-shaped erythrocyte, the use of additional technical devices to facilitate the movement of erythrocytes through the capillaries is necessary to maintain adequate blood flow in various diseases. As diabetes stiffens erythrocytes, causing capillaries to become clogged, so it is necessary to reduce the friction between erythrocytes and capillaries by vibration, halving the static friction coefficient to the kinematic friction coefficient. Thanks to the digital twins, blood flow in capillaries has been studied, and means of activating blood in the lower and upper limbs of humans have been developed and patented. The "Vilim ball", an intelligent human tremor therapy device, has been developed, certified and commercialised after clinical trials. Electromagnetic devices for heart rate stabilisation, acoustic therapy and spinal activation have been developed. A customised methodology and technology for reconstruction of circulatory system flows has been proposed.

© The Author(s) 2025
V. Ostasevicius et al., *Noninvasive Therapeutic Technologies*, Synthesis Lectures on Biomedical Engineering, https://doi.org/10.1007/978-3-031-79025-6_3

3.2   Investigation of the Vibration Influence on Blood Velocity in the Capillary

3.2.1   Capillary Blood Flow Response Assessment

As capillary's displacement coincides with the surrounding soft human tissue movement, it has been decided to measure fluid velocity inside the capillary induced by external low-frequencies vibrations. A virtual 2D model with the settings of the vibrating microchannel of the capillary has been designed to simplify the testing of the influence of different parameters. The aim of the virtual microchannel model was to substitute and to reduce the demand of experimental setup for further studies. The virtual model enables time to be saved and costs are reduced due to the variability of different parameters that can be changed easily. COMSOL Multiphysics software has been used to perform operations with coupled systems of partial differential equations. At each computational step, the fluid flow field and the structure have been evolved as a coupled system. The flow and structure interaction forces were immediately accounted, and their resultant motions enforced in each step. Before designing the model, the research studies of microchannels analysis [1] were overviewed, as well as the built-in blood vessel model being deeply analyzed.

The first, simplified 2D model (Fig. 3.1) was created to investigate alterations of fluid properties affecting it on various vibrational actions. The channel model of 1 mm length and 8 μm diameter was built with reference to the vascular graft tubes that are planned to be used for the experimental setup. Part of the channel of 0.15 mm length was placed in the human tissue properties imitating model. The microchannel was filled by liquid containing blood material properties. The density of 1060 kg/m^3 and the dynamic viscosity of 0.005 Ns/m^2 has been defined. The fluid–structure interaction study has been selected as the most compatible according to the model and its parts. The usability of this study is recommended when modelling the interaction of deformable structure with flowing fluid. Some fluid–structure interaction applications include cell bio-mechanics modules as cell deformation, fluid dynamics, ciliary beating, etc. This type of study enables researchers to observe fundamental physics on the sophisticated numerical calculations between fluids and solids.

The fluid–structure interaction problem can be defined by Ω, including structural domain Ω_s and the fluid domain Ω_f, with an external boundary Γ. The fluid–structure interaction is defined by $\Gamma_s = \Omega_s \cap \Omega_f$. Fluid and structure dynamics can be defined because of the D'Alembert's principle [2]:

$$\rho v_i - \sigma_{ij,j} + f_i = 0 \tag{3.1}$$

where f_i is the body force, ρ is the mass density and $\sigma_{ij,j}$ represents the stress component. In the structural domain, the equation is defined as

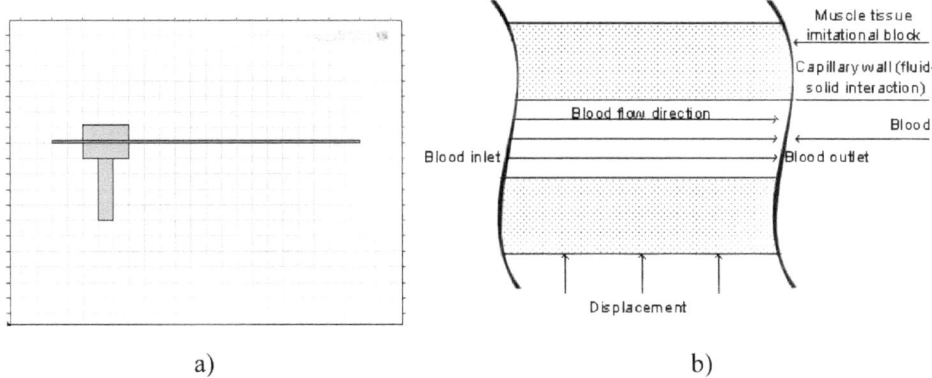

Fig. 3.1 a 2D COMSOL Multiphysics software models of fluid filled microchannel placed in human tissue; **b** schematic drawing

$$\rho^s v_{ij,j}^s + f_i^s = 0, \quad \text{in} \quad \overline{\Omega}_s \tag{3.2}$$

where the superscript, s, labels the amount linked with the structure. The velocity, v_i^s is the material (or total) time derivative of the displacement field u_i^s, i.e., $v_i^s = \dot{u}_i^s$.

Equation (3.2) is usually used to describe the Lagrangian theorem. The first term of the Eq. (3.2) is linked with inertia and the second one—with internal stresses. In the case of describing the material as linear elastic, the structural stress will be described by Hooke's law, i.e.,

$$\sigma_{ij}^s = \lambda \delta_{ij} \varepsilon_{ij} + 2G\varepsilon_{ij} \tag{3.3}$$

where the structural stress σ_{ij}^s is a function of the strains, ε_{ij} and the Lame constants λ and G,

which are determined by

$$\varepsilon_{ij} = \frac{1}{2}(u_{i,j} + u_{j,i}), \tag{3.4}$$

$$G = \frac{E}{2(1+\upsilon)}, \tag{3.5}$$

$$\lambda = \frac{E\upsilon}{(1+\upsilon)(1-2\upsilon)} \tag{3.6}$$

where E is the Young's modulus and v is the Poisson's ratio.

In the fluid domain, the equation is written as

$$\rho^f v_i^f - \rho_{ij,j}^f + f_i^f = 0, \quad \text{in} \quad \overline{\Omega}_f \tag{3.7}$$

which usually stands for the Eulerian description. In the inertia term, equation is given by,

$$v_i^f = \frac{dv_i^f}{dt} = \frac{\partial v_i^f}{\partial t} + v_i^f v_{i,j}^f \tag{3.8}$$

In the case of incompressible Newtonian fluid model, the fluid stress σ_{ij}^f is given by,

$$\sigma_{ij}^f = -p\delta_{ij} + \tau_{ij} \tag{3.9}$$

where p is the static pressure used to enforce the incompressibility condition, $v_{i,i}^f = 0$,

$$\tau_{ij} = 2\mu \left(e_{ij} - \frac{\delta_{ij}e_{kk}}{3} \right) \tag{3.10}$$

$$e_{ij} = \left(v_{j,i}^f + v_{i,j}^f \right) \tag{3.11}$$

The no-slip state on the fluid–structure interaction Γ_s is maintained by defining Dirichlet and Neumann conditions as:

$$v_i^s = v_i^f, \quad \text{on} \quad \Gamma_s \tag{3.12}$$

$$\sigma_{ij}^s n_i = \sigma_{ij}^f n_i, \quad \text{on} \quad \Gamma_s \tag{3.13}$$

The Eq. (3.13) is in fact the differentiation of the displacement condition that both fields share the same interface,

$$x_i^s = x_i^f, \quad \text{on} \quad \Gamma_s \tag{3.14}$$

In some cases, the Eq. (3.14) is being used instead of (3.12).

The displacement of $0.1 \div 8$ mm on the Y-axis and sine waveform function to imitate oscillations varying from 1 to 6 Hz have been determined for the human tissue imitational model. Different angular frequency values of sine waveform enabled the variability of oscillations of the material, imitating the human tissue mechanical properties. The fluid material with reference to the experimental setup was imposed. The prescribed mesh displacement of the fluid material of 0 mm on the X-axis for the inlet and the outlet of the microchannel have been set. The prescribed mesh displacement of 0 mm on the Y-axis was imposed for longitudinal microchannel boundaries excluding fluid–solid interface boundaries. In further studies, Moving-mesh physics has been used. This type of study enables researchers to track the deformation of the fluid mesh. The boundaries of contacting solid and fluid area were prescribed in this study. The two-way coupling conditions can be defined from the equations below:

$$v_{Fluid} = v_{Solid} \tag{3.15}$$

$$v_{Soid} = \frac{\partial u_{Solid}}{\partial t} \tag{3.16}$$

$$(\sigma \cdot n)_{Fluid} = (\sigma \cdot n)_{Solid} \tag{3.17}$$

where v is the velocity vector, u is the displacement vector, σ is the stress tensor, and n is the normal vector to the FSI boundary.

The roller movement restriction of the oscillating part of the model was chosen. The material properties of the oscillating part of the model were set with reference to the human body tissue parameters. Vibrational movement of the oscillating part has been described by the sine waveform function where angular frequency, amplitude and phase were variable parameters. Sine wave function has been considered as the most compatible to define the prescribed oscillations (Eq. (3.18). A 3D model with the same properties was designed for more precise calculations (Fig. 3.1b).

$$f(t) = A \sin(\omega t + \varphi) \tag{3.18}$$

Incompressible Newtonian fluid flow physical model and Laminar Navier–Stokes equations were used to define blood fluid physics.

$$\rho \frac{\partial u}{\partial t} + \rho u \cdot \nabla u - \nabla \cdot \left(-p\mathrm{I} + \eta\left(\nabla u + (\nabla u)^{\mathrm{T}}\right)\right) = F \tag{3.19}$$

$$\nabla \cdot u = 0 \tag{3.20}$$

where ρ is the density, $u = (u, v)$ is the fluid velocity, p is the pressure, I is the unit diagonal matrix, η is the dynamic viscosity and F is the force.

This helps to define the load with a prominent pressure distribution. Open fluid boundaries were defined. The inlet boundary has been selected by prescribing normal inflow fluid velocity of 0.00065 m/s. The biological tissue related domains are included in the mechanical analysis of the study. This type of study is advanced because of the behavior of the materials. Dramatically large strains, nonlinear stress–strain connection and the incompressibility property of hyper-elastic material are the main issues that must be considered when properties of biological materials are involved. It is essential to properly define stress and strain measures. The assumptions of infinitesimal displacements are not acceptable. Geometrical nonlinearity could be prescribed when the strains are larger than a few percent and the loading of the body depends on the deformation. In the case of dealing with these issues, the Nonlinear Structural Material Module has been used. In the case of small displacements and strains, the linear elastic material model can be used. According to these assumptions, muscle material properties of 1200 kg/m^3 density, coefficient μ of $6.20*10^6$ N/m^2, bulk modulus of 20 μ, Poisson's ratio ν of 0.45 and elastic modulus of $1.16*10^6$ N/m^2 have been prescribed. The time domain and stationary studies can be selected for an analysis of fluid dynamics. The further boundary conditions of the model are described below.

A no-slip boundary condition was designated on all walls. The displacement of the Y-axis (at 2D model) and the displacement of the X-axis (at 3D model) with the waveform function to imitate oscillations were used. Time dependent study duration of 10 s with the step of 0.1 s was specified for all the calculations. The structure imitating capillary covering human tissue was a flexible material with the following parameters: density of 30 kg/m^3, Young's modulus of 25 MPa and Poisson's ratio of 0.5 [3].

On the COMSOL Multiphysics model, the cross-section changes of the velocity values were investigated after effecting the fluid on different frequencies' values. The changes of fluid velocity were monitored in the middle of the microchannel. The results were obtained by using the model of a microchannel of 8 μm diameter. The peak fluid velocity of the oscillating model on 4.3 Hz vibrations was 2.74 mm/s, while the maximum value of all the gathered data reached 3.23 mm/s (Fig. 3.2). The average blood flow velocity during the oscillations of 4.3 Hz frequency was 0.98 mm/s. The initial velocity increased by 66.3%. The results show the raised average and peak velocity values on each mean of the given low frequencies.

It was also observed that at some moments the direction of the fluid velocity was negative. In some cases, the turbulent flow marks could be seen. This depends on the amplitude of the oscillating part and the frequency value. This phenomenon can be observed in Fig. 3.3a and b when the velocity curve form at certain time moments is close to horizontal.

Different microchannel diameters require different frequency and amplitude values to reach the same result of velocity changes and turbulent flow marks. These results were

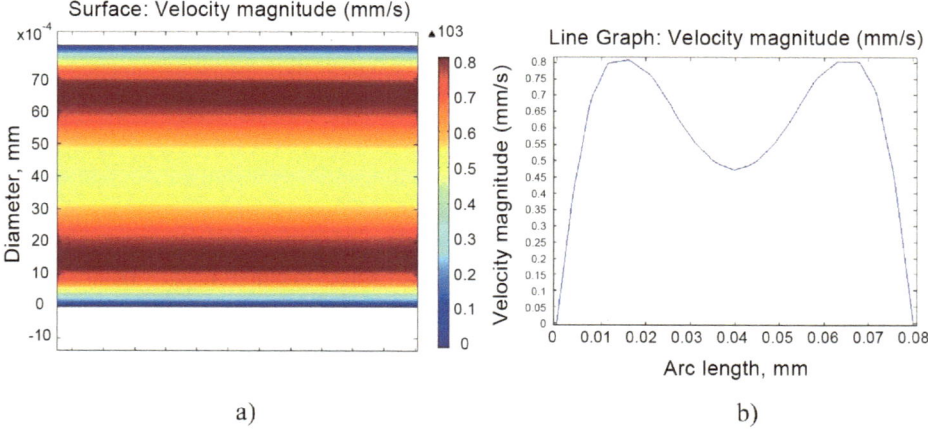

Fig. 3.2 Fluid velocity spectrogram (**a**) and field (**b**) during 4.3 Hz vibration exposure

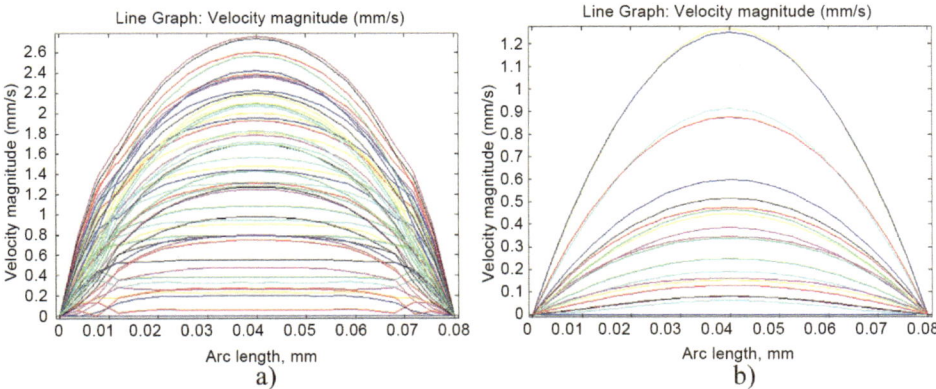

Fig. 3.3 Fluid velocity fields during the vibration exposure of 4.3 Hz (**a**) and oscillating part amplitude of 6 mm during the vibration exposure of 5.8 Hz (**b**)

detected in the enhancing microchannel diameter up to 8 mm. Therefore, it is necessary to identify the purpose where the improvement of blood flow velocity would be the most effective and adapt the model to these findings.

COMSOL Multiphysics was the proper choice for the simulation of the liquid flow in micro-channel imitating capillaries. The study made in [4] notes an increase of blood cell velocity of the femoral artery by 33% on 10–30 Hz. Moreover, based on the findings of this study, it was mentioned that a vibration amplitude of 2.5 mm coupled with vibration frequencies in the order 5–20 Hz produced significant increases in leg blood flow. Our study obtained results that indicated the increase of momentum fluid flow velocity of more than 4 times on 4.3 Hz oscillations and 6 mm displacement. It could be argued that proper vibrations enhance blood circulation on separate vessels of human limbs and could be used as a method to enhance blood flow on diabetic limbs. No significant change in the fluid velocity was recorded on higher frequencies of 49 Hz with low displacement amplitude of <1 mm. The velocity field diagrams and spectrograms were comparable for oscillating micro-channels on the same frequencies and displacement values in both the experimental and computer modelling results. Similar results therefore lead researchers to use virtual models instead of experimental investigations in future studies. It was defined that the different micro-channels' diameters require different vibration values to enhance fluid flow rate. It is essential to choose proper frequencies on stimulating human limb capillaries. A computer modelling platform enables researchers to make investigations on shifting parameters with a less time-consuming method. The human tissue analysis method [5] will be implemented with the purpose of individual excitation frequency identification.

The ability to increase blood flow velocity could be essential in solving blood circulation problems caused by diabetes mellitus. Momentum and average velocity increases were noted at the tube affected by the external vibrations. Studies in [6] show a significant decrease in red blood cell velocity in capillaries in diabetic mice. Considering that further investigations of the flowing RBC in the vibrating arteriole and capillary are foreseen to be carried out. Different material properties of erythrocyte will be used with reference to biochemical changes in the membrane structure in type 2 diabetes mellitus [7] and unaffected erythrocyte.

Previous vibrational training influence studies were performed using vibrating plates with amplitudes ranging from 2 to 6 mm and frequencies ranging from 20 to 50 Hz [8]. In most cases it is noticed that further studies on amplitude selection influence should be done. In [9] it was made a study investigating high and low amplitude effects on the development of strength, mechanical power of the lower limb, and body composition. They have found that high amplitude (4 mm) whole body vibrational training is a useful tool when looking for improved fitness and a full workout. Our study shows an increase in fluid flow velocity on major amplitudes as well, starting from 3.4 mm amplitude up to 8 mm. During the experiment, the highest velocity changes were obtained on measurements of 4.3 Hz and 6 mm, 5 Hz and 5.4 mm, 5.4 Hz and 8 mm, 4.8 Hz and 3.4 mm, 5.8 Hz and 6 mm. The studies, by using higher frequencies than 20 Hz coupling with low displacement amplitude (up to 1 mm), showed the results with non-significant velocity changes. Based on these findings, further analysis was not conducted on higher frequencies.

3.2.2   Determination of Eigenfrequency of Red Blood Cells

The red blood cell (RBC) or erythrocyte is a biconcave shape cell, and its mechanical properties mostly depend on membrane mechanical properties (Fig. 3.4). RBC contains a constant volume of cytosol which is protected by the membrane. The high deformability of the membrane allows the RBC to float through the capillary, which has smaller diameter. The mean value of diameter of a healthy patient's RBC is 7.5 μm and thickness ranges from 1.4 to 2.4 μm. The thickness of the membrane is 2 μm [10]. The most reviewed studies analyze RBC as a structure consisting of membrane and cytosol liquid. In our case, a similar model has been designed and analyzed. λ and μ are the Lamé constants that describes the elasticity of the isotropic composite membrane. Generally, these parameters describe the viscoelastic response of the composite membrane to in-plane deformation [11].

There are various studies where RBC's deformability is analyzed [12] but the mechanical behavior of the membrane is not clearly defined. Thus, the material properties of RBC's membrane can be found defined as Linear or Hyperplastic in several papers. Furthermore, different material models, like Neo-Hookean or Yeoh, are used. However, most material properties are almost the same in most studies. The erythrocyte mechanical model

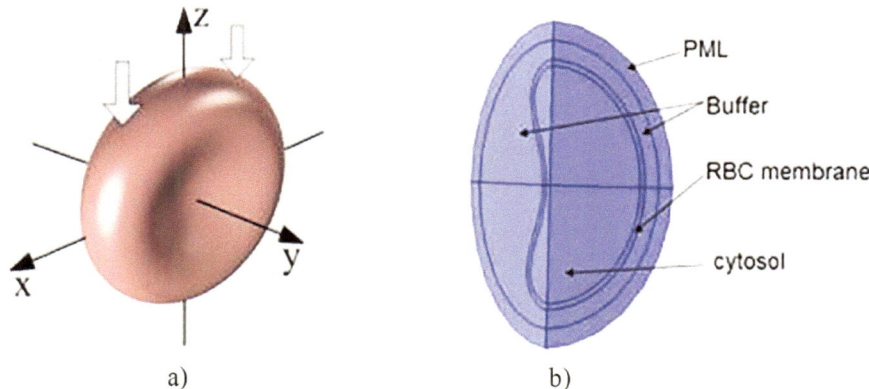

Fig. 3.4 Erythrocyte mechanical model (**a**) and composition (**b**) [11]

has been designed by using SolidWorks software and then imported to COMSOL Multiphysics software (Fig. 3.5). The membrane is considered as a two-dimensional elastic continuum having two equal Lamé constants $\mu = \lambda$ [13]. Membrane as linear elastic material has been analyzed because there are no findings that could clearly define its material properties and behavior. The material properties of the membrane are listed in Table 3.1. Initial pressure of 5333 Pa has been prescribed pursuant to the blood pressure in the capillary (40 mm Hg). According to various papers, the density of cytosol liquid is equal at 1200 kg/m^3 and the viscosity at 0.006 Pa s. In some papers, it is considered as eight times higher compared to water viscosity [14]. Thus, the water material has been defined and the parameter of dynamic viscosity has been multiplied by eight. In the case of the study where RBC was placed into the liquid, the blood material properties have been defined for a surrounding liquid.

Several different types of calculations have been used. First, Solid mechanics physics has been used for the analysis of the RBC's membrane natural frequencies. This type of study excludes the influence of fluid that reduces the natural frequencies of a solid body. Therefore, the Acoustic-Solid Interaction Frequency domain module has been used for the Eigenfrequency analysis of the fluid consistent model where cytosolic liquid has been taken into consideration. The desired number of eigenfrequencies calculations initially was set to 30, but according to the results this number was reduced to 20 for further calculations. After all, the RBC has been placed into the blood liquid to identify the changes of Eigenfrequency values depending on the medium. The cytosolic fluid has been considered as viscous fluid and the Bulk viscosity had to be prescribed. In the literature, it is noted that it may vary from 0.1 to 0.8 Pa s. The mean value of 0.4 Pa s has been prescribed. Blood's (37 °C) Bulk viscosity parameter was taken equal to 3.4 10^{-3} Pa s at the environmental temperature of 36.6 °C. The physics-controlled \mesh of an extremely fine grid has been selected.

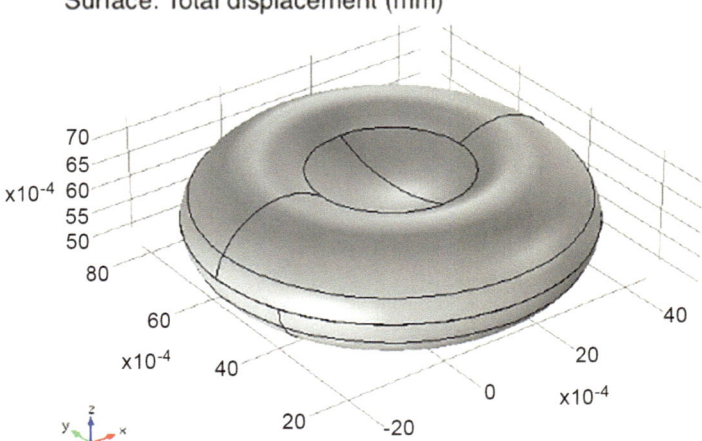

Fig. 3.5 Red blood cell model

Table 3.1 RBC membrane's
material properties [15, 16]

Parameter	Value
Density	1100 kg/m^3
Poisson ratio	0.49–0.499
Young's modulus	4500 Pa

The number of studies where RBC's rigidity was investigated provide findings of increasing rigidity of erythrocyte membrane in the case of diabetes mellitus or other diseases. The consensus is unequivocal that the Young's modulus increases on diabetics. Thus converts the erythrocyte, as hardly deformable material, especially in the case of entering a capillary. The deformability is significantly lower as Young's modulus is much higher in diabetics compared with healthy patients [17]. In one study, an atomic force microscope has been used to investigate changes of Young's modulus on blood samples affected by diabetes mellitus. The results show that Young's modulus can increase greater than 3 times in diabetics patients compared with healthy ones [18]. The healthy patient RBC can enter the microchannel of 3 μm considering that its non-deformed diameter is 7.5 μm (Fig. 3.6). Understanding the behavior of the RBC's shape deformability (Fig. 3.6c) it was decided to investigate its natural frequencies and define displacements of the cell's membrane that would enable RBC to enter the capillary more fluently.

First, the eigenfrequency analysis has been performed on RBC's membrane, excluding the cytosolic liquid and the environmental parameters. The purpose of this study was to identify the deformability of the membrane, depending on the natural frequencies. It is known that the erythrocyte enters the capillary by bending and changing its disc

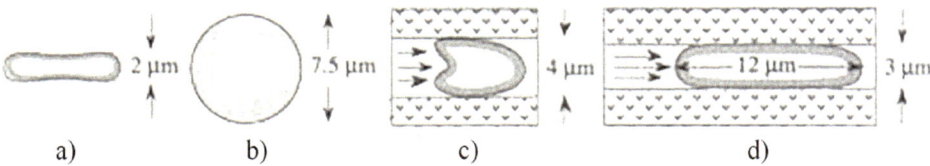

Fig. 3.6 RBC deformability: **a** RBC top projection (thickness); **b** non-deformed RBC, front projection (diameter); **c** partly deformed RBC (parachute form); **d** fully deformed RBC in the narrowest capillary channel [19]

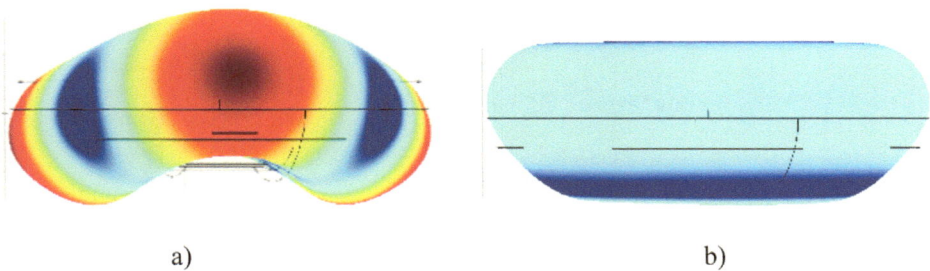

Fig. 3.7 Shapes of deformed RBC at 2.01×10^5 Hz (**a**) and 1.11×10^5 Hz (**b**)

form. The natural frequencies of the same or similar shape have been an objective of the Eigenfrequency analysis.

The results of the RBC's membrane natural frequencies have been analyzed. The shapes of deformed membrane could be compared to one at the moment of entering the capillary. These shapes have been identified on the frequency value of 2.01×10^5 Hz (Fig. 3.7a) and 1.11×10^5 Hz (Fig. 3.7b). No appropriate shape deformations were identified on lower frequency range values.

Further analysis has been conducted by using the acoustic-solid interaction frequency domain study. The model of this study contained cytosolic liquid, thereby the obtained results of frequencies and deformations of the membrane were different. First, the healthy patient's RBC has been analyzed and the highest displacements of actual areas were obtained at 1.47 Hz (Figs. 3.8 and 3.9).

The higher values of the Young's modulus parameter increase the natural frequencies values. It can be obtained that the RBC may be deformed more fluently by affecting it with an external vibrational excitation of low frequencies. However, these results had to be compared with the immersed model that is more adequate to the natural environment. When the mechanical structures are immersed in a fluid, their natural frequencies are reduced. The fluid, as a source of damping, induces changes of the mode shapes, thus it

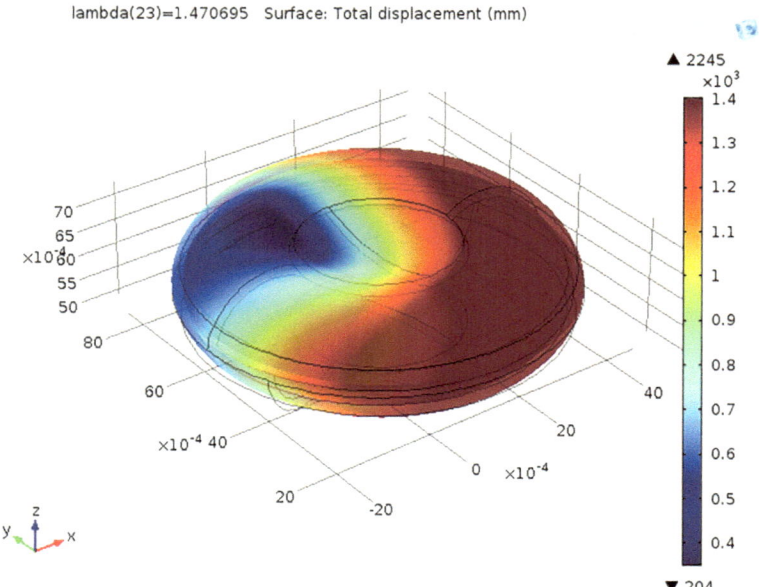

Fig. 3.8 Deformations of healthy patient RBC at 1.47 Hz

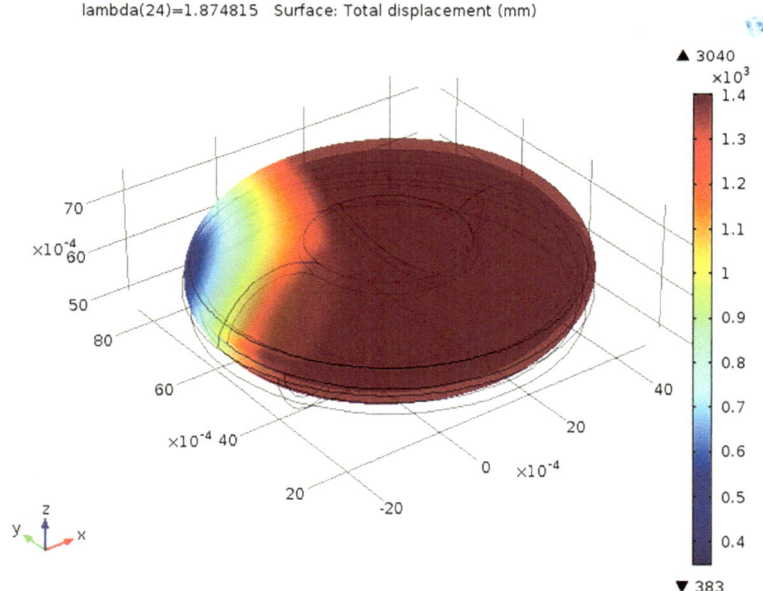

Fig. 3.9 Deformations of disease affected patient RBC with 3 times higher Young's modulus at 1.87 Hz

Fig. 3.10 RBC immersed in blood

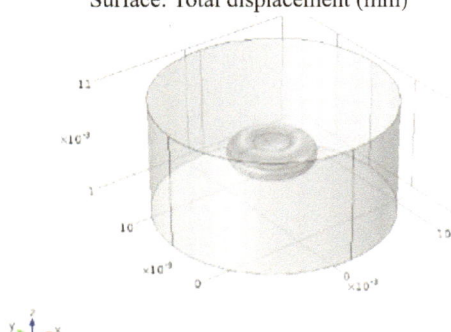

Surface: Total displacement (mm)

was crucial to conduct this type of study. The problem was defined as a coupled acoustic-structure eigenvalue analysis and the damping was accounted due to the fluid viscosity by including a viscous loss term.

The model of RBC comprising cytosolic liquid and immersed in blood has been designed (Fig. 3.10). A cylinder shape, imitating part of blood vessel, has been designed in which the erythrocyte model has been immersed.

First, the analysis of natural frequencies has been conducted on a healthy patient erythrocyte. Next, the eigenfrequency study was performed for a prescribed model with three times higher Young's modulus of 13,500 N/m^2 [17]. The natural frequencies of 2.34 Hz (Fig. 3.11) were defined for a healthy patient RBC as the most appropriate, by deforming RBC for a more fluent entrance to the capillary. The eigenfrequency of 4.02 Hz (Fig. 3.12) of damaged erythrocyte with membrane material of a three times higher Young's modulus has been obtained. The natural frequencies of the disease affected patient RBC vary from 0.4 to 48 Hz according to calculations by changing the Young's modulus and Poisson's ratio.

The results of the eigenfrequency study have showed the RBC's areas of deformation at the lower frequency ranges. Basically, the outer area of the membrane is mostly affected. This phenomenon could be compared to the natural deformations of RBC's by entering the capillary. The increase of deformability of the RBC during the vibrational excitation on low frequencies could be an effective way of rehabilitation for various diseases. Vibrational exposure is suggested as an approach of reduced friction in dynamics of the RBC's movement through the capillary. Therefore, further related investigations have been conducted.

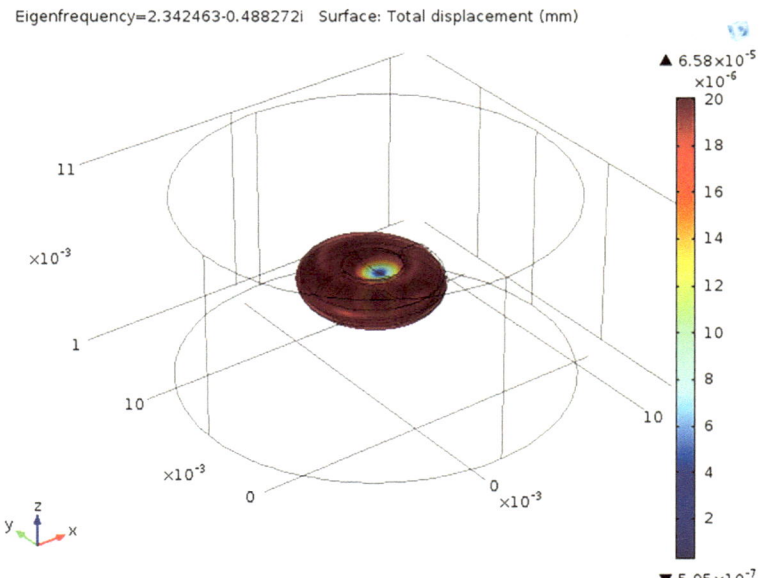

Fig. 3.11 Healthy RBC's displacement at eigenfrequency of 2.34 Hz

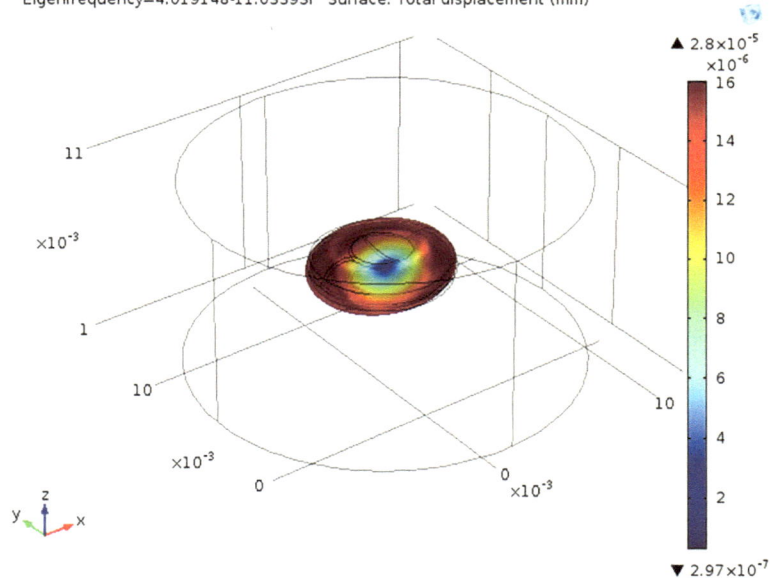

Fig. 3.12 Damaged RBC's displacement at eigenfrequency of 4.02 Hz

3.2.3 Influence of Vibrations on the Mechanical Properties of Red Blood Cells

The RBC's flow by entering capillary has been analyzed. Static and dynamic analysis has been conducted. A 2D model of immersed erythrocyte has been designed and a fluid–structure interaction study was performed. The RBC's membrane material property of Young's modulus has been changed during the different stages of investigation. A healthy patient erythrocyte of 4500 N/m^2 and three times higher of 13,500 N/m^2 for disease affected RBC has been used. In most papers, the erythrocyte's membrane is defined as hyperplastic material while in others as a linear elastic one. Studies of both different types of material of RBC's membrane has been conducted. To initiate RBC's deformability on the tapering channel, the contact pair parameter has been defined between the membrane's outer boundaries and capillary's walls. Inlet and outlet fluid boundaries were defined on the right and left sides of the model respectively. Yeoh mesh smoothing type and fluid as an incompressible flow was prescribed for this type of study. The RBC's movement through the channel was defined by the function of prescribed displacement and using a displacement parameter to identify the steps of the stationary study. The RBC model has been immersed in the model of fluid with material properties of blood. Initial experiments were made without oscillating the whole model. The maximum contact pressure parameter was observed on the contact pair RBC membrane-capillary wall surface. Contact pressure analytically can be defined as a function on the x axis by the equation [20]:

$$P = \sqrt{\frac{F_n E'}{2\pi R'}} \times \left(1 - \left(\frac{x}{a}\right)^2\right) \tag{3.21}$$

$$a = \sqrt{\frac{8 F_n R'}{\pi E'}} \tag{3.22}$$

where F_n is the applied load per unit length, E' is the combined elasticity modulus, and R is the combined radius.

The equations of combined Young's modulus and radius are listed below:

$$E' = \frac{2 E_1 E_2}{E_2 \left(1 - v_1^2\right) + E_1 \left(1 - v_2^2\right)}, \tag{3.23}$$

$$R' = \lim_{R_2 \to \infty} \frac{R_1 R_2}{R_1 + R_2} = R_1 \tag{3.24}$$

Young's modulus of RBC's membrane and capillary wall are defined by E_1 and E_2 respectively and R_1 is the radius of the RBC upper part. The Penalty contact method has been used to assess the applied load at the contact boundary. This parameter can be expressed by using the local value of the contact gap distance variable g, constant penalty factor δ and an estimated contact pressure T_0:

$$T_n = \begin{cases} T_O - Eh_{\min}\delta g \ \ if\,(g \leq 0) \\ T_{Oe}^{-\frac{Eh_{\min}\delta g}{T_O}} \quad otherwise \end{cases} \qquad (3.25)$$

If the interference (g < 0) occurs, the applied load is linearly increased using a penalty stiffness, the minimum element size on the contact pair boundary and a penalty factor δ. Using this method is not necessary to define an extra variable for the contact pressure.

The experiments with prescribed oscillating movement of the liner elastic part of the model had been conducted. Displacement of the oscillating part had been defined in the range of 5 mm to 2 cm with 5 mm steps. The main results are listed below (Figs. 3.13, 3.14, 3.15 and 3.16). The deformability of healthy patient RBC during the stage of entrance to the capillary has been investigated. The maximum contact pressure on the surface of the RBC was observed. In Fig. 3.13, the entrance of healthy patient RBC is shown with the value of a maximum contact pressure of 29.8 N/m^2. After increasing the stiffness of the RBC by three times, the maximum contact pressure increased by three times also, up to 89.4 N/m^2 (Fig. 3.14).

The same parameters were investigated during the disease affected patient RBC's flow, by inducing vibrational oscillations to the model. First, the vibrations of 3 Hz frequencies and 5 mm displacement were prescribed. The maximum contact pressure has increased up to 95.9 N/m^2 (Fig. 3.14) at the same moment as entrance. The displacement has been increased by 5 mm. The mean of contact pressure increased up to 96.2 N/m^2.

After increasing the displacement up to 15 mm, the monitored value had decreased and was equal to 87.3 N/m^2. This means it is lower compared to the non-vibrating model. Furthermore, enhanced displacement of the moving model by 20 mm had the lowest value of maximum contact pressure of 64.1 N/m^2, which is nearly twice higher compared to the healthy patient erythrocyte and 28.2 N/m^2 lower in proportion to disease affected patient RBC (Fig. 3.15). However, by increasing the amplitude higher than 5 mm, negative

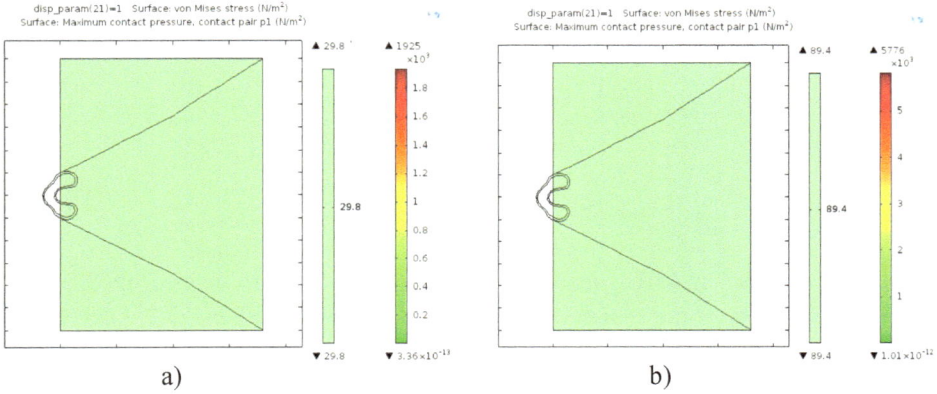

Fig. 3.13 Healthy (**a**) and disease affected (**b**) patient RBC without vibrational oscillations

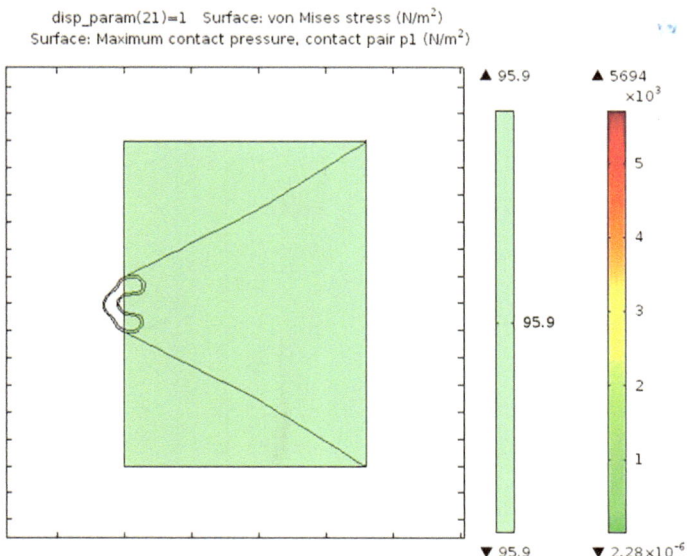

disp_param(21)=1   Surface: von Mises stress (N/m²)
Surface: Maximum contact pressure, contact pair p1 (N/m²)

Fig. 3.14 Disease affected patient RBC on vibrational exposure of 3 Hz with 5 mm displacement

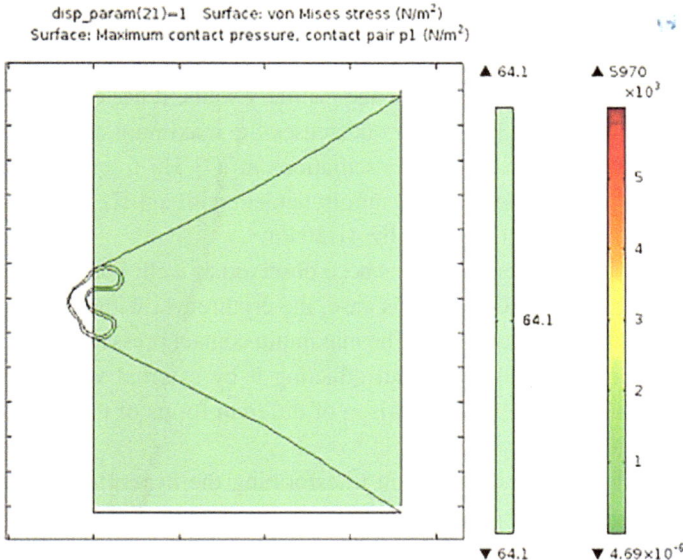

disp_param(21)=1   Surface: von Mises stress (N/m²)
Surface: Maximum contact pressure, contact pair p1 (N/m²)

Fig. 3.15 Disease's affected patient RBC on vibrational exposure of 3 Hz with 20 mm displacement

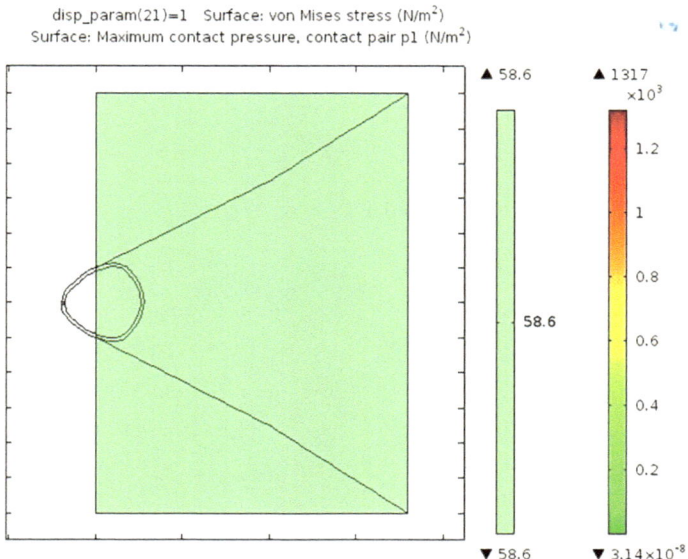

Fig. 3.16 Different form RBC entering capillary without affecting by external vibrations

results where contact pressure increased up to 104 N/m^2 were achieved. The monitored values of increased displacement up to 50 mm did not show any reduction of maximum contact pressure between the erythrocyte and capillary walls. It has been observed that the displacement ranging from 13 to 22 mm decreases the maximum contact pressure value and is desirable during the vibrational oscillations at a 3 Hz frequency. Moreover, the displacement in the range from 0.6 to 2 mm in tandem with a 4 Hz frequency obtained a decrease of maximum contact pressure by 41.2 N/m^2.

Another form of RBC deformation has been observed as well. Sometimes, pathological disorders affect the form of RBC. In this case, the erythrocyte without indentation in the middle of the body has been analyzed. The maximum contact pressure values were higher, even during the natural entrance without affecting it by external vibrations (Fig. 3.16). Further analysis must be done in comparison of different forms of the RBC and influence of vibrational excitation.

Similar results have been obtained on transforming the hyperplastic material properties to the Linear Elastic. The values of the maximum contact pressure of stiffer RBC decreased in the range of 10–22 mm of displacement at the 3 Hz frequency. However, the decrease was significantly lower in all cases.

As it was noted before, the low-frequency vibrational excitations could be used for an improvement of human blood flow. However, there is a lack of numerical analysis studies made on investigating the cause of positive effect. Thus, meeting the objectives of research; the blood flow on the microchannel of capillary and RBC's deformability analysis has been made by using the COMSOL Multiphysics software. Designed models of micro channel and RBC enables researchers to make an analysis of the external mechanical vibrations influence on blood flow velocity and deformability of the body structure. Furthermore, the deeper mechanical analysis of micro cells can be executed by investigating Eigenfrequencies and their dependence on various input parameters of the model.

The numerical simulations performed throughout the research may be grouped in a few case studies: (i) Evaluation of fluid flow improvement in the micro channel due to vibrational excitation; (ii) Evaluation of RBC's natural frequencies depending on changes of material properties of rigidity; iii) Evaluation of RBC's deformability improvement by using external vibrational oscillations.

Main conclusions drawn from the numerical simulation results are the following:

- COMSOL Multiphysics modelling results of the blood flow through the results enables reliable use of computer models for further studies. Numerical analysis showed that low frequency (from 4 to 8 Hz) and higher amplitude (from 3.4 to 8 mm) of external vibrations could significantly increase blood flow. However higher frequencies combined with lower amplitudes did not give similar results. The beating phenomenon method could be used for creating the prescribed vibrations on a human's limbs.
- Analysis of three types of natural frequencies' analysis has been done for the erythrocyte's membrane: as a solid model without interaction with liquid; as a solid containing cytosol and as an immersed solid containing cytosol. The Eigenfrequencies' studies of immersed RBC have shown that lower frequencies could be used in the case of deformability of morbid RBC. The frequencies of 4.02 Hz affect the outer areas of the cell, thus providing higher deformability of the membrane with enhanced rigidity. Further analysis should be done in case of clearly defining the erythrocyte's material properties.
- Healthy and disease affected RBC's entrance to the capillary study has been conducted. The results showed that vibrational excitations of 3 Hz frequency, coupled with the displacement ranging from 13 to 22 mm, lowered the maximum contact pressure value by 28% at the contact of the RBC and capillary's wall in the study of RBC with three times increased stiffness. The maximum contact pressure increased when higher displacement than 22 mm occurred during the same frequency vibrational excitation. The lower displacement in a couple with 4 Hz frequency obtained a decrease of the maximum contact pressure by 54%.

According to the results of the experiments, it was decided to develop a vibrating bracelet for experiments on a human's hand. Identified motor regimes will allow researchers to generate the correct vibrations when using them on a human's limbs. This would allow researchers to gather the physiological parameter changes. Next, it is planned to make an investigation of blood circulation with a leg vibrating machine.

3.3   Intensification of Blood Flow in Capillaries

An overview of the existing applications of vibrational technologies in the healthcare field has provided an understanding of the needs and manner to solve problems of blood flow disorders. Accessible means are designed for different problems, but all have relations with issues of insufficient blood circulation. In most cases, vibratory movement of higher than 20 Hz frequency is used. This is the most significant difference separating the suggested approach from the existing solutions. Side effects to long-term vibration exposure to the internal organs are well known. Considering this, it was decided to develop devices by using locally adopted technological solutions. With the importance in mind of sufficient blood flow, especially in limbs, devices have been developed for these human body parts actuations.

The importance of safety issues must be considered in the case of development of human body interacting devices. Low voltage electrical components have been selected, ensuring assessment of possible injury issues. The accessibility dimension for people with disabilities was estimated in the cases of Arthritis or Diabetes mellitus.

From the technical point of view, sufficient and directly transferred force were the main issues to solve. Low-frequency vibrational excitations by generating considerable displacement was the main aim. Furthermore, the vibrational actuation should be transmitted directly to the limb, avoiding any losses so the source components should be coupled motionlessly with the excited part of human body.

Size and weight of the developed actuators were also relevant. The importance of usability at home, as well as transportation, was extremely high. Transportation matters are crucial because the treatment of circulatory disorders should be performed daily. Furthermore, the device control must be simple, without the need for any specific knowledge. Safety issues should be considered; therefore, the rotating and electrical parts must be covered to eliminate human interaction.

The aim of previously conducted numerical research was to define the proper working range of vibrational exposure devices for a solution of specific problems of blood flow disorders. The extraction of concentrated axial vibrations through the interaction with specific parts of the human body, which have various degrees of freedom, has been taken into consideration as the most important issue. The variability of weights of human body parts has been calculated and estimated in the case of providing sufficient vibrations. Improvement of the quality of life for people with diseases of circulatory disorders is the main purpose of the developed actuators.

3.3.1 Activation of Blood Circulation in the Upper Limbs

Stimulation of blood circulation by external vibration should be from one to two minutes. As it was noted previously, low frequencies are considered more efficient to improve blood flow than high frequencies. But the additional higher frequency component on the main low frequency is suitable in many cases. As capillaries are considered as the "second heart" the mechanical vibrations could be useful for the human limb's actuation and the intensification of the blood circulation in the human body. Sufficient force must be generated in the case of vibrational excitation on human limbs. To ensure low frequency vibrations and higher than 1 mm limb amplitude, the beating phenomenon has been considered as the most appropriate. Otherwise, high voltage and heavy motors have to be selected in the case of aspiration of low frequencies.

The beating phenomenon [21] occurs when two harmonically oscillating pendulums (signals of their vibrations are shown in Fig. 3.17, of slightly different frequencies are impressed on a body. They are a periodic variation in vibration at a frequency that is the difference between two frequencies.

The beating phenomenon enables the transfer of energy into the system where low-frequency vibrations could be induced by coupling two high-frequency sources. The beating phenomenon is part of the classical theory of mechanical vibrations, but its beneficial facilities are not widely used in contemporary technologies. The equation of motion of the pendulums without damping can be acquired from the equation [22]:

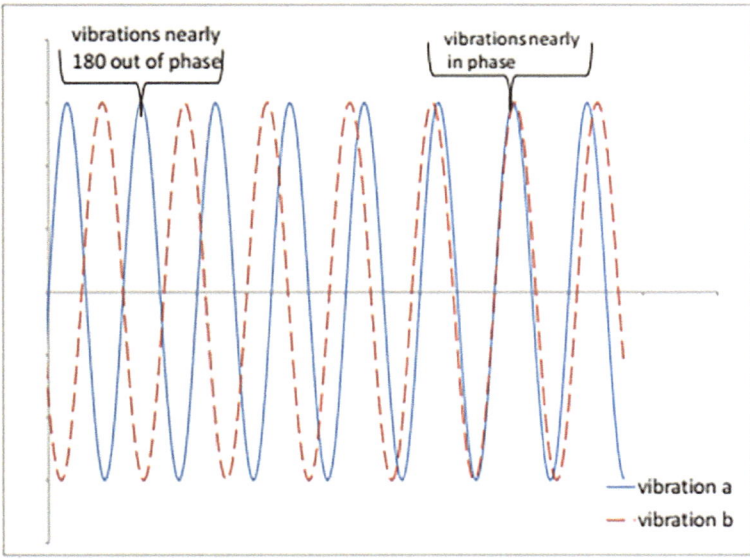

Fig. 3.17 Beating phenomenon occurrence [21]

$$\begin{bmatrix} 1 & \mu\alpha\mu \\ \alpha & 1 \end{bmatrix} \begin{bmatrix} \ddot{x}_1 \\ \ddot{x}_2 \end{bmatrix} + \begin{bmatrix} \omega_1^2 & 0 \\ 0 & \omega_2^2 \end{bmatrix} \begin{bmatrix} x_1 \\ x_2 \end{bmatrix} = \begin{bmatrix} 0 \\ 0 \end{bmatrix} \tag{3.26}$$

where, μ mass ratio, ω_1—natural frequency of the structure and ω_2—is the natural frequency of the damper, x_1 and x_2—systems' displacements,

The modal frequencies of this system are given by:

$$\overline{\omega}_{1,2} = \sqrt{\frac{\omega_1^2 + \omega_2^2(1 + \mu) \pm \Pi}{2(1 + \mu - \alpha^2\mu)}} \tag{3.27}$$

where $\Pi = (\omega_1^2 - \omega_2^2(1 + \mu))^2 + 4\omega_1^2\omega_2^2\alpha^2\mu$, the parameter α is responsible for the beat phenomenon.

If the primary and the secondary systems are damped, equation of motion applies:

$$\begin{bmatrix} 1 & \mu\alpha\mu \\ \alpha & 1 \end{bmatrix} \begin{bmatrix} \ddot{x}_{\prime\prime 1} \\ \ddot{x}_2 \end{bmatrix} + \begin{bmatrix} 2\omega_1\zeta_1 & 0 \\ 0 & \omega_2^2\zeta|\dot{x}_2|/4g \end{bmatrix} \begin{bmatrix} \dot{x}_1 \\ \dot{x}_2 \end{bmatrix}$$
$$+ \begin{bmatrix} \omega_1^2 & 0 \\ 0 & \omega_2^2 \end{bmatrix} \begin{bmatrix} x_1 \\ x_2 \end{bmatrix} = \begin{bmatrix} 0 \\ 0 \end{bmatrix} \tag{3.28}$$

where ζ is the head loss coefficient and g gravitational acceleration.

This equation can be numerically integrated at different levels of the ζ coefficient. The graphical interpretation of the differences between the beat response and head loss coefficient is shown in Fig. 3.18.

In the case of low-vibration exposure on the human limbs, the induction of the beating phenomenon has been chosen as the most suitable approach. To generate sufficient force in the limbs, the proper apparatus had to be chosen. In this case, the force induced while beating was calculated before selecting the electromechanical motors and designing unbalanced masses. It was considered that the average weight of handbreadth of the human hand is about 400g, therefore the sufficient generated force must be at least twice as high. As the proper vibrating motors with unbalanced masses were not found on the market, it was decided to choose an existing motor and to design the unbalanced mass. In this case, two vibrating motors for beating phenomenon and the calculated mechanical parameters were divided into two. Avoiding possible harm to the human body, high frequencies of the rotating unbalanced masses have not to exceed 100 Hz.

It was considered that a spring-mass system was constrained to move only in a vertical direction and excited by unbalanced rotating mass (Fig. 3.19). Here x is the displacement, m is the mass of the eccentric and r is the distance from the motor shaft to the center of the eccentric mass (r is usually called eccentricity e), ω is the angular velocity, M is bulk mass of the whole system and F_0 is the constant load. Then the equation of motion is:

$$(M - m)\frac{d^2x}{dt^2} + c\frac{dx}{dt} + kx = F_0\sin(\omega t) \tag{3.29}$$

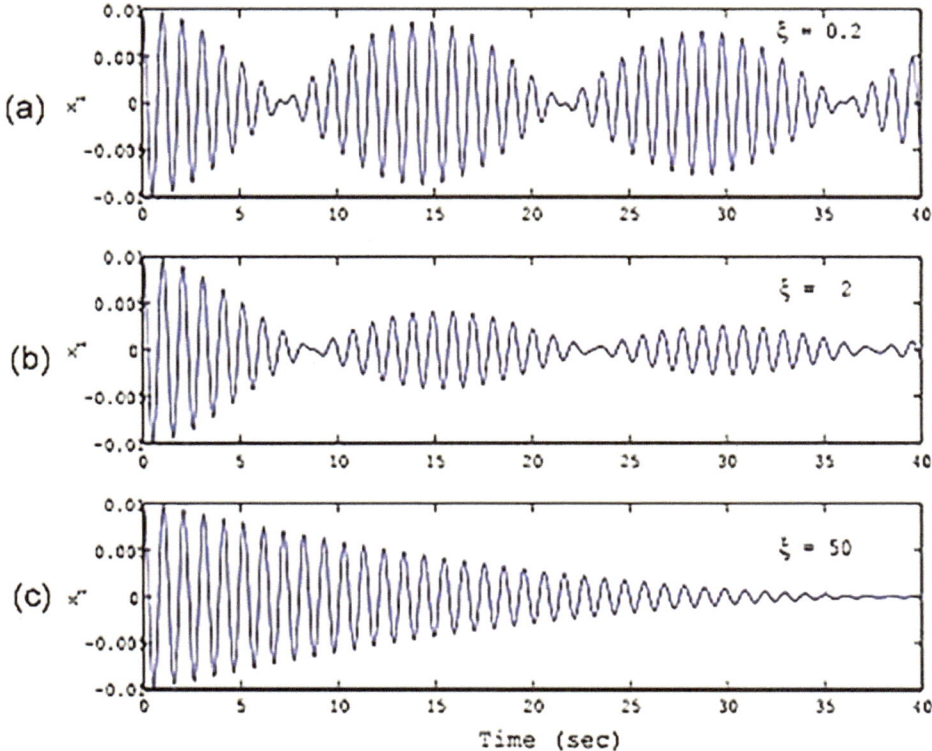

Fig. 3.18   Time histories of response for ξ = 0.2 (**a**), 2 (**b**) and 50 (**c**)

The generated force can be calculated from the simple equation below:

$$F = mr\omega^2 \tag{3.30}$$

It has been calculated that the angular speed of the motor should be equal or higher than 2000 rpm. The upper limit of this speed is desired up to 5700 rpm. In this range of operation, the force induced by the beating phenomenon can be ranged from 6 to 42 N.

According to the calculations, overall dimensions and electrical parameters, the Johnson 20,703 electromechanical motors were chosen as most eligible. Below, the main parameters of this motor are given (Table 3.2).

For human handbreadth excitation the vibrating bracelet was developed for disabled people as a tool for executing this exercise without any muscle effort. It could be useful for healthy people to simplify this exercise and enhance concentration on vibrational training in eliminating actuation of muscles. The main part of the vibrating bracelet consists of two small size, low voltage vibrating motors with unbalanced masses creating the beating phenomenon.

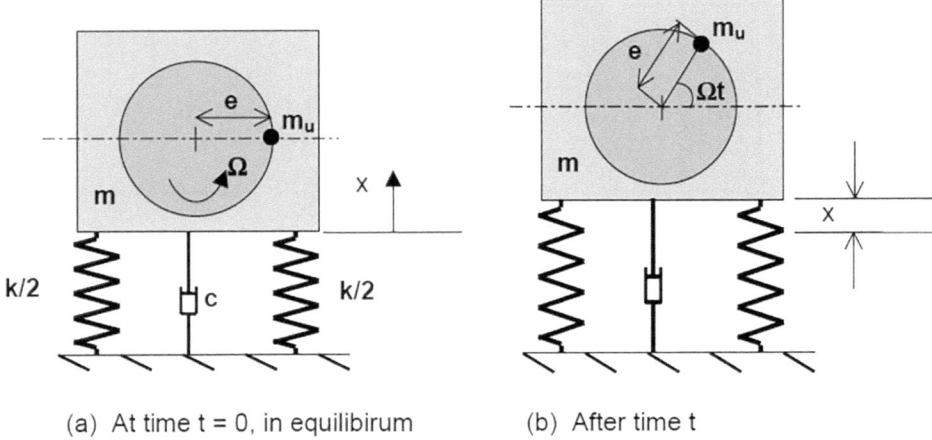

(a) At time t = 0, in equilibirum   (b) After time t

Fig. 3.19 Scheme of the motor with unbalanced mass system on the shaft [23]

Table 3.2 Johnson 20,703 motor parameters

Name	Value
Voltage	3–13 V
Current	0.24 A
RPM	2989–5977
Rotor dimensions	13 × 2 mm
Motor dimensions (L × Ø)	31 × 24 mm

Beats were observed when two sine functions with near-equal frequencies were superimposed. When frequency ratio $r \approx 1$, the forced solution for two superimposed frequencies is approximately [21]:

$$x(t) = \frac{2F_0}{m} \frac{1}{\omega_n^2 - \omega^2} \sin\left(\frac{\omega - \omega_n}{2}t\right) \cos\left(\frac{\omega + \omega_n}{2}t\right) \qquad (3.31)$$

where ω frequency, t time, F_0 force amplitude, m—mass, x(t)—mass displacement.

Therefore, no data was given according to the motor's RPM dependence on voltage. These parameters are crucial in the case of calculating the force created by the rotating unbalanced mass. Furthermore, the load of the unbalanced masses modifies the factory provided parameters. To identify these parameters a short experiment was made, and RPM values have been registered at different voltages. The means were registered with photo tachometer / stroboscope Lutron DT-2259 [24].

Table 3.3 Unbalanced mass parameters of hand actuator

Parameter	Value
Bulk mass	14.86 g
Mass without unbalance	5.95 g
Unbalance mass	8.91 g
Whole diameter	7.5 mm
Diameter without unbalance	4.5 mm
Diameter by the middle of unbalance	6 mm

The vibrational oscillations can be created by making unequal allocation of mass around an axis of the rotor. It is called a rotating unbalance when the center of mass does not match the geometric axis. The moment caused by unbalance initiates a vibratory movement thus generating oscillations and displacement of the rotations' source. To initiate this phenomenon, two identical masses were made to be mounted on the rotors of the selected electromechanical motors. Unbalance mass was designed by using SolidWorks software and was made from AISI 1020 steel. The aim of the beating phenomenon was to create a force higher than 7.85 N by using small sized and lightweight electromechanical motors. Therefore, masses were limited by the free area next to the second unbalanced mass. The main parameters of the unbalanced masses are given below (Table 3.3).

For the evaluation of eligibility, a special experimental set up was made whose structural scheme is presented in Fig. 3.20. Two motors were fixed together linearly on the cantilever without any possibility to move relatively to each other's direction, even at high level vibrations. The motors were screwed on the glass-cloth laminate cantilever. The cantilever's fixing holes were drilled at different lengths (50 and 100 mm) to observe alterations of vibrations regarding the cantilever length. Motors were attached at the free end of this cantilever in a position to generate a vertical force. Primary experiments were made without using any damping element. Later, a damping box package of water and air was created for further experiments to eliminate any possibility of cantilever resonance (Fig. 3.21). Inductive sensor IFM IG6084 was used to measure the cantilever's frequency and displacement (gradient: 1,389 V/mm). The data was registered by using the Oscilloscope Pico scope 3424 and the PC software 'Pico Scope 6'. Motors and vibrations measuring sensors were fed by three power suppliers.

The rotor's RPM alterations on the supplied voltage were investigated. The experiment was conducted by starting the motor's rotations at 4 V with registered 1370 rpm. The value of RPM has been registered at every 0.5 V. Angular speed was increased by approximately 200 rpm. At the peak value of 16.5 V, the motor's rotor had reached nearly the highest mean that is noted in the datasheet—5960 rpm (Fig. 3.22). The collected data enabled researchers to make calculations of the generated force during the beating phenomenon. These parameters are essential for the evaluation and selection process of the availability of electromechanical motors.

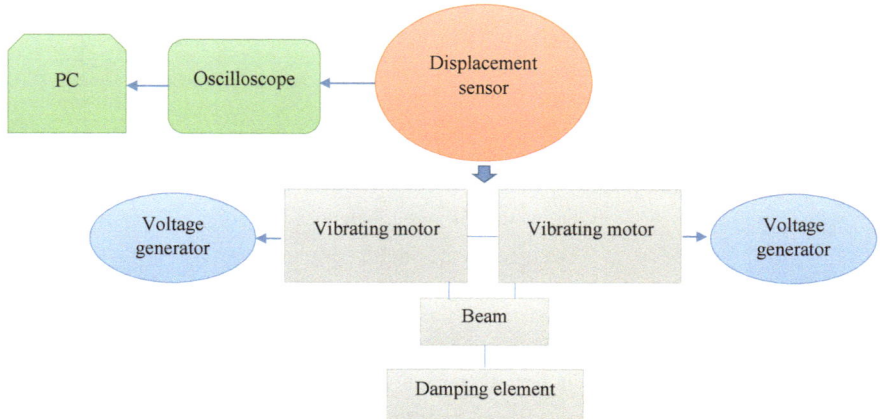

Fig. 3.20 Structural scheme of the vibrating platform and measuring elements

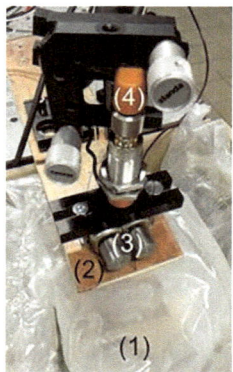

Fig. 3.21 Vibrating motors (3) on the cantilever (2) with damping element (1) and displacement sensor (4) on the top

Next, an experiment with one motor fixed on the cantilever was made with the purpose of investigating its generated force. The gathered data on different voltage values disclosed that the vibrating frequencies remain stable independently from the supplied voltage and RPM values. The value of 25 Hz was calculated by using a shorter cantilever (50 mm length) at a voltage range from 4 to 6.5 V (Fig. 3.23). In the case of using a damping element and when the system is out of resonance, one motor was not able to generate sufficient force that would be high enough to cause cantilever vibrations. The values of the measured vibrational frequencies were different with the longer cantilever (100 mm length), but they were not analyzed deeply because of the presence of resonance. Therefore, the usage of one motor is insufficient for wrists excitation purposes.

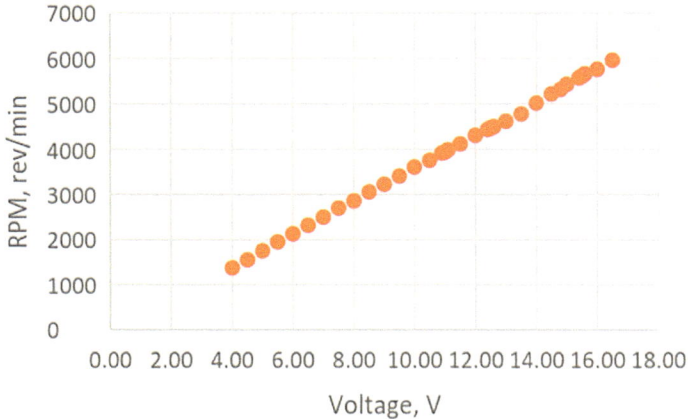

Fig. 3.22 Electrical motors RPM dependence on voltage

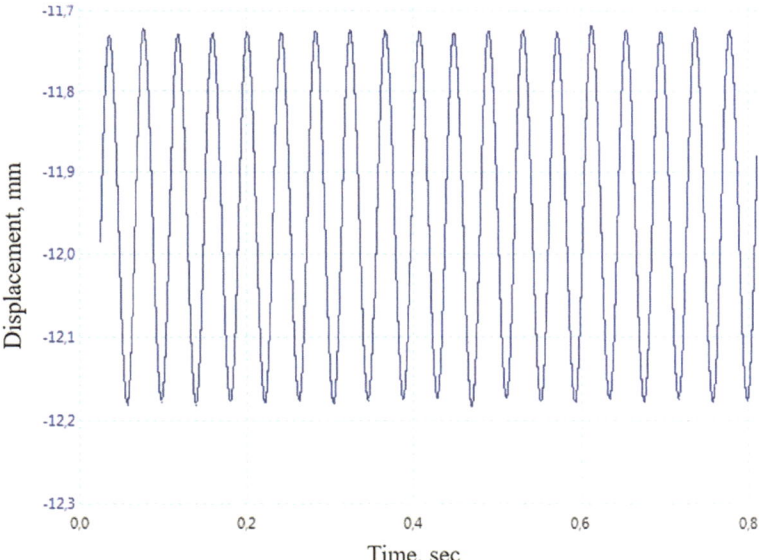

Fig. 3.23 The cantilever vibrations excited by one motor without beat phenomenon at 24 Hz frequency

After the completion of experiments with one motor, another motor was fixed on the top of the cantilever. The most appropriate results were collected during experiments with two motors and using higher than 10 V voltage values (Fig. 3.24). Supplied lower voltage values were insufficient to exceed the cantilever's resonance. The cantilever without the damping element was actuated in the range of displacement of 13 mm on the beating phenomenon. The oscillations frequency from 2 to 10 Hz was obtained. The beating phenomenon is clearly noticeable from the curves below. This phenomenon occurred after the vibrating motors had generated enough force to surpass the cantilever resonance.

However, it has to be taken into consideration that the human wrist is made from various connections, joints and tissues, which causes damping. Especially if wrist is held raised and has no fulcrum except the shoulder joint. Therefore, it is necessary to investigate the cantilever's frequencies by using a damping element. It is essential to find a working regime that would allow the device to generate oscillations independently on the wrists position or weight. Further experiments with a damping element have shown that electromechanical motors with unbalanced masses generate sufficient force to overcome the damping force and the system was not allowed to enter the resonance stage (Fig. 3.25). All observations were obtained only when the beating phenomenon occurred. During the measurements on the beating phenomenon, the amplitude of the cantilever's movement

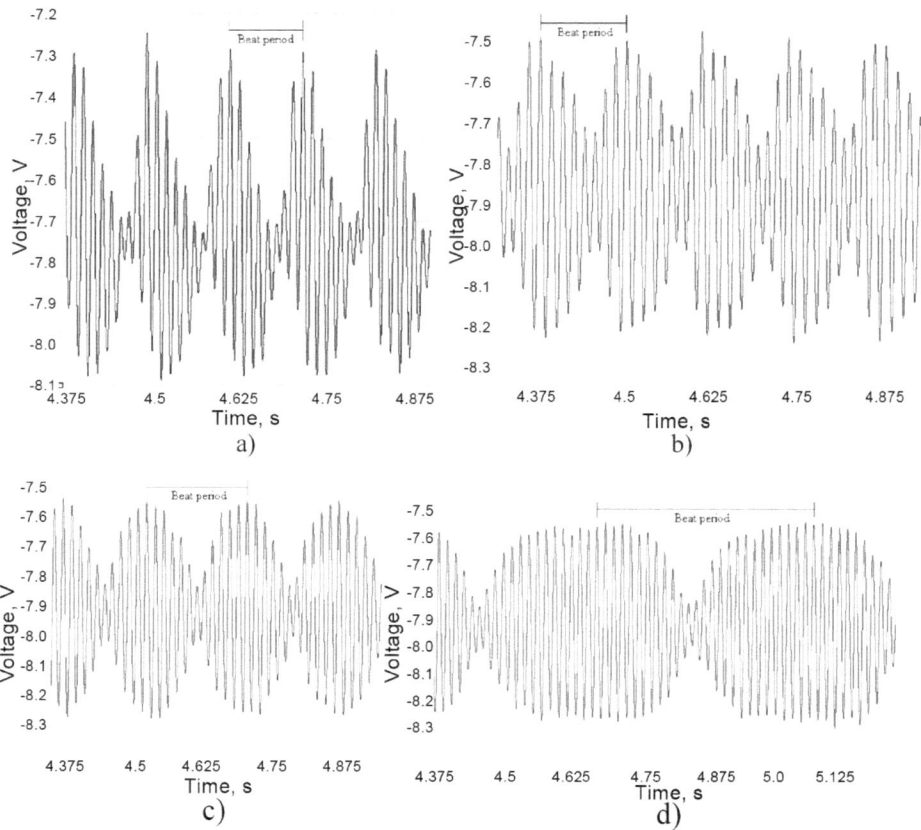

Fig. 3.24 Two motors vibrations without damping: **a**—at 10 Hz (14.5–11 V); **b**—at 8 Hz (12.5–10 V); **c**—6 Hz (12–10 V); **d**—2 Hz (11.5–10 V)

reached 5 mm. This value is even higher compared to the existing solutions. Investigations into the influence on displacements and frequencies must be done subsequently. However, these results have confirmed the assumptions that the designed cantilever platform could be used for further experiments without the necessity of using human body parts.

Furthermore, exciting force calculations have been conducted for each voltage combination in studies when the damping element was used. The values were divided into three groups according to the higher frequency value that could be used without harm to a human's internal organs or separate body parts [25]. The first group of values were up to 50 Hz, second—from 51 to 80 Hz and third, from 81 to 100 Hz. The calculated range of vertically generated force for the first group is from 3.31 to 11.54 N by using two vibrating motors. The force values for the second group started from 12.32 N and increased to 28.08 N. The third group values were distributed in the range from 26.29 to 41.48 N. Values from the first, safest group are high enough to generate vibrational oscillations on a human's wrist. The means were defined as sufficient to select the motors for the

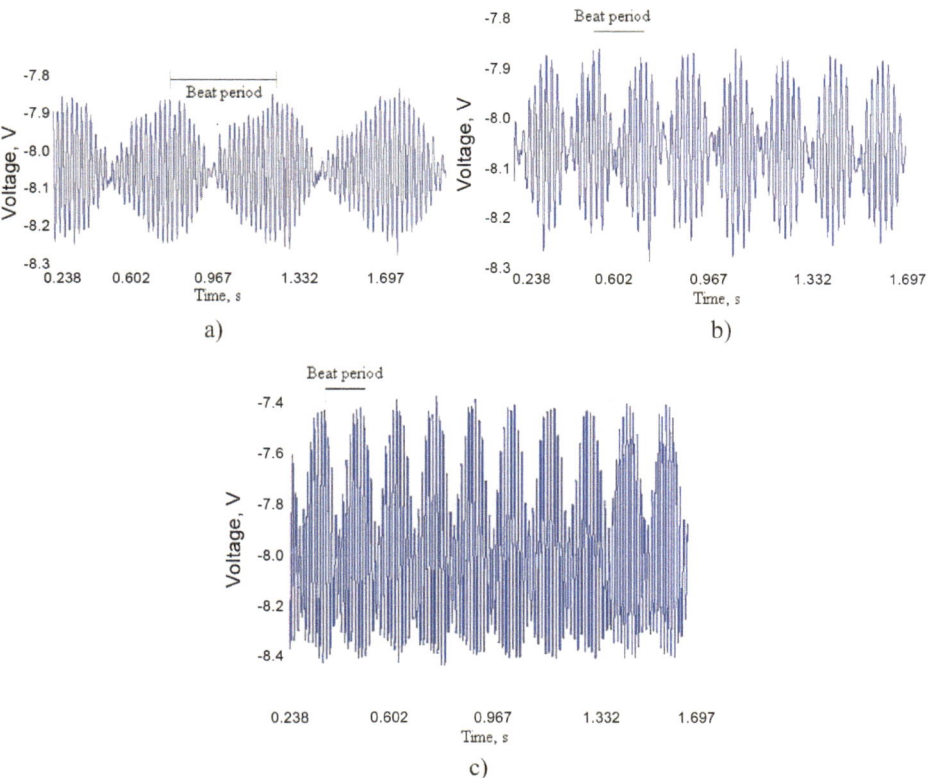

Fig. 3.25 Two motors vibrations with damping: **a** at 2 Hz (8–8 V); **b** at 6 Hz (9.5–8.5 V); **c** at 8 Hz (14.8–14.8 V)

Fig. 3.26 Virtual model of
vibrational bracelet prototype
fixed on the human
handbreadth: (1)—vibration
actuator and control panel;
(2)—human skin interacting
soft material

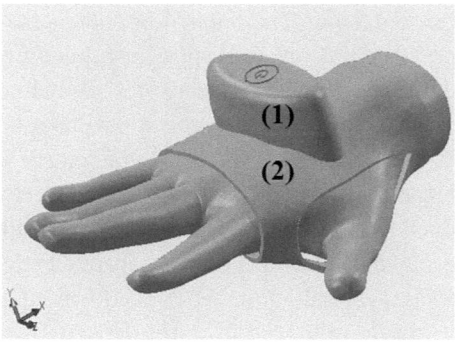

development of a vibrating bracelet prototype. This is a new approach of implementation
of low frequency vibrational methodology with the purpose of stimulating blood circulation in human wrists. Similar technology of using two electromechanical motors has
been claimed in previously described patent US 4,570,616 A [26]. The main difference
of the application of the beating phenomenon in these cases is that the patented object
consists of connected unbalanced disks, unlike the suggested approach. Furthermore, the
proposed methodology enables the shift between different frequency values without the
need of changing the unbalanced masses. At the end, the patented device was designed
specifically for massage purposes.

The prototype of a vibrating bracelet device has been designed with the purpose of
transferring the vibrational force perpendicularly to the palm and fingers of a human hand.
The position of the vibrational actuator has been selected to minimize biomechanical
damping elements (for example, wrist joint) and induce maximum oscillations to the
palm and fingers. The virtual model of the prototype is shown in Fig. 3.26. The bracelet
comprises of two vibrating motors with inwardly rotating motors relative to one another.
Consequently, this approach enables the device to induce vertical vibrational movement
at the Y axis.

The terms of reference of the vibrating bracelet control panel have been prepared
according to the needs and application purposes. The aim of testing the device prototypes
development for medical trials was the main reason. The control panel has been designed
to control each motor individually with a step of 0.1 V and displaying the voltage on the
screen. The voltage can be changed by pushing a button up or down. For experimental
purposes, manually tuned voltage enables the motors to work continuously. A button for
the prescribed working time intervals has been implemented. The purpose of this button
is to set the motors to work for a defined time of 30, 60 and 90 s and continuing until
300 s with 30 s intervals, respectively with one push. The motors and control panel are
fed by a li ion battery and can work continuously for at least 60 min. Charging can
be done via a standard micro-USB connector. Red and green LED indications define the
battery capacity, charging process, turning on and off the motor's prescribed time regimes.
The terms of reference for the control panel have been designed with the purpose of the

adoption to the different parameters' motors, thus the replacement of motors will not require changing the control panel. The electrical scheme has been designed with the possibility to integrate a Bluetooth module for data transmission. Selected microprocessor MSP430F2272IRHAT with 16 MHz CPU speed and 32KB program memory size would be sufficient for more sophisticated calculations [27]. This enables the refinement of the control panel if there is a need.

Preliminary tests disclosed the need of pressing the vibrating motors by hand to eliminate leaping by the induced force. During the preliminary tests, this issue was solved by using plastic straps as shown on the left image of Fig. 3.27. According to this problem, the case of the bracelet has been designed (Fig. 3.27b) with the SolidWorks software. The case prototype, comprising three separate parts, was printed with a 3D printer. The main box with a 1 mm thick wall and two covers (top and bottom) comprises of a plastic printed case. The vibrating motors are placed in the bottom part of the case, which is pressed to the hand by using the Velcro strap that passes through the specially designed rectangular hole. A non-elastic strap enables the force to be more fluently transmitted. The upper part of the case consists of a control panel and a cover. The battery, with a capacity of 500 mAh, is placed in the bottom part of the case [28].

The patented vibrating bracelet [29] fulfils all the previously defined needs. The autonomous energy supply, control panel and adjustable strap enable research and clinical trials to be made. Furthermore, after the identification of the patients' needs, the case size can be reduced to about 20–50% of volume.

3.3.2 Activation of Blood Circulation in the Lower Limbs

The demand for treatment of blood circulatory disorders in legs is considerable, especially in Diabetes mellitus patients. Considering the legs' weight, different components have to be used to obtain the same frequencies and at least the same displacements as provided by the prototype of the vibrating bracelet. Therefore, more powerful electromechanical motors must be selected. A new constructional approach of leg vibration exposure also must be designed.

For this reason, glass epoxy material has been considered as the most appropriate to transmit vibrational oscillations because of its flexibility and high cycle fatigue properties. The plate's length of 485 mm and width of 400 mm were chosen because of comfortability and ergonomic reasons. It was decided to make a constructional solution with an option of changing the longitudinal position of the plate where the legs have to be located. Thus, the machine must be comfortable for a person of any height. Four fixing points are located at both sides of the end part of plate. Therefore, the plate is considered as a cantilever, where one end is fixed, and the other end has displacement freedom at the Y-axis. A cross tube has been attached to reduce the plate's shear deformations. Considering a human's legs position, the electromechanical motors were screwed at the free end of

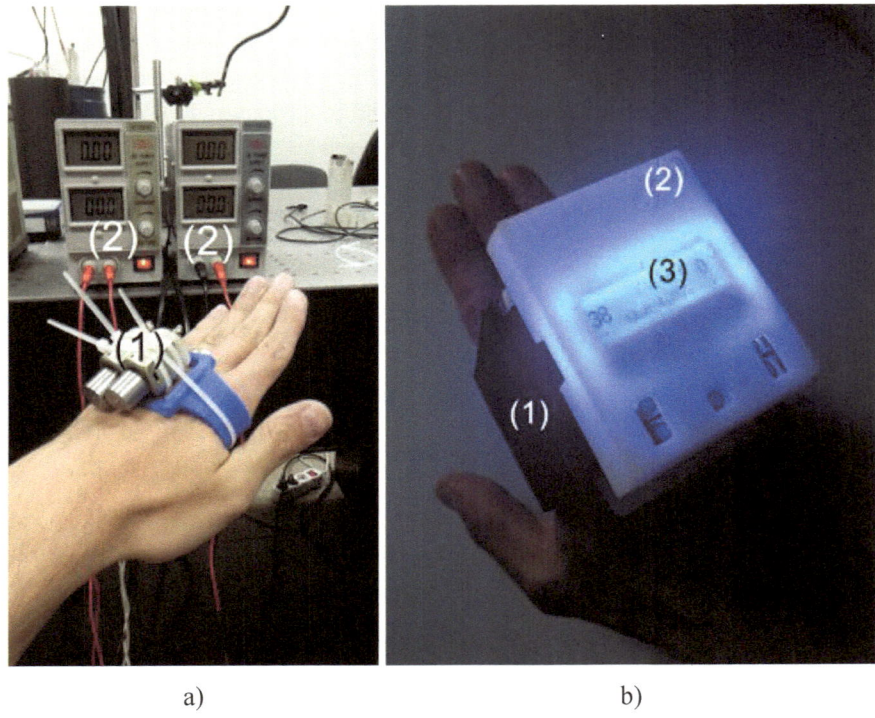

a)   b)

Fig. 3.27 Vibrating bracelet prototype development: **a**—primary prototype where vibrating motors (1) were fed by stationary voltage suppliers (2); **b**—autonomously working 3D printed (2) prototype comprising control panel (3), vibrating motors, battery, and adjustable strap (1))

the cantilever plate. The mount construction has been designed for the reason of fixing two motors motionlessly. The plate's fixing points enable users to reduce the unacceptable shear deformations and provide concentrated vertical vibrations at the local axis of the plate to achieve the maximum effect. The plate was coated by a thin foam to make it more comfortable.

In most cases, existing ready-made vibration motors are specified and adopted for various systems, and it would be hard to find a suitable motor for the defined research. For this reason, unbalanced mass was designed by using SolidWorks software with parameters given in Table 3.4. Two identical steel imbalances were manufactured to be mounted on the rotors axis of the electromechanical motors to induce vibrations during the rotational movement, thus generating a vertical direction (perpendicular) force to the glass epoxy cantilever plate.

Doga D.C. electromechanical motors were selected because of the suitable dynamic properties. Both motors (Table 3.5, Fig. 3.28) with mounted unbalanced masses were used to induce the beating phenomenon and higher amplitude oscillations compared to

Table 3.4 Unbalanced mass parameters of leg actuator

Parameter	Value
Bulk mass	616,8 g
Mass without unbalance	212,92 g
Unbalance mass	403,88 g
Diameter	66 mm
Diameter without imbalance	36 mm

Table 3.5 Doga D.C. motor parameters

Parameter	Value
Bulk mass	2.6 kg
Nominal voltage	24 V
Nominal Torque	0.75 Nm
Nominal speed	1000 rpm
Nominal current	5.5 A

one vibration motor. Each motor's angular speed parameter was controlled by a shifting voltage on the power supply. Two rotating unbalances with slightly different frequencies (supplied voltage values) induce the beating phenomenon.

It is known that the beats occur when two frequencies are close together. The frequency of the beating phenomenon can be controlled by raising or lowering each motor's supplied

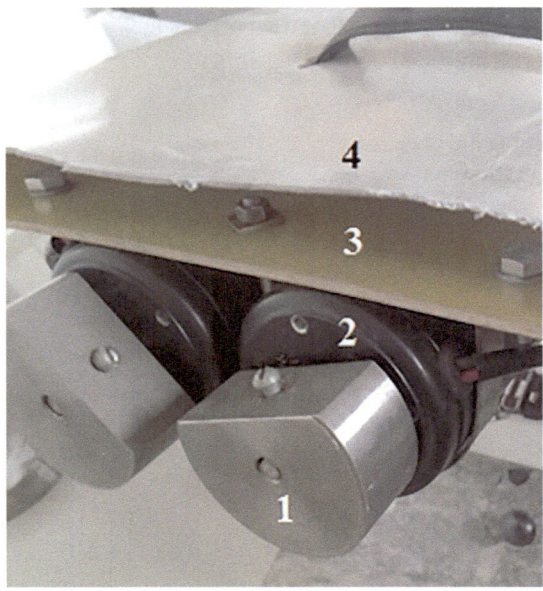

Fig. 3.28 Doga D.C. electromechanical motors with unbalanced masses: 1—unbalanced rotor; 2—motor; 3—glass epoxy plate; 4—foam cover

voltage. Transfer of energy takes place in the coupled system which could induce vibration in the primary system instead of suppressing them. The coupled equations of motion without damping in both systems can be obtained from Eq. 3.1, by setting the damping in each system equal to zero.

One of the main tasks of the leg vibrational actuator (Fig. 3.33) is to solve blood circulation disorders for people with disabilities. The facility of changing the slope of the plate's position enables the accessibility and variability of usage in different environments for the different state of patients. The first prototype version has been designed with a facility to change the angle manually, but it is foreseen to automate this process. Furthermore, it is well known that raised legs increase blood flow and reduces poor circulation the in human body.

Leg mass calculations have to be done before the investigation of the cantilever plate natural frequency. The data was collected according to the findings in [30] studies. The total legs weight is equal to 16.68% of a total males' weight and 18.43% of a total females' weight. Identification of leg mass in dependence of different body weight was accomplished and presented in Table 3.6. These values are necessary for the material selection process of the vibrating plate and for Eigenfrequency analysis with COMSOL Multiphysics software.

Similar principles of vibrational exposure as in the vibrating bracelet have been considered in the use of developing the legs actuator. Thus, COMSOL Multiphysics software with the structural mechanics module has been used for the calculations of the cantilever type vibrating plate. The Structural Mechanics Module was tailor-made to model and simulate applications and designs in the fields of structural and solid mechanics. The module is dedicated to the analysis of mechanical structures that are subjected to static or dynamic loads. The Eigenfrequency analysis was made for the natural frequencies of both unloaded and loaded structures.

Table 3.6 Leg mass identification

Body weight	Leg mass
55 kg (female)	20.273 kg
60 kg (female)	22.116 kg
65 kg (female)	23.959 kg
70 kg (female)	25.802 kg
75 kg (male)	25.02 kg
80 kg (male)	26.688 kg
85 kg (male)	28.356 kg
90 kg (male)	30.024 kg
95 kg (male)	31.692 kg
100 kg (male)	33.36 kg

A computational model of the cantilever plate has been used to assess its natural frequencies and response to the applied load. The cantilever plate, according to the engineering mechanics, is a component that is designed to support transverse loads that act perpendicularly to the longitudinal axis of the cantilever. The bending load is supported by the cantilever only, without external bracing. It is assumed that the cantilever has a longitudinal plane of symmetry and is fixed at only one end. Glass epoxy plate of the leg's actuators 2D calculations has been performed.

A rectangular shape solid model of 0.485 m length and 0.004 m thick was designed. The length has been selected according to the ergonomic parameters of the human calf. Glass epoxy material properties with a density of 2000 kg/m^3, Young's modulus of 17 kPa and Poisson's ratio of 0.32 was assigned to the model (Fig. 3.29). Resonance frequency could be used if higher displacement values are required. The model was fixed at the left end and the motors' weight load was set on the right end with vertical direction and on the top of the human legs weight imitating load. Loads of leg mass of 25.02 kg and the motors bulk mass of 6.43 kg were added to the cantilever model at relevant places on the vibrational actuator.

The designed model could be easily adjustable considering variations of input parameters such as length, width, or load material. The model is simplified and requires minimal time resources for making large amounts of calculations. This model will be used for further studies for the purpose of identifying Eigenfrequency values of different heights of vibrating glass epoxy cantilever plates. A 3D model was not admissible due to the low efficiency of the use of time for calculations.

The Eigenfrequency analysis of the epoxy glass cantilever plate was accomplished with COMSOL Multiphysics software. Primary calculations were without adding leg mass and after then tapping in the legs mass of 75 kg weight male (equal to the tested person). The

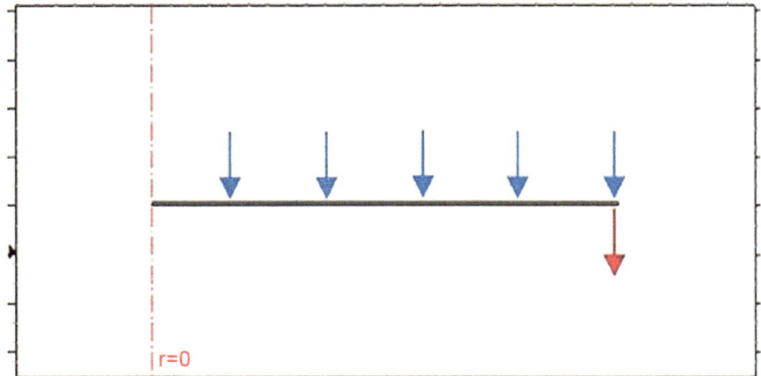

Fig. 3.29 Glass epoxy cantilever plate model with legs mass load (blue arrows) and motors mass load (red arrow), fixed edge is indicated by dotted red line

Eigenfrequency of the glass epoxy cantilever without leg mass load was equal to 9.05 Hz (Fig. 3.30a). After adding leg mass of 25.02 kg and the motors bulk mass of 6.43 kg, the Eigenfrequency value decreased to 3.28 Hz (Fig. 3.30b).

Further calculations with the aim to identify frequency range of different weights of male and female were made by changing the legs' mass load on the cantilever plate are reflected in Table 3.7. Frequency values were chosen from 3.47–3.25 Hz for females at 55–70 kg weight range and frequency range from 3.28–3.02 Hz for males at 75–100 kg range.

The leg vibrational actuator was developed with the aim of eliminating the negative effects of standing human vibrations that are described in various studies and recommendation papers (Fig. 3.31). For example, in ISO 2631-1 guidelines on Mechanical vibration and shock—"Evaluation of human exposure to whole-body vibration" is written, which

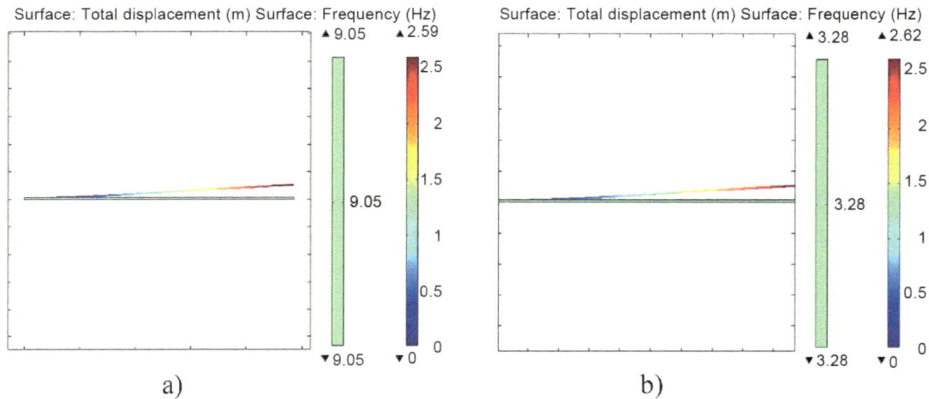

a)   b)

Fig. 3.30 Eigenfrequency value of the main vibration mode without (**a**) and with (**b**) load

Table 3.7 Eigenfrequency values differ depending on body mass and gender

Body mass (kg)	Gender	Eigenfrequency (Hz)
55	Female	3.47
60	Female	3.39
65	Female	3.32
70	Female	3.25
75	Male	3.28
80	Male	3.22
85	Male	3.17
90	Male	3.11
95	Male	3.06
100	Male	3.02

Fig. 3.31 Leg's actuator:
1—glass epoxy vibrating
cantilever type plate; 2—legs
fixing belt; 3—plate's fixing
points, 4—slope selection
holes

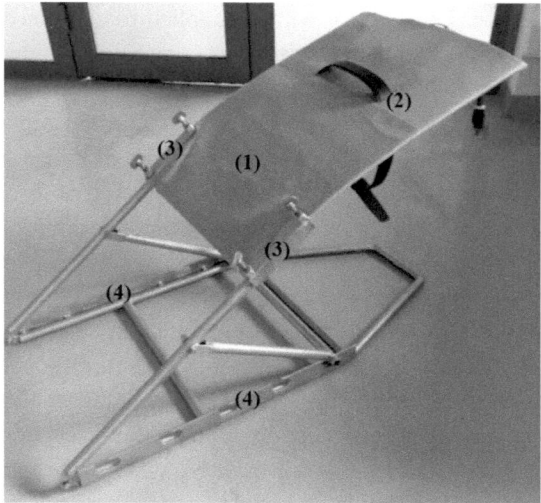

considers that long-term high-intensity whole-body vibration indicates an increased health risk to the lumbar spine. It is noted that this may be due to the biodynamic behavior of the spine: horizontal displacement and torsion of the segments of the vertebral column. Furthermore, whole-body vibration exercise may worsen certain endogenous pathologic disturbances of the spine. The approach of local exposure at the developed legs' actuator eliminates the negative vibrational excitation effects that are caused by the standing position. Further studies are planned for the measurements of physiological parameters after affecting a human by the prescribed protocol of vibrations by using the prototype of a legs' actuator.

The need to fix the legs on the plate has been obtained considering the movement disorders for people with disabilities. A belt has been attached for this purpose, but in this case the need for a second contributory person exists. Therefore, in a newly designed construction it is foreseen to replace this persons' function with an easily maintained construction [31].

The construction strength calculations have been made with SolidWorks Simulation software. The additional frame of a trapezia shape has been added in the front of the construction to ensure stability and keep a vertical velocity vector inside the build. An initial prototype has been made from stainless steel tubes and it is foreseen to update this construction by manufacturing it from aluminum. This will make the machine lighter and more easily transportable.

The constructional solutions of the assembled parts provide an ability to test it in various environments. Testing of human interaction with a prototype may present suggestions of constructional changes, therefore the main purpose of the designed prototype was to provide a device for a suggested approach. The same control panel as the vibrating bracelet is used for the leg's actuator. In this case, the main difference will be the voltage source. The actuator will be supplied from a power socket because the motors' voltage is too high for the use of a compact and lightweight portable power source.

The vibrating devices are recommended to be used on raised limbs to gain the maximum effect. In this figure the legs actuator is placed on a special table, but it could be used by placing it on the floor or just on a bed. The devices can be used separately or together, dependent on the purpose or type of disease. Prototypes are designed to be used separately because there are no communication modules integrated in any of them. This function is foreseen in further steps of development. Generally, these devices may be used for different purposes and different diseases.

Products on the market use different vibrational frequencies (mostly higher than 30 Hz) and different amplitudes (up to 5 mm) of the oscillations, therefore the purpose of its applicability is different. Many vibrational therapy devices are made for athletes for the purpose of enhancing muscle performance, bone density or just a warm-up before any physical activity. For this reason, a decision was taken to design and manufacture the prototypes by focusing on blood flow disorders and improvement possibilities. Therefore, the devices of low-frequency and higher vibration amplitude have been designed. The beating phenomenon has been induced to create a sufficient force and oscillations frequency ratio. Comprehensive conclusions of this section are listed below:

- Experimental stand of glass epoxy cantilever comprising of vibrational actuators has been designed for experimental investigations. The working regimes of a sufficient force and low-frequency vibrations have been defined during the studies. A vibrating bracelet has been designed as an experimental tool to investigate blood flow improvement by using different vibrational frequencies. An autonomous device, comprising vibrating motors, control panel and adjustable strap was developed for clinical trials. The prototype is mainly intended for arthritis patients because the pain occurrence is mostly in the hands.

- Vibrating machine for legs has been developed with a purpose of making investigations of blood flow improvement in legs, by changing the working frequencies, slope and human body position. The prototype was created considering the needs of people with disabilities and diabetics. Furthermore, constructional changes are foreseen in the case of improving accessibility and comfort level.

- Numerical calculations considering the vibrating plate as a cantilever have been conducted. The natural frequencies without the leg's weight load were equal at 9.05 Hz and after assessing a 75 kg male's legs weight 3.28 Hz. This value is close to the determined frequency range from the earlier experiments where the highest impact of cardiovascular parameters and liquid (blood) property changes were obtained.

- Eigenfrequency values of 3.47–3.25 Hz for females (weight: 55–70 kg) and 3.28–3.02 Hz (weight: 75–100 kg) for males were calculated for a cantilever of a glass epoxy material. These values prescribe the working regimes and supply voltage means depending on human weight and will be implemented in the device control algorithm.

3.4 Experimental Studies on Intensification of Limb Blood Flow

The following section defines the experimental investigations of the vibrational excitation influence on blood flow parameters. The main aim of these studies was to identify the most influential vibrational frequency and amplitude range. The experimental setup of an imitational blood circulation system consisting of the peristaltic pump, artificial blood vessel, pressure sensor and vibrational actuator has been designed. The aim of this study was to identify the influence of vibrational excitation within the range of frequencies of 0.5–30 Hz to the fluid pressure parameters and to identify the most influencing values. This was followed by deeper analysis of the processes in fluid during the vibrational bouts being investigated by using the micro-particle image velocimetry method. The analysis of fluid velocity vectors and abstraction of different velocities' streaming lines inside the channel has been conducted.

Considering the process when external vibrations are affecting the human body, the body tissue could be assumed as a damping system. Thus, the presumption of possible frequencies' difference between the source (vibrational actuator) and receipt (micro blood vessels) needed to be investigated. The analysis of the human body tissue response on the vibrational influence has been done with the purpose of identifying the differences of frequencies between the source and finger marker in the range of 1–10 Hz vibrational bouts. Furthermore, validity studies were conducted by monitoring cardiovascular parameters and temperature changes in limbs before and after vibrational excitation. The studies were carried out with the designed prototypes of vibrating bracelet and legs actuator. The effect on oscillating limbs was monitored by changing input parameters of electromechanical motors. Furthermore, the cardiovascular parameters (electrocardiogram, heart rate, respiration rate) have been analyzed against the effect of vibrational exposure. These studies were necessary to validate the developed prototypes and to define proper working regimes for further investigations on disease affected patients with circulatory disorders.

3.4.1 Limbs Blood Pressure Monitoring

Investigation of blood flow pressure response on the vibrational excitation was performed with an assembled experimental setup, consisting of a peristaltic pump and fluid filled medical tubes that were fixed by a vibrating beam (Figs. 3.32 and 3.33). The aim of this experiment was to identify the vibrations' influence on fluid pressure and to determine the proper working regimes for the designed prototypes. Moreover, this study provides an understanding of how the external vibrations influence a human's blood vessels. The medical peristaltic pump has been used to imitate the blood's exhaust from the heart. Furthermore, in later studies, plastic tubes were replaced by an artificial blood vessel (Table 3.8) that related to the output tube of the pump. The artificial blood vessel's part

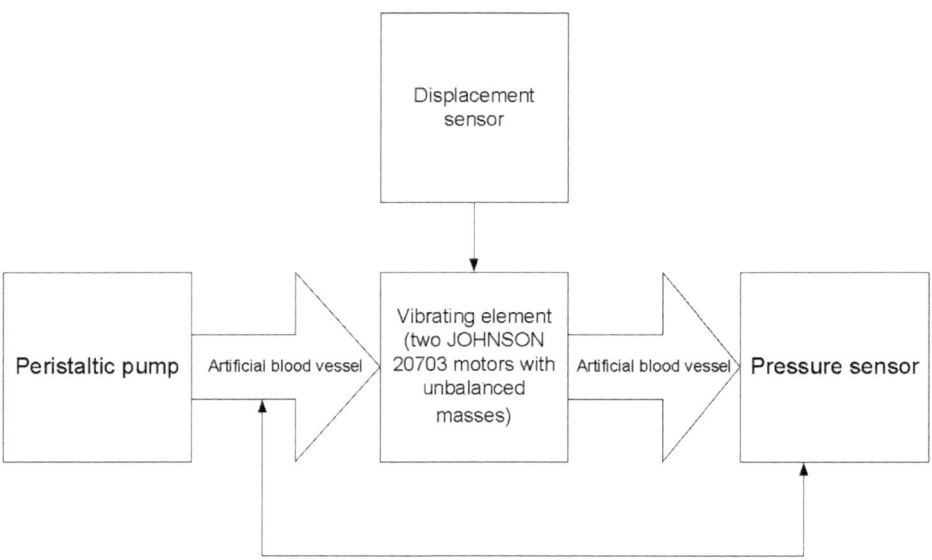

Fig. 3.32 Principal scheme of the experimental set-up

was mounted on the vibrational actuator comprising of two electromechanical motors to initiate the beating phenomenon. The vessel was surrounded by foam to imitate human body tissue. A displacement sensor has been attached at the top of the actuator. Pressure changes were registered by the pressure sensor during the generation of different frequencies.

Motor and vibration measuring sensors were fed by three laboratory power suppliers. Inductive displacement sensor IFM IG6084 was used to measure the beam's vibrations (gradient: 1,389 V/mm). All data was registered by the Oscilloscope Pico scope 3424 and was stored and analyzed by using the PC software Pico Scope 6. Motors characteristics (revolutions per minute) have been registered with a photo tachometer/stroboscope Lutron DT-2259. Therefore, the measurement of the motors' revolution par minute (RPM) on different voltage values by using the damping element was conducted during this experiment. RPM values were measured in regimes of tachometry and stroboscope to get validated data. First, the experiment was conducted without the damping element. Next, the experiment was repeated by adding the damping element consisting of air and water packages. The damper has been placed at the bottom of a vibrating beam with the actuator. The damper was designed with the purpose of eliminating the resonance frequencies of the beam and to reproduce similar characteristics such as human body tissue rheological characteristics. The inlet and outlet tubes were immersed in the fluid tanks.

The fluid pressure parameter was monitored by the developed pressure sensor. The pressure sensor (Fig. 3.34) comprising of pressure gauge Mpx5010gp, voltage stabilizer 7805 TO220 (2) and compensator 2200μF was created for this experiment. The pressure

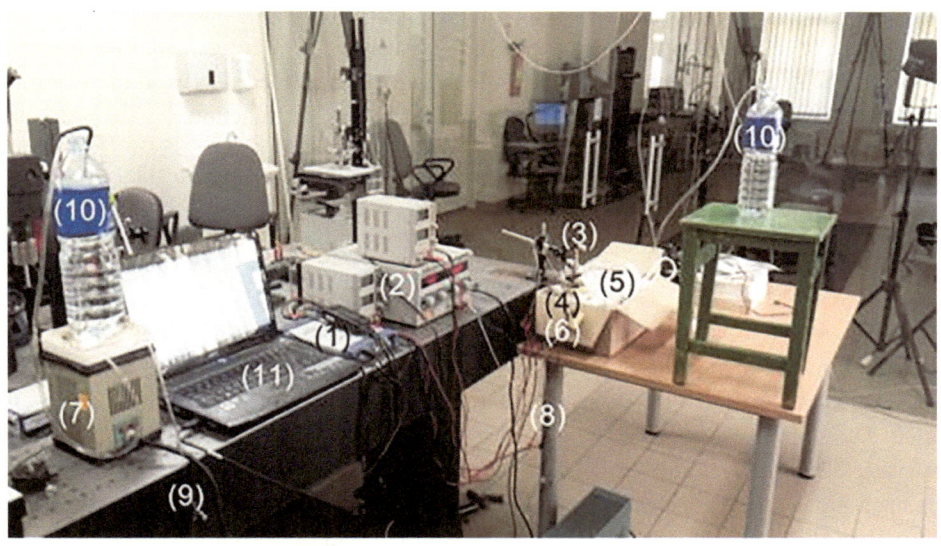

Fig. 3.33 Experimental set-up: 1—oscilloscope; 2—DC supply; 3—inductive sensor; 4—vibrating motors; 5—damping element; 6—pressure sensor; 7—peristaltic pump; 8—artificial blood vessel (Table 3.2); 9—medical tubes; 10—water tanks; 11—PC with Pico scope software

Table 3.8 Physical and mechanical properties of the artificial blood vessel made from expanded polytetrafluoroethylene [32]

Physical properties	Metric	Mechanical Properties	Metric
Density	0.700–2.30 g/cm^3	Ball indentation hardness	27.0–37.0 MPa
Apparent Bulk Density	0.360–0.950 g/cm^3	Tensile strength, ultimate	10.0–45.0 MPa
Water Absorption	0.000–0.100%	Tensile strength, yield	0.862–41.4 MPa
pH	9.5	Modulus of elasticity	0.392–2.25 GPa
Viscosity	19.0–25.0 cP	Flexural modulus	0.490–3.36 GPa
	1.00e + 13–1.00e + 15 cP	Flexural yield strength	14.0–27.6 MPa
	Temperature 340–380 °C	Compressive yield strength	1.50–23.4 MPa

gauge was selected because of the accuracy (4.413 mV/mm H$_2$O) and range of pressure monitoring (0–10 kPa). Output signals of the pressure sensor were gathered by an oscilloscope. The sensor was connected by a trident tube that was placed beyond the vibrating beam. Pressure was calculated by using the following transfer function:

$$V_{out} = V_S \times (0.09 \times P + 0.04) \pm (\text{Pressure Error} \times \text{Temp. Factor} \times 0.09 \times V_S).$$
$$V_S = 5.0V \pm 0.25Vdc.$$

$$(3.31)$$

where V_{out}—output voltage, V_s—supply voltage, P—pressure, Pressure error—± 0.5 kPa, Temp.Factor—temperature factor.

At the beginning, an experiment with one motor was conducted by altering the voltage value. The supplied voltage ranged from 3 to 16 V with 0.1 V step and without using any damping element. The next experiments with two motors were performed. The voltage for each motor had been altered in the same range, starting from 3 to 16 V with 0.1 V step. Then, the damping element was added with the purpose of eliminating the natural beam's frequencies. Motors were supplied with the same range of voltage as in earlier experiments. The same experiments were repeated after substituting the medical plastic tube with an artificial blood vessel. Pressure alterations were registered at the beginning of the experiment and during it, together with the beam's displacement.

The fluid pressure in the fulfilled channel has been registered. The value of 4.5 kPa was recorded, which is close to the mean of pressure in human capillaries. The peristaltic pump working regime of 1 Hz was set, which is equal to a heart rate of 60 beats per minute. The initial experiment was conducted with one motor. The highest-pressure changes of about 1 kPa were noted when the motor was supplied by 6 V and 11 V voltages respectively.

Fig. 3.34 Designed pressure sensor: 1—pressure gauge Mpx5010gp; 2—capacitor 2200 μF; 3—positive-voltage regulator 7805 TO220

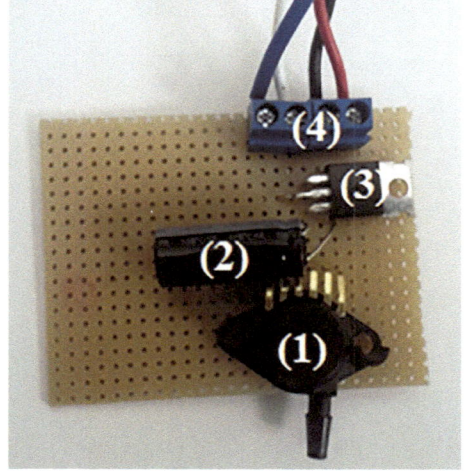

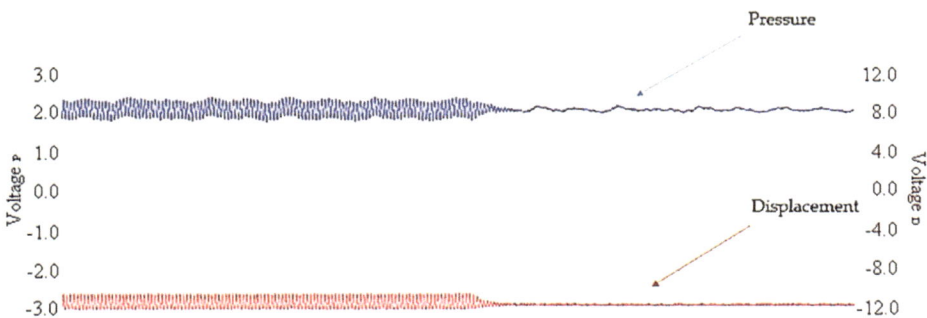

Fig. 3.35 Pressure rise of 2 kPa affecting artificial blood vessel by 6 Hz frequencies

The artificial blood vessel and damping element have been added for experimentation. Damped beam vibrations of 6 Hz frequency were noted when the motor was supplied by 5 V voltage. A pressure rise of 2 kPa was registered (Fig. 3.35).

The beating phenomenon was induced by starting the second motor with unbalanced mass. The two motors were supplied by voltages of 5 V and 5.8 V respectively to generate the beating phenomenon (Fig. 3.36). The results of pressure and displacement measurements are represented in one line to show the dependency. In the graph below it is clearly visible that the fluid pressure is directly dependent on the beam's oscillations. An overlapped view of diagrams shows that reliance. The pressure rises during the vibrational excitation and decreases dramatically when displacement amplitude was close to zero. These results were similar when comparing the medical plastic tubes and the artificial blood vessel.

The later experiments were conducted with an artificial blood vessel in the experimental setup instead of the medical plastic tube. Moreover, higher pressure rise was noted in the case of two motors. In comparison, the highest rise of pressure means, using one motor that was supplied by 9 V, gained a 3 kPa increase in value. Furthermore, two motors supplied by 5.1 V and 4.9 V respectively, generated a rise of 8 kPa (Fig. 3.37). The processed results showed that the pressure changes have increased in parallel with the oscillating

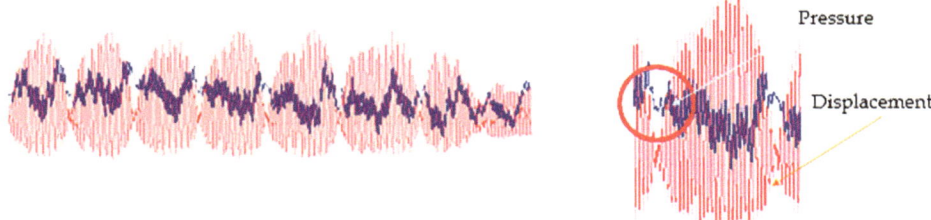

Fig. 3.36 Overlapped pressure and displacement graphs during the beating phenomenon

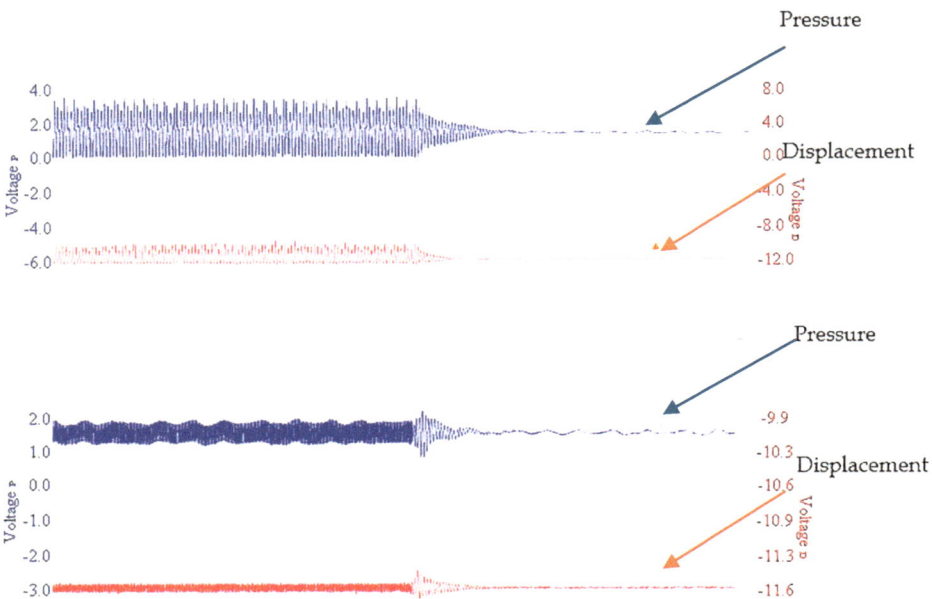

Fig. 3.37 Results of using artificial blood vessel: two motors' induced beating phenomenon and 8 kPa pressure rise (upper graphs); one motor vibrations and 3 kPa pressure rise (lower graphs)

beam's displacement amplitudes. It was also observed that at higher frequencies than 10 Hz, pressure change amplitude becomes lower and the momentum value changes become more frequent. The most influential frequencies of the beating phenomenon were noted in the diapason from 2 to 5 Hz. As it was observed during the study, the displacement amplitudes ranging from 4 to 20 mm are the most desirable. The values are coherent with the results of numerical calculations.

The results of pressure monitoring provide only momentum alterations, but longer-term pressure increase was not monitored. The peristaltic pump exhausts the same amount of volume of fluid; therefore, it was unable to monitor the fluid volume alteration per time unit. However, the significant increase of fluid pressure enables researchers to assume that low-frequency vibrations could be used with the purpose of improvement of blood flow in human limbs.

3.4.2 Monitoring of Limb Blood Flow Velocity

Experimental results of previous studies have shown demand for deeper analysis of fluid parameter changes during the vibrational bouts. Observation of the fluid velocity distribution streamlines and vectors' field was made by monitoring the movement of particles in fluid. The previously described experimental stand consistent of peristaltic pump, vibrational actuator and artificial blood vessel has been coupled with a micro particle image velocimetry (μPIV) system. The article [33] describes the methods of velocity analysis of a fluid excited by vibrations.

Experiments of the flows in microchannels were made at the Lithuanian Energy Institute. A unique experimental setup (Fig. 3.38) consists of a μPIV system vibrational excitation and measurement equipment part. μPIV system (Fig. 3.40) consists of Nd: YAG laser (Dantec Dynamics), laser control system LPU 450 (Dantec Dynamics), 2048×2048 pixels Flow Sense EO CCD camera (Dantec Dynamics) that was fixed on an inverted Leica DM ILM microscope (Leica Microsystems). The prescribed fluid flow was generated by a syringe pump (Aladdin AL4000, World Precision Instruments) with connected medical blood tubing lines. The tubing line length starting from the syringe pump to measurement microscope was 1.5 m long. About 30 cm away from the syringe pump, the tubing line was placed in a material imitating human tissue that was fixed by an oscillating epoxy glass cloth laminate beam. A special electromechanical actuator consisting of two small size, low voltage and high RPM electric motors (Johnson 20,703) each with attached unbalanced masses of 14.86 g was used for generating the beating phenomenon and proper frequencies. These motors were screwed to the epoxy glass cloth laminate. As it was defined on an earlier study of the author, the electric motors could generate a force on beating phenomenon up to 41.48 N depending on the supplied voltage. Oscillations and movement amplitude of the beam were measured by an inductive displacement sensor IFM IG6084 that was stationary fixed right above the beam. The output signal was collected by an oscilloscope Pico scope 3424 and processed by the corresponding software on the PC. The measurements of the fluid parameters were made after a minute of the vibrational effect of every frequency value and amplitude. The input voltage of the motor was chosen considering the real-time generating frequency response. The voltage values, ranging from 2 to 5.5 V for one motor and from 6.0 and 6.1 V to 8.0 and 11.1 V with 0.1 V step for two motors accordingly were selected to induce the beating phenomenon. The monitoring point was 1 m of channel away from the vibrational actuator.

The scheme of the μPIV system separately is presented in Fig. 3.39.

The microchannel used for experiments was made from special vascular graft, produced by the USA Gore Company. Here, Gore hybrid vascular graft is made of an expanded polytetrafluoroethylene vascular prosthesis that has a section reinforced with nitinol. The nitinol reinforced section is partially constrained to allow easy insertion and deployment into the human body. The Gore hybrid vascular graft has a continuous lumen with a Carmeda Bioactive surface consisting of a stable covalently bonded, reduced molecular weight heparin of porcine origin.

The solution, having similar technical specifications as real blood, was used as a fluid. The velocity of the fluid flow is measured by applying spatial flow lightning and registering the movement of the indicating particles. The velocity vectors' field of the particles

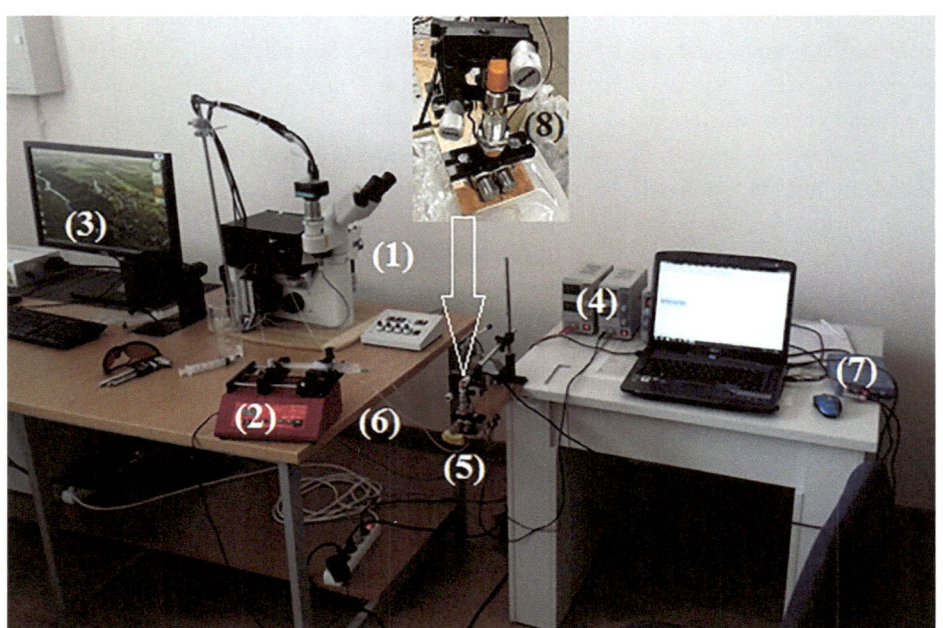

Fig. 3.38 Experimental set-up: 1—Leica DM ILM microscope; 2—syringe pump; 3—YAG laser; 4—DC power supply; 5—vibrating beam with two electric motors and attached unbalanced masses; 6—medical tubes; 7—oscilloscope Pico scope 3424; 8—inductive displacement sensor IFM IG6084

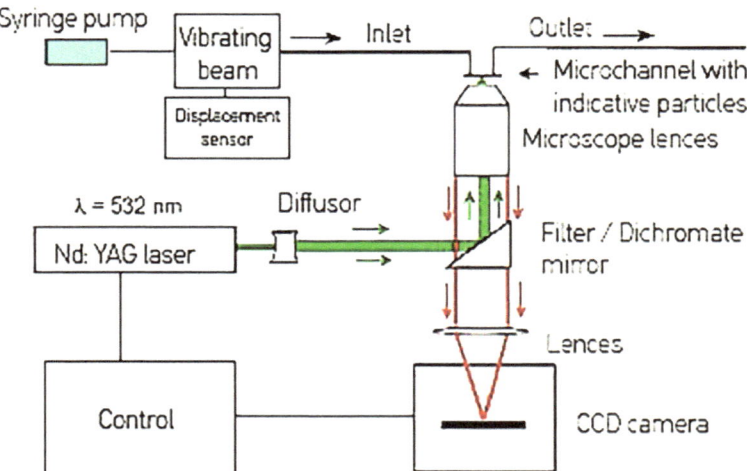

Fig. 3.39 Schematic drawing of μPIV system

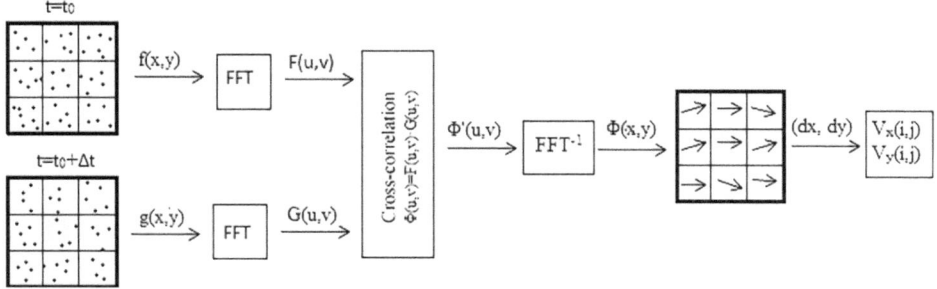

Fig. 3.40 Principal scheme of μPIV correlation establishment

were determined by μPIV measurements. Knowing the time interval between taking pictures Δt and the displacement of the particles Δx, the velocity could be calculated by the Eq. (3.1):

$$v = \frac{\Delta x}{\Delta t} \tag{3.32}$$

The fluorescent particles of 1.0 μm (3.94×10–5 in) diameter were used for the measurements. The density of the particles in space was close to fluid density and the size was chosen to avoid Brown flow influence, as well as getting a strong enough fluorescent signal.

The principal scheme of image analysis is shown below (Fig. 3.40) where the image intensity function in the fast Fourier transforms, and cross-correlation was established. The image intensity function was performed by inverse Fourier transform and the result was displayed by the velocity vector field and the velocity components.

The displacement was calculated for all particles. The calculations were made by the cross-correlation method [34] using the Fast Fourier Transform method. Calculating the Φ value

$$\Phi(x, y) = \sum_{x=1}^{p} \sum_{y=1}^{q} f(x, y) \cdot g(x + m, y + n) \tag{3.33}$$

where p and q—net window dimensions in x and y directions, f (x,y) and g (x,y)—the image intensity functions on the first and the second frames, m and n—the displacement coordination, Φ (x,y)—the correlation function between two windows of the net (p x q size) with mutual displacement (x,y),

During the research, turbulence was observed in the channel with oscillations and amplitudes of a certain frequency range (Fig. 3.41). The entire range of shear creates a cross-correlation plane, which features the largest value indicate of the displacement of the particles [35]. At individual time points (with 4.3 Hz oscillations), the flow velocity increases to 2.7 mm/s, when the initial velocity is equal to 0.65 mm/s without external oscillations. When the tests used 4.9 Hz, 5 Hz, 5.7 Hz beat frequency, the average speed during the measurements increased to 0.8 mm/s. During the other measurements, the average speed increase was lower and reached 0.7 mm/s. The short pulses in the opposite direction of 1.5 mm/s velocity were observed at 5, 5.3, 5.4 and 5.8 Hz oscillations, which cause turbulence in the channel and increase the fluid pressure.

During the analysis, clear changes in the fluid velocity were recorded in the presence of low-frequency vibrations and corresponding movement amplitudes (Figs. 3.42 and 3.43). This allows us to assume that mechanical vibrations can be used to intensify human blood flow.

The μPIV experimental analysis showed a significant influence of vibrational bouts on the fluid velocity in the microchannel. Again, the low-frequency oscillations with higher amplitude of displacement provided the more significant findings. In most cases of vibrational exposure, the average increase in fluid velocity has been observed (Fig. 3.43).

The correlation of the simulation results (Fig. 3.44) with the experimental results confirms the adequacy of the model and the possibility of using mathematical models in further research, reducing the need for expensive experiments.

These results prove the vibrational influence on fluid parameters, and it could be assumed that properly selected vibrational expose to the human body could affect the blood flow. It was agreed that further analysis has to be done by using the developed vibrating bracelet and legs actuator prototypes, and monitoring cardiovascular parameters coupled with temperature changes of limbs.

3.4.3 In Vivo Testing of a Vibrating Bracelet and Legs Actuator

Experimental investigations of vibrational exposure on the human cardiovascular system by using the developed prototypes has been defined as a crucial validation process of the suggested approach. Therefore, various cardiovascular parameters needed to be monitored before and after vibrational excitation. Furthermore, the thermal imaging monitoring method was obtained as the most appropriate in the evaluation process of blood flow disorders and improvement means. For this reason, thermal photos of hands and legs were taken before and after vibrational exposure.

First, the device with a tri-axial accelerometer [18] was used to identify the bandwidth of naturally vibrating limbs (hands). The accelerometer model LIS331DLH was selected to satisfy the needs for the measurement range and bandwidth. The accelerometer cannot operate on its own, so the previously developed device was used (Fig. 3.45).

The device contains a Micro Controller Unit to hold all the logic, LIS331DLH MEMS accelerometer to measure 3D accelerations, MicroSD card to save measured data samples, battery to power everything, some light emitting diodes to display the state the device is in and a USB connector so the data can be downloaded to a personal computer for further

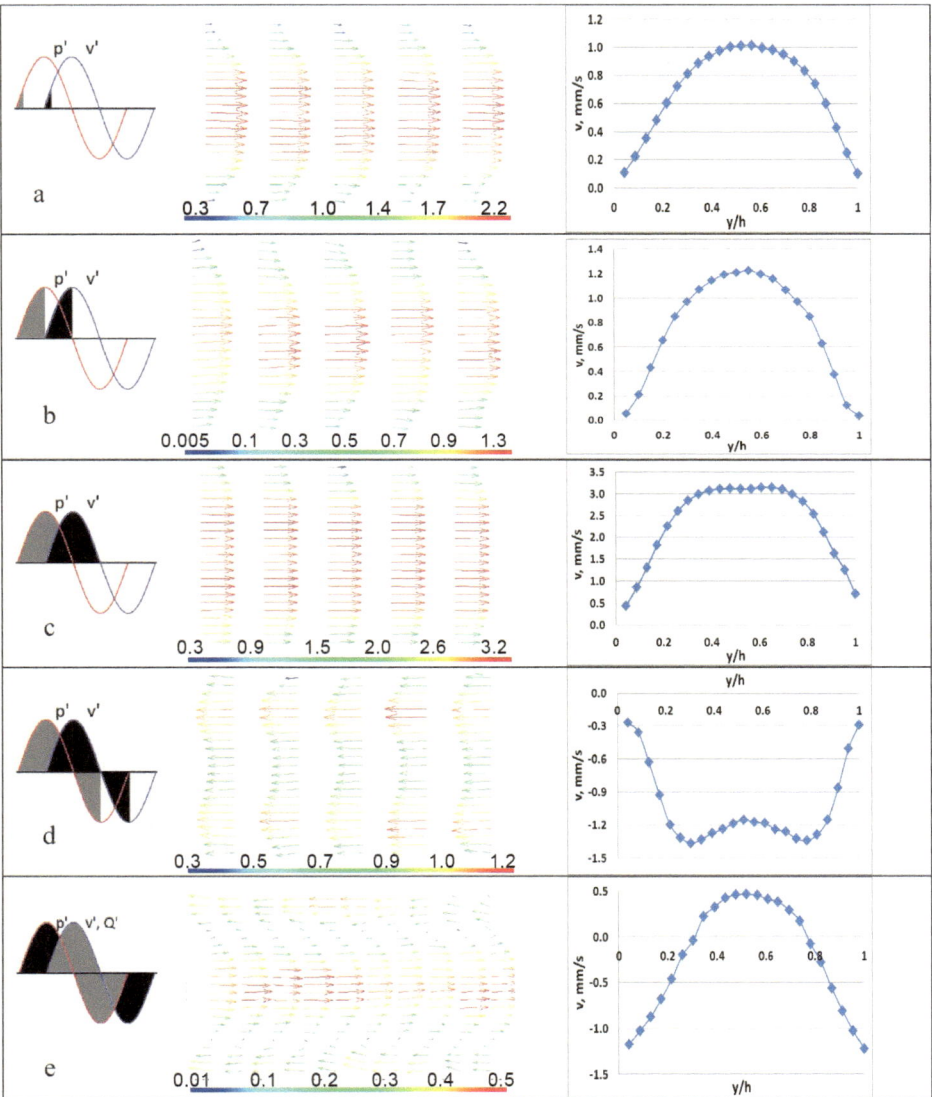

Fig. 3.41 Instantaneous velocity vectors in different phases of the cycle, in the presence of vibrations with a frequency of 4.3 Hz and an amplitude of 6 mm: **a**—beginning of the cycle, increased pressure gradient (maximum speed equal to ~1 mm/s, and ReDh ~ 0.15); **b**—increasing pressure gradient, expanding profile of the velocity graph; **c**—at the end of the positive increasing pressure gradient phase, the flow has the highest acceleration and obtained a wide profile of the velocity graph, which reflects a discontinuous flow; **d**—an instantaneous change in the direction of the velocity is recorded in the phase of negative pressure; **e**—the flow in the initial and opposite directions is observed in the last phase

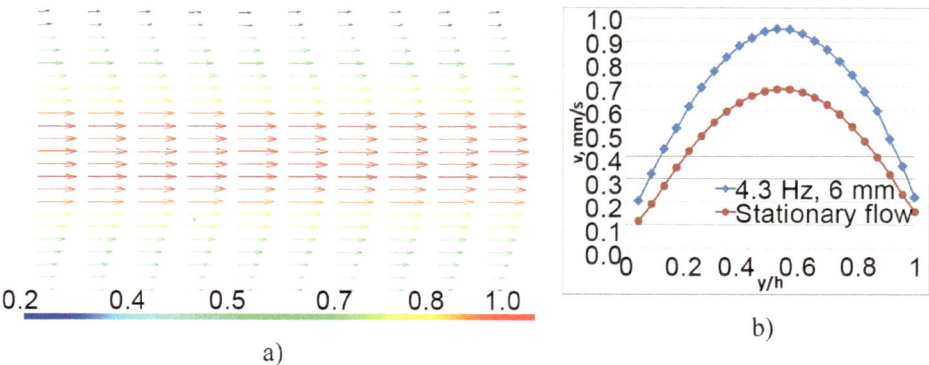

Fig. 3.42 **a** Average velocity vector field at 4.3 Hz and 6 mm; **b** average velocity profile at 4.3 Hz and steady flow

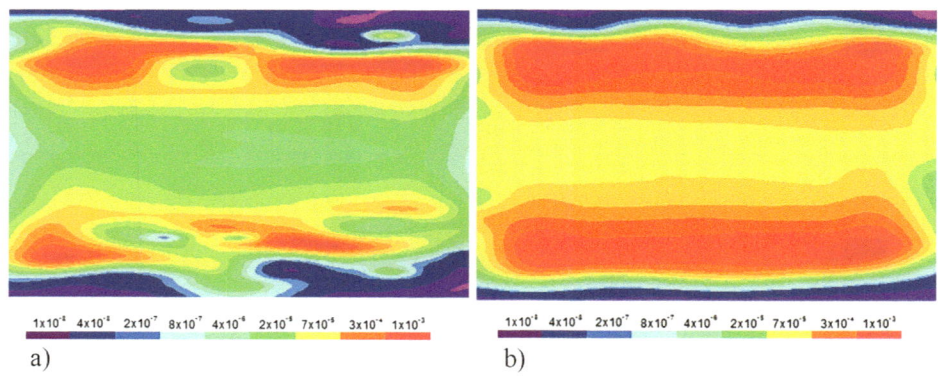

Fig. 3.43 **a** Spectrograms of fluid velocities at a frequency of 4.3 Hz and an amplitude of 6 mm; **b** spectrograms of fluid velocities at 5.8 Hz oscillations and 6 mm amplitude

processing. The final acceleration range requirement was selected to be $\pm 8g$. Naturally, the initiated limb frequencies during the suggested Katsuzo Nishi exercise [36] while lying on the back with legs and arms raised and shaking were observed as high as 4 Hz. Therefore, the close values of frequencies have been argued as the most appropriate for further study with patients.

First, blood pressure monitoring was performed before and after exercise to identify the effect of external vibrations on the human body. Blood pressure monitor Microlife BP A100 [37] was suggested by the clinicians, because of its high accuracy. Other physiological parameters were monitored with a Schiller MT-101 2-channel Cardio Logger [37] device. The device monitors electrocardiogram and heart rate from 4 points of body. Specified computer software was used for observation of collected signals.

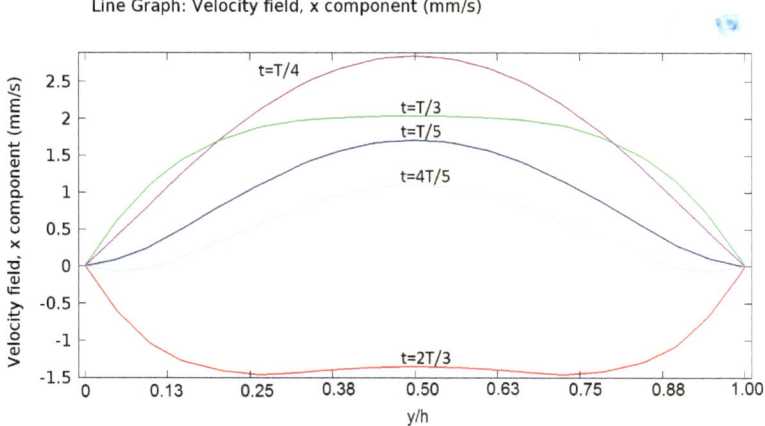

Fig. 3.44 Simulation results showing similarity of phase profiles compared to experimental results at different cycles at 4.3 Hz, 6 mm

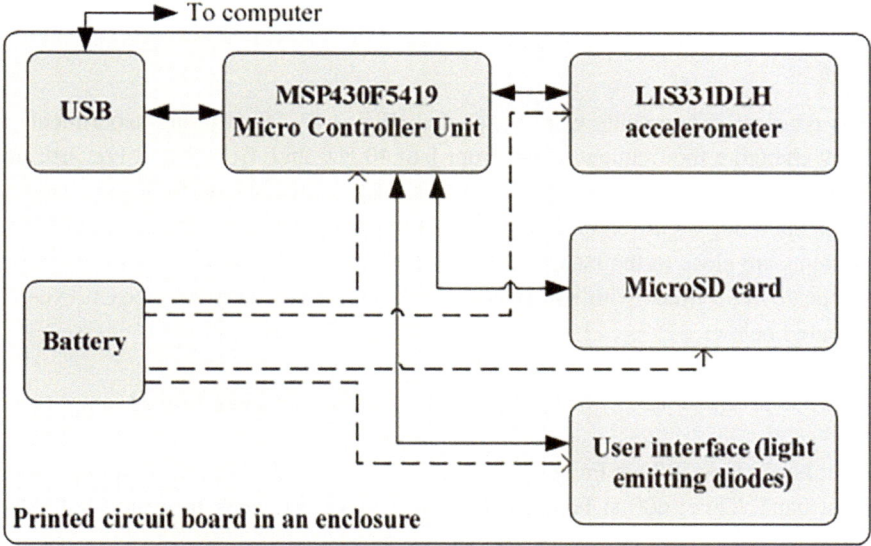

Fig. 3.45 Principal scheme of the acceleration measurement device

Experiments testing a human's body reaction on vibrational effect were conducted in the Institute of Mechatronics at Kaunas University of Technology. The experimental set-up is shown on Fig. 3.46. The vibration stand has been used to initiate the prescribed vibrations on a human hand. Displacement has been observed with the Keyence LK-G82 laser.

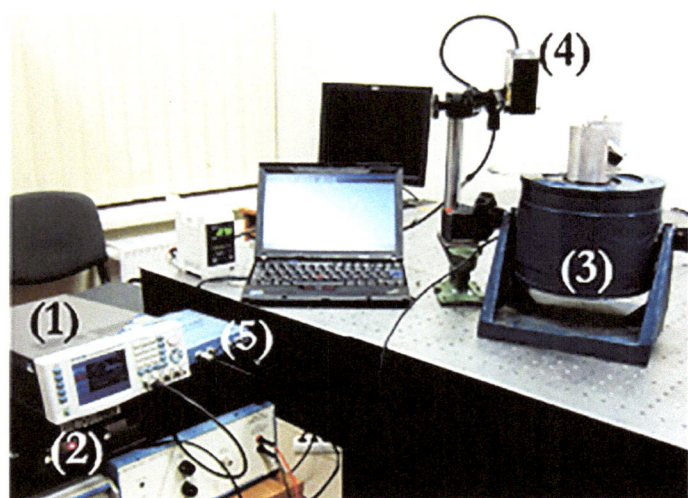

Fig. 3.46 Experimental set-up: 1—waveform generator Tabor Electronics WW5064 50 Ms/s; 2—power amplifier EPA-104; 3—vibrational stand Veb Robotron Type 11,077 with developed device mounted on top; 4—displacement measurement unit laser Keyence LK-G82 with controller Keyence LK-GD500; 5—ADC Pico scope 3424

Two types of experiments were conducted (Fig. 3.47). Firstly, the experiments were made by changing the frequency (1st: from 1 to 40 Hz; 2nd: from 1 to 8 Hz; 3rd: from 2 to 12 Hz). The second type of experiment was made with constant frequency values of 3 and 4 Hz operating on different time periods. Frequency values used at the second type of experiments are close to the means that were observed as the most efficient. Experiments were repeated two times with two patients. The detailed description of each experiment is presented below:

- Right hand. Time: 120 s; Frequency: from 1 to 40 Hz; Peak to peak amplitude 300 mV.
- Right hand. Time: 120 s; Frequency: from 1 to 8 Hz; Peak to peak amplitude: 500 mV.
- Right hand. Time: 600 s; Frequency: from 2 to 12 Hz; Peak to peak amplitude 300 mV.
- Right hand. Time: 120 s; Frequency: 3 Hz; Peak amplitude: 1 V.
- Right hand. Time: 120 s; Frequency: 4 Hz; Peak amplitude: 1 V.
- Right hand. Time: 600 s; Frequency: 3 Hz; Peak amplitude: 1 V.
- Right hand. Time: 600 s; Frequency: 4 Hz; Peak amplitude: 1 V.

Fig. 3.47 Human's body reaction on vibrational effect experiment: 1—vibration stand; 2—human hand with acceleration sensor; 3—cardiology device

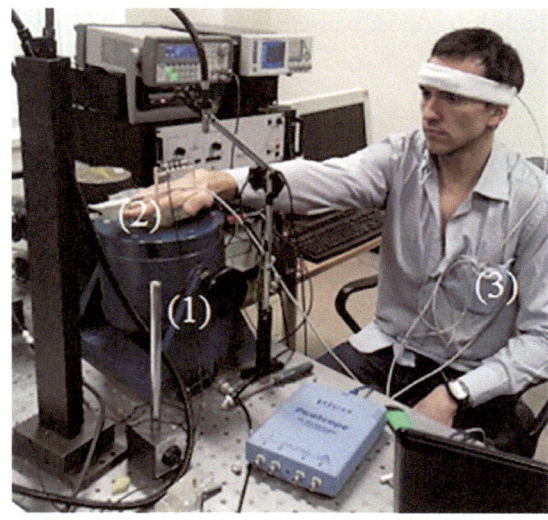

Table 3.9 Blood pressure changes before and after experiment

Time period	Alteration of average systolic blood pressure (mm Hg)	Alteration of average diastolic blood pressure (mm Hg)
Before the experiment	–	–
5 min. after the experiment	−0.75%	16.39%
10 min. after the experiment	4.51%	16.39%

Blood pressure was measured before the vibrational excitation and two times after the experiment: 5 and 10 min later (Table 3.9). A significant change of diastolic blood pressure value was recorded.

The experiment with vibrational oscillations of static frequency has shown different results (Table 3.10). The change of systolic pressure value was found right after the experiment. However, the average value of diastolic blood pressure has decreased. The alterations of blood pressure show the impact of vibrational excitation, but a larger quantity of subjects was considered necessary in the case of proving correlation between values of vibrational frequencies and blood pressure.

The 10-min duration peak to peak experiment has shown some significant changes in the respiration rate and electrocardiogram curves (Fig. 3.48). The major amplitudes have been observed on the highest frequency values. The "uncomfortable feeling" of high frequency vibrations was outspoken by both patients. The higher frequencies values were eliminated from further studies.

Another separate investigation by registering heart rate has been performed. The subject's average and maximum mean of resting heart rate during the 5-min time before an

Table 3.10 Blood pressure changes before and after the 10 min. experiment on vibrational stand

Time period	Alteration of average systolic blood pressure (mm Hg)	Alteration of average diastolic blood pressure (mm Hg)
1 min. before the experiment	–	
Right before the experiment	9.34%	−1.28%
2 min. after the experiment	2.54%	−7.69%

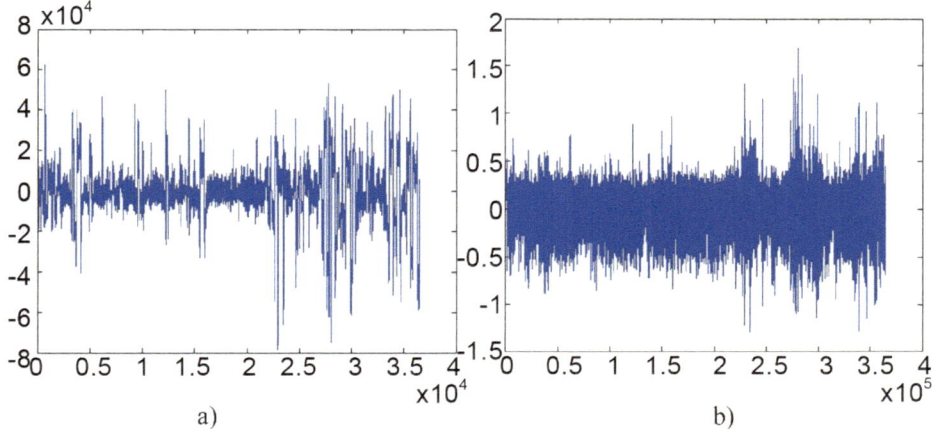

a)   b)

Fig. 3.48 Respiration frequency (**a**) and electrocardiogram (**b**) changes during the 10 min. peak to peak experiment with hand on vibrational stand

experiment was registered. Then the heart rate was observed with a Polar HRM heart rate monitor at 2 min interval by holding the right hand raised. Values of the average and maximum heart rate were registered. Next, the heart rate measurement in the same position but with a vibrating bracelet was made. The beat frequencies of 3 Hz were induced for 2 min. The same physiological parameters defining blood output were registered. Tests were performed 5 times with a one-day break between.

Heart rate measurements showed that the pulse decreases when the hand was affected by vibrations compared to measurements with the bracelet turned off (Fig. 3.49). The average margin of measured average heart rate (MHR) was 59.25 (without vibrations) compared to 57 (with vibrations). The average maximum heart rate (AHR) difference of 64.5 (without vibrations) and 61.25 (with vibrations).

Furthermore, the following experiment's results showed a higher difference between vibrating bracelet and without vibrations. The average difference of average heart rate value was 71.5 (without vibrations) compared to 69 (with vibrations). The average maximum heart rate was 78 (without vibrations) compared to 74.25 (with vibrations) (Fig. 3.50).

Fig. 3.49 First measurement of heart rate values: red line—MHR without vibrations; yellow line—MHR during vibrational exposure; blue line—AHR without vibrations; green line—AHR during vibrational exposure

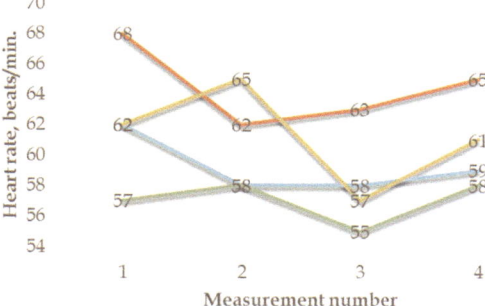

Fig. 3.50 Second measurement of heart rate values: red line—MHR without vibrations; yellow line—MHR during vibrational exposure; blue line—AHR without vibrations; green line—AHR during vibrational exposure

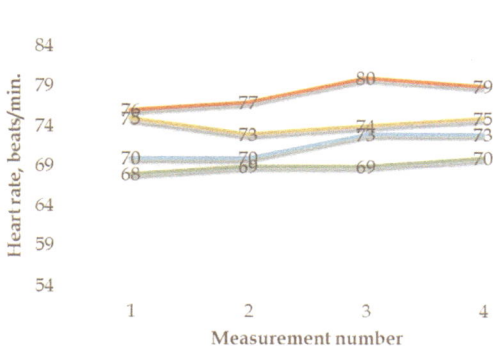

A significant difference of heart rate value in the vibrational exposure effect has been noted. This can be explained by an assumption that increased blood flow with the effect of vibrational excitation reduces the need of the heart's effort to pump the blood. This shows that vibrational therapy could be used as a relaxation method for athletes after a physical load. Temperature monitoring is one of the most common methods of identifying blood flow disorders or changes in separate parts of the human body. An investigation into monitoring temperature changes in the fingers were made after giving vibratory movement at the beating phenomenon frequencies ranging from 1 to 6 Hz with a step of 1 Hz. Each experiment was conducted for a time of two minutes. The temperature measurement results were collected before and after the experiment. Temperature changes were registered with a FLIR t62101 thermal imaging camera. The images were captured on both sides of the hand, on three points of two fingers, before and after the experiment. The vibrational excitation has been induced with the prototype of the vibrating bracelet that was defined in the chapter before.

The highest increase of temperature was obtained after 4 and 4:30 min of vibrational exposure. The most significant alterations of 0.8 °C (Fig. 3.51) were on the palm after a vibrational exposure of a 6 Hz frequency and 0.7 °C raise on the other side of the hand after the vibrational excitation of 3 Hz were noted. Increases in temperature were obtained after all tests of vibrational excitation. Experiments were repeated ten more times, and the results were very similar. In some cases, the temperature increase after

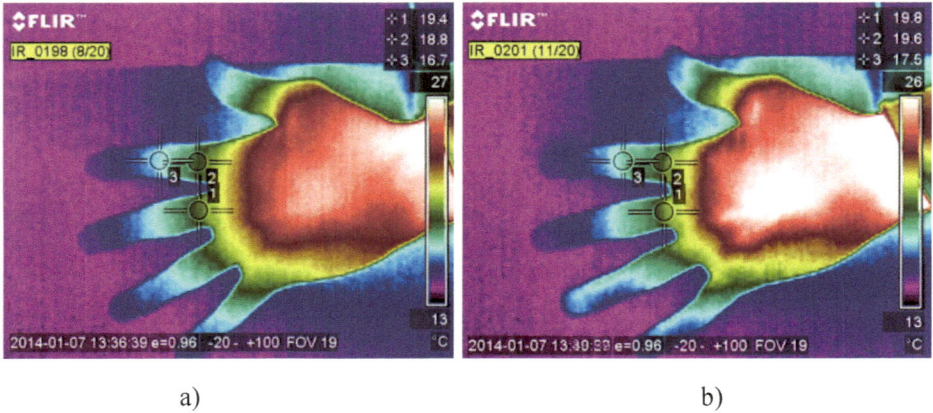

a)   b)

Fig. 3.51 Handbreadth temperature measurement results at three points of palm: **a**—before the experiment; **b**—after the experiment

the vibrational exposure was lower compared to the numbers monitored before, but it increased after a period of a few minutes. The remaining cases showed almost the same increase of temperature of 0.1 to 0.2 °C rise after the exposure.

Temperature increases of 0.3 to 0.5 °C have been registered after a 5-min period in all the remaining experiments of vibrational excitation. These results show that the beating phenomenon frequencies of coupled motors with unbalanced masses could be used for the improvement of blood flow in human limbs. The increase of temperature is significant in most cases and low frequencies are appropriate with the purpose of improvement of blood flow in handbreadth (Fig. 3.52).

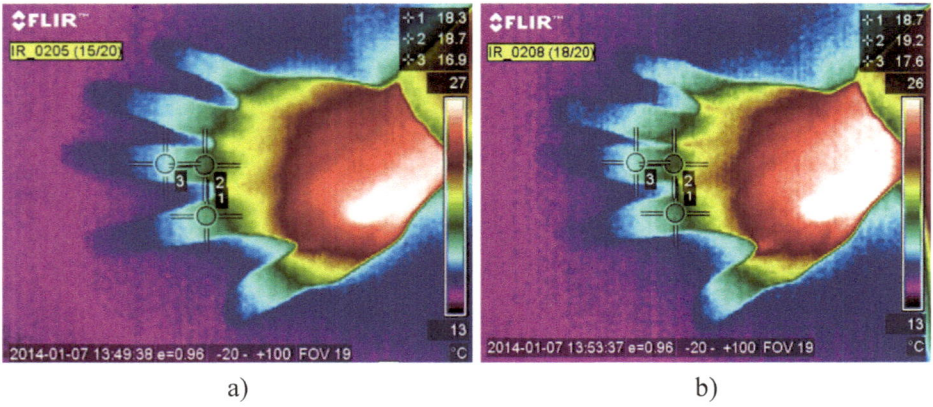

a)   b)

Fig. 3.52 Temperature measurement results at three points of the outer part of handbreadth: **a**—before the experiment; **b**—after the experiment

It was decided to create a vibration actuator for feet exclusively to improve blood circulation in the feet, which is especially relevant for diabetic patients. Considering the fact that the weight of the legs is greater compared to the hands, it was necessary to create a separate device. In this case, to meet the need for greater force, it was decided to use higher power electromechanical motors that could be attached to a flexible plane on which the test subject's legs would be positioned. After calculating the theoretical leg mass in the test weight range from 55 to 100 kg, an analog leg was designed in the 2D environment of COMSOL Multiphysics. After loading it with the masses of the legs and motors, the natural frequencies were determined. In this case, the mass of the legs (25.02 kg) was chosen taking into account the planned tests with the test subject in a real environment, adding the mass of the engines (6.43 kg) together with the unbalanced masses. After loading the drum with these masses, its natural frequency was calculated to be equal to 3.28 Hz. Next, identical calculations were performed, varying the load generated by the legs depending on the mass of the test subject. The calculated eigenfrequencies for test women from 55 to 70 kg weight were in the range of 3.47–3.25 Hz, and for men from 75 to 100 kg weight were from 3.28 Hz to 3.02 Hz. The leg vibration actuator (Fig. 3.53a) was developed taking into account the recommendations contained in the ISO 2631-1 guidelines on the effects of vibrations on the human body, eliminating the negative effects of vertical vibrations on the spine when a person is standing on a vibration source. Taking into account the potential areas of use of the simulator, it was decided to improve the design of the device, which would allow for comfortable blood circulation activation in the limbs. The leg attachment part has also been improved, which allows the patient to adjust the pressure of the legs against the plate. These solutions enable disabled patients to use the equipment as well (Fig. 3.53b).

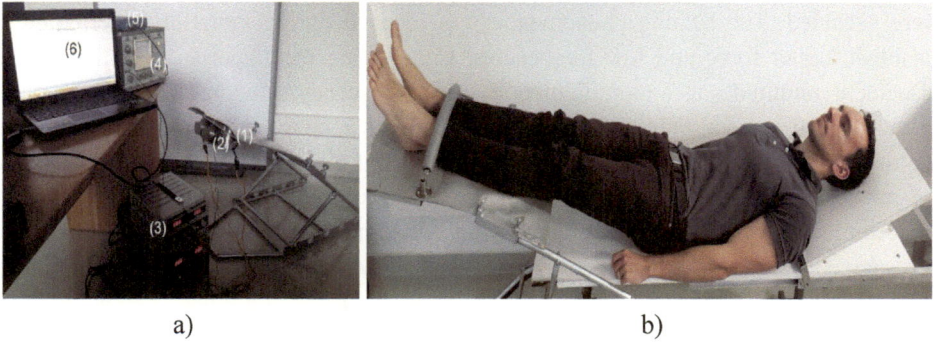

a)   b)

Fig. 3.53 **a** Experimental set-up for legs actuation: 1—legs actuator with motors and unbalanced masses; 2—acceleration sensor KB12; 3—power suppliers (0-30 V/20A, adjustable); 4—Robotron 00,032; 5—Pico scope 3424; 6—PC with Pico scope 6 software; **b** simulation of therapy with experimental set-up

Considering previously described findings with upper limbs, the experiment by monitoring the leg temperature has been conducted too. Moreover, the vibrational frequencies of Glass epoxy plate were registered with the aim of validating the results of numerical modelling. The prototype of the legs actuator that was previously described in detail was a main part of the experimental setup presented in Fig. 3.56. The prototype of the leg's actuator (Fig. 3.53) was developed with the ability of changing the plate's inclination angle while the tested patient's legs are fixed. An angle of 45° degree was selected for this experiment. The glass epoxy cantilever type plate was chosen as the vibrating part because of its high cyclic durability of the flexural strength. The plate was covered with foam for better comfort reason. The plate's length can be adjustable depending on the human's height or leg length. Motors were fixed motionlessly next to each other and adjusted to give an opposite rotation to unbalanced rotors, so creating a force in the vertical direction. Slightly different voltage values create the beating phenomenon that enables it to induce sufficient force by using low voltage and small size motors for making vibrational movement of adequate displacement. Vibration data was gathered with a Robotron 00,032 with a low frequency acceleration sensor KB12 and a sensitivity of 300 mV per 1 m/s^2, then processed with a Pico scope 3424 with Pico scope PC software. Motors were supplied by Digimess HY3020 power suppliers (1ch, 30V, 20A, adjustable).

Vibrational excitation influence is widely defined in previous studies and was mentioned in the first chapter. Various techniques of measurement can be used. In this paper's case, the high-sensitivity infrared thermal imaging camera FLIR-t62101 was used to identify the vibrational excitation influence on foot blood flow. Four points on the right foot (Hallux toe, Long toe, right point on the foot and left point on the foot) were monitored before and after experiments. Temperature differences were registered by making thermal images immediately after the exposure and capturing images 3 and 5 min later.

The experiments with the legs vibrating machine on identifying working frequencies were executed. The beating phenomenon was induced during vibrational excitation to establish higher force and low frequencies. Considering the importance of higher displacement amplitudes as a more influential effect, frequency value has been chosen close to the Eigenfrequency value of Glass epoxy plate as a possible for each experimented leg mass. The experiment was conducted with a 75 kg weight patient with considered leg mass of 25.02 kg and motors bulk mass of 6.43 kg. The calculation of the leg mass has been made according to the previously described methodology of statistically defined percentage ratio from the body mass. Voltage values were chosen according to the results of the numerical study and tested a person's vibrational excitation impact feeling. Beating phenomenon frequencies ranging from 0.5 to 4.8 Hz were registered during the experiment (Fig. 3.54 and 3.55). Furthermore, the generated force values of vibrating motors have been calculated. These values are given in the figure captions of the graphs below.

Low voltage causes low angular speed and a lower acting force. The resistance force of legs starts from approximately 200 N. Higher amplitudes of oscillations were obtained with the highest force values. The flexibility properties and calculated Eigenfrequency

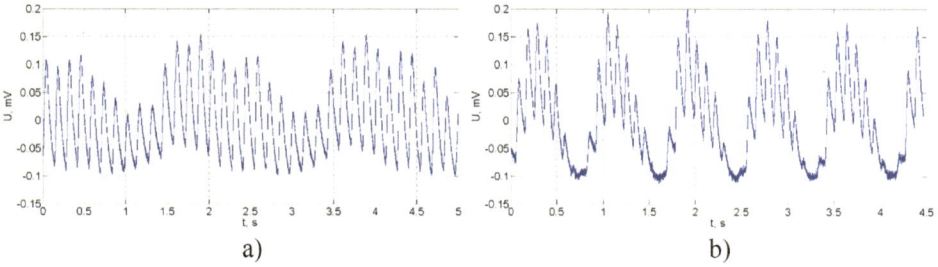

Fig. 3.54 Cantilever plate excitation voltage: **a** 7.8–7.4 V; beating frequency: 0.5 Hz; force to legs: 44.68 N and **b** 10.7–9.6 V; beating frequency: 1.168 Hz; force to legs: 78.12 N

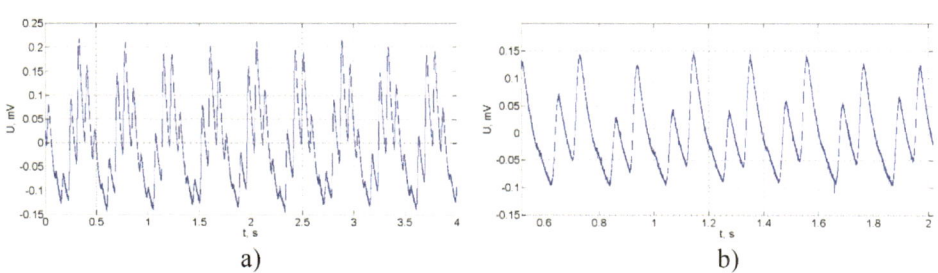

Fig. 3.55 Cantilever plate excitation voltage: **a** 11.2–13.8 V; beating frequency: 2.217 Hz; force to legs: 117.78 N and **b** 15.1–10 V; beating frequency: 4.844 Hz; force to legs: 137.10 N

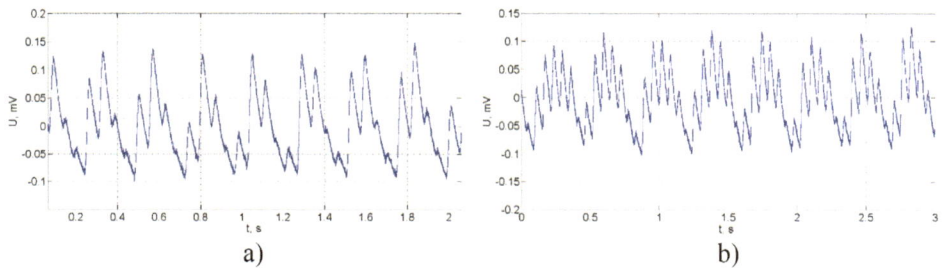

Fig. 3.56 Cantilever plate excitation voltage: **a** 16.9–12.4 V; beating frequency: 4.152 Hz; force to legs: 116.30 N and **b** 16.9–13.9 V; beating frequency: 3.311 Hz; force to legs: 180.2 N

value of the vibrating plate enables research to induce sufficient vibrations with lower values of generated force. In the graphs at Fig. 3.54, glass epoxy plates and feet oscillating frequencies are significantly smaller compared to Eigenfrequencies values that were calculated numerically. This means that the influence of blood flow stimulation should be minor. Therefore, higher voltage values were used for further investigations (Fig. 3.55) with the purpose of generating a higher force. Beating phenomenon has been induced by adjusting the input voltage of each motor. The beat phenomenon could be defined from all diagrams listed below. It should be noted that natural frequencies of the motors have not been felt by the tested patients.

The voltage values of 16.9 and 13.9 V (Fig. 3.56) were chosen for further experiments to register the vibrational excitation influence on blood circulation at the foot. The frequency of 3.311 Hz was the closest value to eigenfrequency, which was calculated with COMSOL Multiphysics software. Motors with unbalanced masses working on this regime generate 180.2 N force. The force is enough for sufficient displacement and the greatest among the other values of beat frequencies (2.217, 4.844, 4.152 Hz,).

Temperature monitoring has been conducted on four points: two on different toes (Hallux and Long) and two points on the foot (one on the left and one on the right). The emissivity means of 0.98 has been prescribed on the camera settings for monitoring human skin temperature. Temperature changes were recorded just after the exercise and 3 and 5 min later. Peak temperature increase values were registered after resting 3 min after the vibrational excitation. A temperature rise of 0.7 °C on the Hallux toe (Fig. 3.57), 1 °C on the Long toe (Fig. 3.58), 0.9 °C on the right foot point (Fig. 3.59) and 1.5 °C on the left foot point (Fig. 3.60) were captured.

Furthermore, additional experiments were undertaken by monitoring temperatures by using a different measurement methodology. First, the temperature was monitored on three points of the Hallux toe, one point of the Long toe and two point on the right and left side of the foot. Second, the lowest temperature point of the foot has been monitored. The results were similar compared to the primary ones. The captured values have been continuously increasing in the period of 5 min after the experiment. At the top point of the Hallux toe the temperature increased by 0.9 °C after the first experiment and by 0.4 °C after the second. In the middle point of the Hallux toe the captured increase was equal to

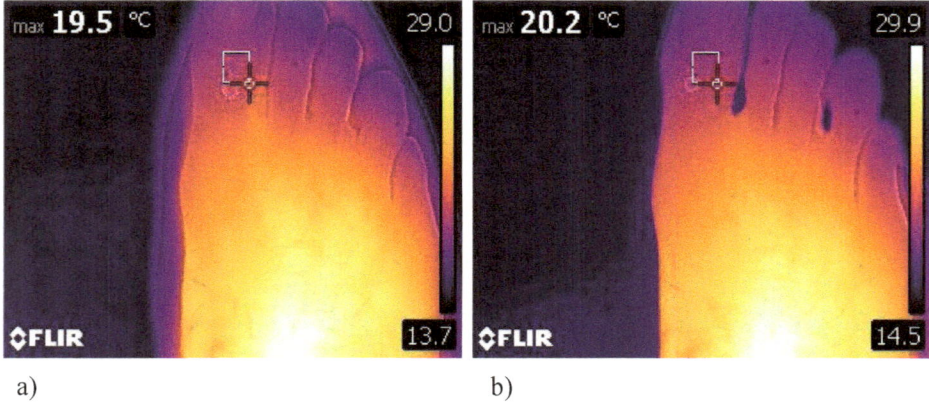

a)   b)

Fig. 3.57 Hallux toe temperature before (**a**) and after (**b**) legs actuation

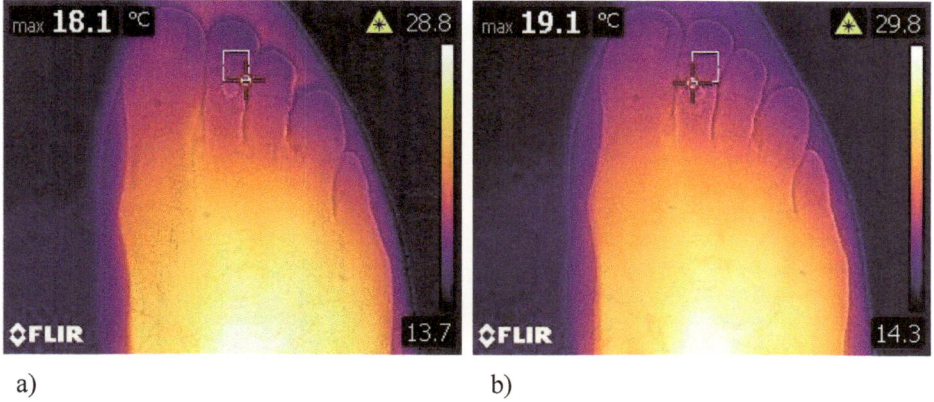

Fig. 3.58 Long toe temperature before (**a**) and after (**b**) legs actuation

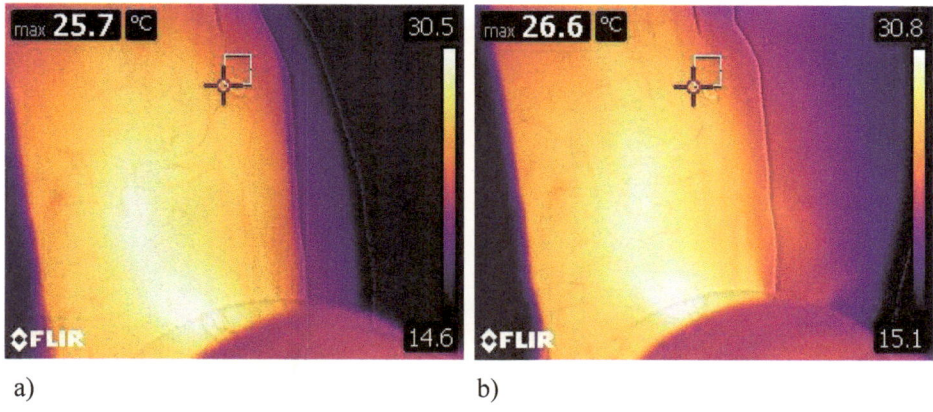

Fig. 3.59 Right foot point temperature before (**a**) and after (**b**) legs actuation

0.7 °C and 0.4 °C respectively. The lowest point's temperature of the same toe increased by 0.9 °C at both measurements. The temperature of the big toe increased by 0.8 °C and 0.4 °C respectively. The right and left points of the foot became warmer at an average of 1 °C. The results of the lowest value measurement have shown temperature increases of 0.4 °C after 5 min after the experiment (Fig. 3.61).

The alterations of temperature are significant; hence the assumption of increased blood flow can be proved. A gentile stitch feeling in the feet after the vibrational exposure was noted by the subject. Further investigations of using capillaroscopy methodology for monitoring blood flow in capillaries is planned to be conducted. Capillaroscopy is the most common approach of examination of capillaries with a microscope. The use

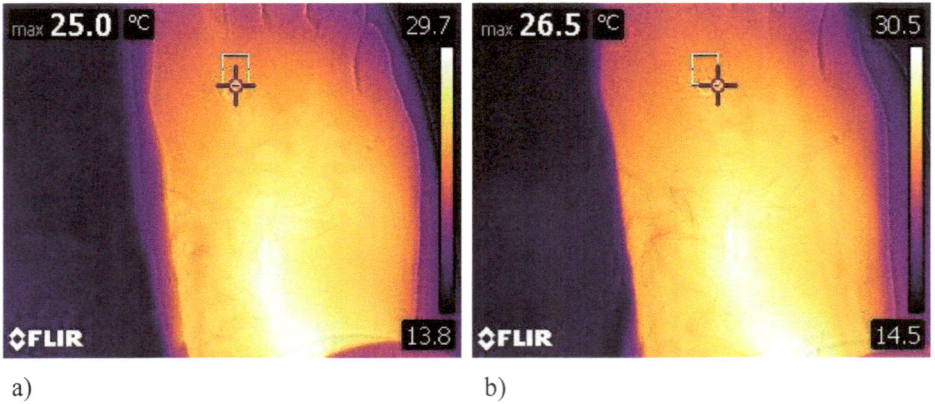

Fig. 3.60 Left foot point temperature before (**a**) and after (**b**) legs actuation

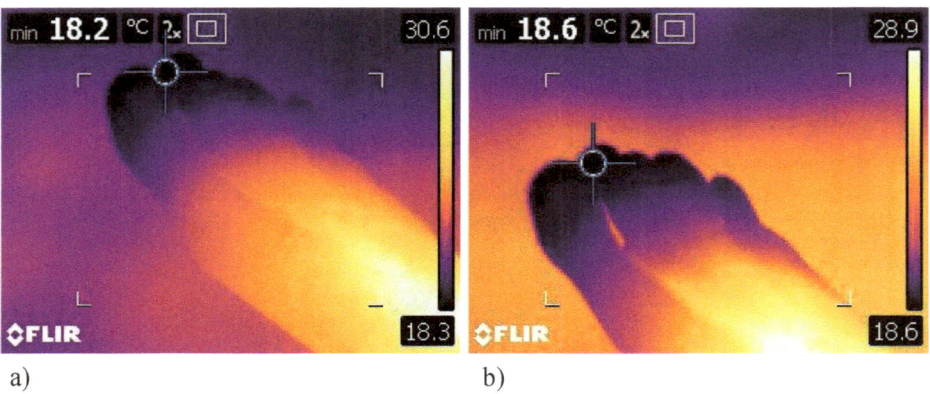

Fig. 3.61 The lowest temperature point measurement: before (**a**) and after (**b**) the experiment

capillaroscopy means has been suggested by colleagues from the Lithuanian University of Medical Sciences.

The study revealed statistically significant differences in heart rate variability before, during and after the use of vibration therapy. The tendency of the heart rate variability to increase shows us that the heart also reacts to the changes taking place when the peripheral circulation of the feet is affected.

After conducting the study and analyzing the results of the functional relationships between heart rate variability and temperature changes, we found that statistically significant differences were found only at the peripheral point of the foot. Statistically significant differences were found in all phases of vibration therapy. Before vibration therapy, immediately after it and 5, 10, 15 min after vibration therapy comparing data with variability before and after vibration therapy. An inverse relationship was found that heart rate variability increases with low foot temperature and decreases with increasing temperature. This can be explained by the fact that the adaptation of the cardiovascular system to thermal stimuli occurs due to the simultaneous activation of the efferent branches of the cardiac autonomic nervous system and the peripheral blood vessels (Flouris, 2009). It was not possible to find studies that would have been conducted to compare the correlations between heart rate variability and changes in human peripheral blood circulation temperature. This could be a topic for future research.

3.5   Trials of a Smart Device for Tremor Therapy

Parkinson's disease is a common neurodegenerative disease of the central nervous system with a possible genetic predisposition that results from the loss of dopaminergic cells in the black matter of the brain [38], and manifests as movement disorders: tremor, rigidity, bradykinesia, and postural instability. These dysfunctions can significantly impact the individual's quality of life, leading to a decline in overall well-being. Tremor is an unintentional rhythmic movement of any part of the body. Shaking or trembling hands is a typical hand tremor symptom. Tremors are usually caused by problems with areas of the brain that control movements. The two main diseases that cause chronic hand tremor are Essential Tremor and Parkinson's Disease [39]. The problem exacerbates when patients try to do something, including simple tasks such as drinking from a glass, eating or tying shoelaces. For these reasons, even if tremor is not a life treating disease, it has a great impact on the patient's life quality, especially considering that essential tremor typically worsens over time: unfortunately, for some patients the intensity of the disease can be as severe as an invalidating condition. Traditional treatment options for tremors, including medication and neurosurgical interventions, are not adequate for many patients. The use of drugs has historically been the primary treatment approach, but it often fails to produce the desired therapeutic response. This is due to the complex interactions between different drugs and the intolerable side effects experienced when using high doses to control tremors. In the case of Parkinson's disease, dopaminergic medications, which are commonly used, only reduce tremors in 50% of patients. For individuals with severe and medically resistant tremors, invasive procedures like deep brain stimulation or magnetic resonance-guided focused ultrasound may be considered. However, these options have drawbacks such as high costs, significant risks, potential for irreversible neurological damage, and consequently, low acceptance rates among patients. Therefore, there is a pressing need for a safe and dependable first-line therapy that can effectively manage Parkinson's disease symptoms without causing the adverse effects associated with pharmacotherapy or the risks associated with invasive procedures [40]. Rehabilitative therapy, such as occupational therapy and exercise, complement pharmacologic treatments [41]. Physical therapy is proven to slow down the progression of Parkinson's disease [42]. Another alternative is vibration therapy. It can be especially helpful in addition to physiotherapy. Applying vibration to the whole body or the upper extremities improves proprioception and relieves the symptoms of astigmatism and tremor. Still, it should be noted that vibration-induced effects provide only short-term improvement [43]. Patented "Vilim ball" device [44] reduces tremors in some Essential tremor patients and is safe to use in that condition. Parkinson's tremor occurs mostly at rest, so it doesn't disturb daily routines as much as essential tremor. As a result, this study was conducted to see if the local hand-arm vibration treatment can improve the outcome of traditional physiotherapy exercises for individuals with Parkinson's disease [45]. The study was conducted with Parkinson's patients who were members of the Kaunas Parkinson's disease society at Kaunas City Polyclinic by physiotherapists, at Kaunas Dainava Polyclinic Youth Center. Research was conducted with the formal approval of the local human subject care committees. The studies were conducted on men and women diagnosed with Parkinson's disease aged 50 to 80 years.

3.5.1   An Identification System for the Early Diagnosis of Parkinson's Disease

Parkinson's syndrome affects more and more people every year. Currently, there are approximately 10 million people in the world. people suffering from this disease. In Lithuania, this number reaches 12,000. Since this disease is slowly progressive, but in its initial stages it is not dangerous or clearly noticeable, it is very important to monitor the health status of the person and apply timely treatment. In order to identify the trajectory of the movement of the hand during tremors and the most suitable position for attaching the diagnostic device, a study was conducted in the biomechanics laboratory of the Institute of Mechatronics of Kaunas Technology University, and the accelerations of different points of the limb (hand) were analyzed and compared with each other. Eight volunteers participated in the study (Fig. 3.62), whose hand tremor profile was analyzed by evaluating the data collected at the points of the fingers, teeth, wrist, elbow and shoulder.

After analyzing the collected data, the tremor frequency and the amplitude of each measured point were evaluated. The results showed that any measurement point can be used to identify the tremor frequency, as the dominant frequency was successfully identified in all cases (Fig. 3.63).

After evaluating the displacements of the measured points (Fig. 3.64) and comfort aspects, the project team developed a wrist-mounted device (Fig. 3.65) for monitoring the kinematics and kinetics of the upper body limbs. When moving the ring, the linear acceleration, angular velocity and orientation of the wrist movement in three axes in space are recorded using a 3D accelerometer. The data is recorded on a micro SD card, which is later analyzed by a medical specialist (Fig. 3.66). By registering the movements of the patient's hand and analyzing the change in the mentioned parameters, it is possible to

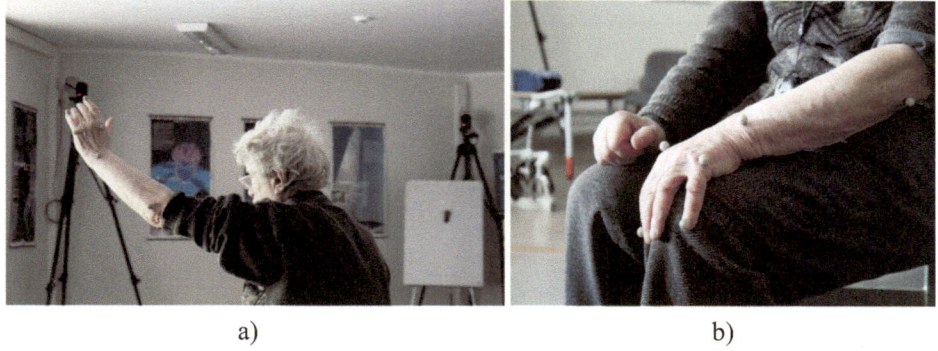

a)   b)

Fig. 3.62 Examination of the limb biomechanics of a Parkinson's disease patient with the Qualisys analysis system: **a** standing, **b** sitting

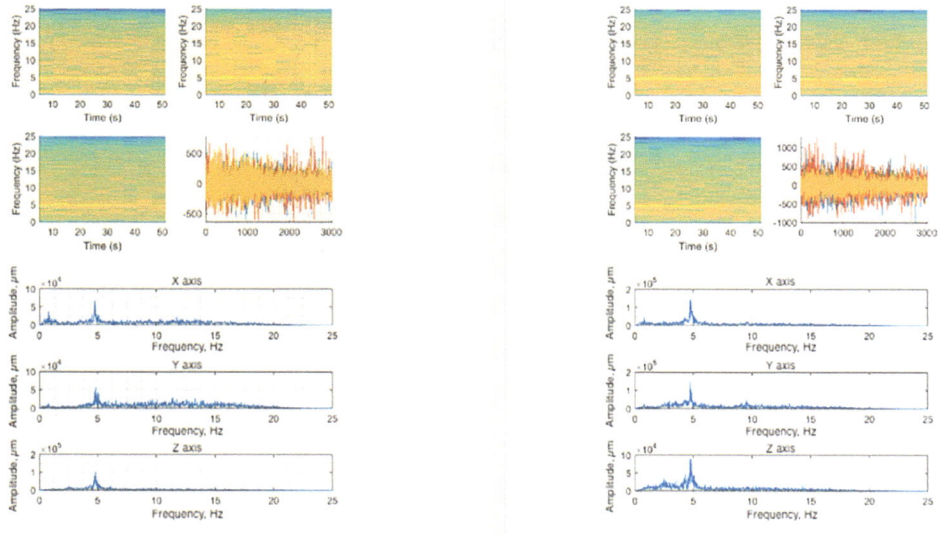

Fig. 3.63 Wrist frequency (left) and knuckle frequency (right) in X, Y and Z axes

follow the state of the disease, its stage, progress or regression. Research has shown that if treatment procedures are not applied, the patient loses the possibility of self-service already eight years after the onset of the disease, while if the symptoms are diagnosed in time, the expected period is doubled.

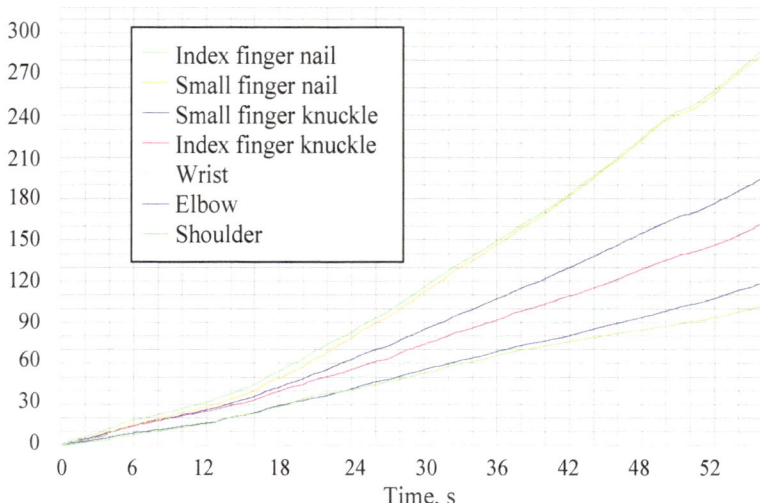

Fig. 3.64 Cumulative displacement of endpoints during 54 s of measurement

Fig. 3.65 Hand tremor
diagnostic device for
Parkinson's patients

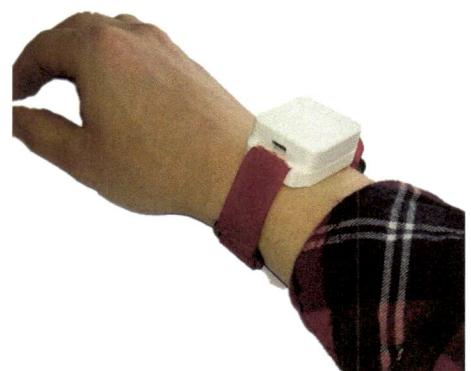

3.5.2 Vibrational Tremor Therapy in Parkinson's Disease

Vibrational therapy was performed with "Vilim ball" (Fig. 3.67) device. The Vilim ball is a certified Class IIa medical non-invasive handheld therapeutic device that reduces hand tremor, provides symptomatic relief, and facilitates activities of daily living. The device incorporates Machine Learning algorithms that use various sensors to analyze tremors, optimize vibrational therapy and interrupt the neurological loop that causes tremors. The "Vilim ball" emits low-frequency mechanical vibrations in the range of 8–18 Hz. The device is intended to be used in homes and clinical environments.

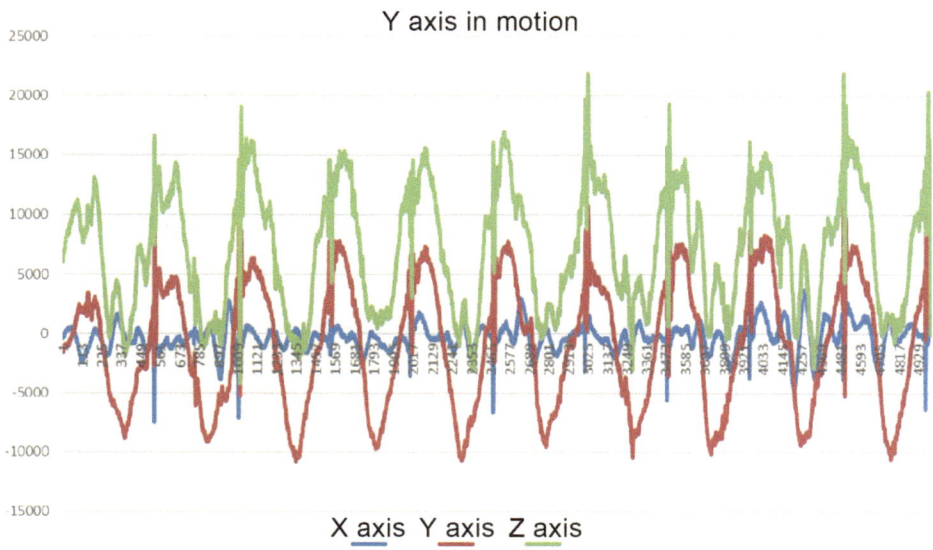

Fig. 3.66 Visualization of data collected by a hand tremor diagnostic device in Parkinson's patients

Fig. 3.67 "Vilim ball" device

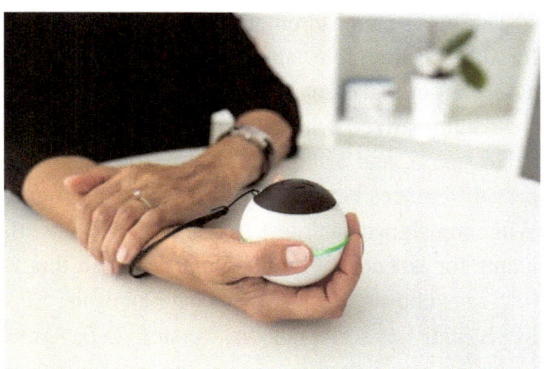

Study subjects were then divided into two groups: the first group (N=12, 7 male, 5 female) that performed only physiotherapy, and the second group (N=12, 7 male, 5 female) that performed physiotherapy and used the "Vilim ball" additionally. The subjects of the first group were aged from 60 to 79 years with a mean of 68.1 years. The second group of subjects were aged from 60 to 76 years with a mean of 67.1 years. The subjects in the first group performed physiotherapy for 50 min, while the second group of subjects used the device before the procedure (10 minutes for each hand) and performed physiotherapy for 30 min. Tremor assessments were performed to assess upper limb abnormalities in people with Parkinson's disease before and after physiotherapy. Hand dynamometer (microFET®2) was used to measure the grip strength—maximum gripping force in kilograms (0–90kg). The subjects were assessed in a sitting position with arms bent at 90° through their elbows angled, tucked to the sides, and not placed on the supporting table. Measurements were performed 3 times in both hands separately. The arm coordination evaluation was performed using Nine-Hole Peg Test [46]. The test measures finger dexterity and hand coordination. During the test the patients were seated in a chair with their arms rested on a table in front of them with elbows in 90° flexion and palms downward. A pegboard with 9 holes was positioned in front of them. The participants were instructed to quickly remove all the pegs from the holes, place them into the container, then take back the pegs from the container, and put them back into the holes on the board. The test scores were based on the time taken to complete the test activity, recorded in seconds with a stopwatch. Hand tremor power was calculated using an accelerometer embedded in a mobile phone. Specialized mobile application "Steady Hands" [47] was used for this purpose. The software logs accelerometer data in all three-movement axis and calculates spectral power density estimates using a Fast Fourier Transform [48]. Acceleration recording time was set to ~1 minute with a 36 Hz sampling rate. All 3 (X, Y, Z) accelerometer axis are summed and a Hanning window of length 2048 was applied before calculating spectral power density. Tremor power in this study is defined as spectral power density integral in a typical Parkinsonian tremor frequency band (4–16 Hz).

During the measurements, the subjects were seated, with their hands placed comfortably on the table, and the mobile phones held gently in their palms. Patients were asked not to make any voluntary movements during the data collection. Quantitative data were summarized with descriptive statistics: median, minimum value (min), maximum value (max), and arithmetic mean. The Mann-Whitney-Wilcoxon test was used to compare differences between two independent groups for not normally distributed data. Also, Wilcoxon signed-rank test to compare two sets of scores that come from the same participants for not normally distributed data. In this work statistical significance level of $p <$ 0.05 was chosen. Software for data analysis: SPSS 25 (IBM Corp. Released 2017. IBM SPSS Statistics for Windows, Version 25.0. Armonk, NY: IBM Corp.).

In the physiotherapy group, the right-hand coordination improved significantly after intervention: median 29.66 seconds at baseline versus median 28.05 seconds post-intervention. In the physiotherapy group that used the vibrational medical device the right-hand coordination was improved significantly from median 30.29 seconds at baseline versus median 29.54 seconds post intervention. There were no significant differences in right-hand coordination between the groups at ($U = 50.00$; $p = 0.204$) or after interventions ($U = 46.00$; $p = 0.133$).

For more information, see Table 3.11 and Fig. 3.68.

In the physiotherapy group the left arm coordination improved significantly after intervention: median 32.29 seconfs at baseline vs. median 31.05 seconds post intervention. In the physiotherapy group that used the vibrational medical device the left arm coordination

Table 3.11 Right hand coordination data

Group	Baseline (Md sec)	Baseline (Min sec)	Baseline (Max sec)	Baseline (A.M. sec)	Post Intervention (Md sec)	Post Intervention (Min sec)	Post Intervention (Max sec)	Post Intervention (A.M. sec)	Z-score	p-value
Physiotherapy	29.66	25.49	32.57	29.43	28.05	24.13	32.15	28.31	−2.28	0.023
Physiotherapy + vibrational medical device	30.29	27.54	37.45	31.81	29.54	27.13	34.12	29.98	−2.90	0.040

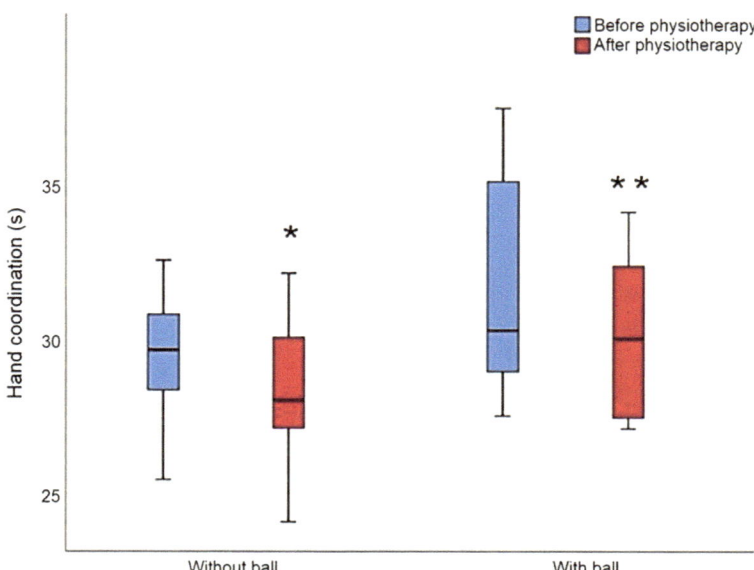

Fig. 3.68 Right hand coordination at baseline and after physiotherapy with or without the vibrational medical device "Vilim ball": *statistically significant difference in comparing the right-hand index in the group of physiotherapy without the use of a vibrating ball before and after the procedure ($p < 0.05$). ** statistically significant difference in comparing the index of the right arm with the use of physiotherapy with a vibrating ball before and after the procedure in the group ($p < 0.05$)

improved significantly after intervention: median 36.33 seconds at baseline vs. 34.35 seconds. There were no significant differences in left-hand coordination between the groups at baseline ($U = 39.00$, $p = 0.057$) or after interventions ($U = 38.50$, $p = 0.053$), see Table 3.12 and Fig. 3.69.

In the physiotherapy group the right-hand tremor power decreased from median 1.135 $(m/s^2)^2$ at baseline to 1.051 $(m/s^2)^2$ after physiotherapy. In the physiotherapy group with the device usage the right-hand tremor power spectrum decreased significantly after the intervention: from median 1.372 $(m/s^2)^2$ at baseline to median 0.712 $(m/s^2)^2$ post intervention. The tremor power spectrum did not differ significantly between the groups either before ($U = 61.00$, $p = 0.525$) or after ($U = 63.00$; $p = 0.603$) the interventions. However, the tremor intensity decreased by 7.38 % after only physiotherapy and by 48.11 % after physiotherapy in addition to the "Vilim ball" (Table 3.13 and Fig. 3.70).

The left-hand tremor intensity assessment revealed different results. In the "only physiotherapy" group, left-arm tremor power was similar before and after intervention: median 0.612 $(m/s^2)^2$ at baseline vs. median 0.635 $(m/s^2)^2$, while a significant decrease in tremor intensity was found in the "physiotherapy and Vilim ball" group post intervention: 0.821 $(m/s^2)^2$ at baseline versus 0.573 $(m/s^2)^2$ post intervention. There was no statistically

Table 3.12 Left hand coordination data

Group	Baseline (Md sec)	Baseline (Min sec)	Baseline (Max sec)	Baseline (A.M. sec)	Post Intervention (Md sec)	Post Intervention (Min sec)	Post Intervention (Max sec)	Post Intervention (A.M. sec)	Z-score	p-value
Physiotherapy	32.29	28.64	39.11	32.95	31.05	27.98	35.78	31.16	−3.06	0.002
Physiotherapy + vibrational medical device	36.33	30.78	43.41	36.11	34.35	29.15	40.03	34.01	−3.06	0.002

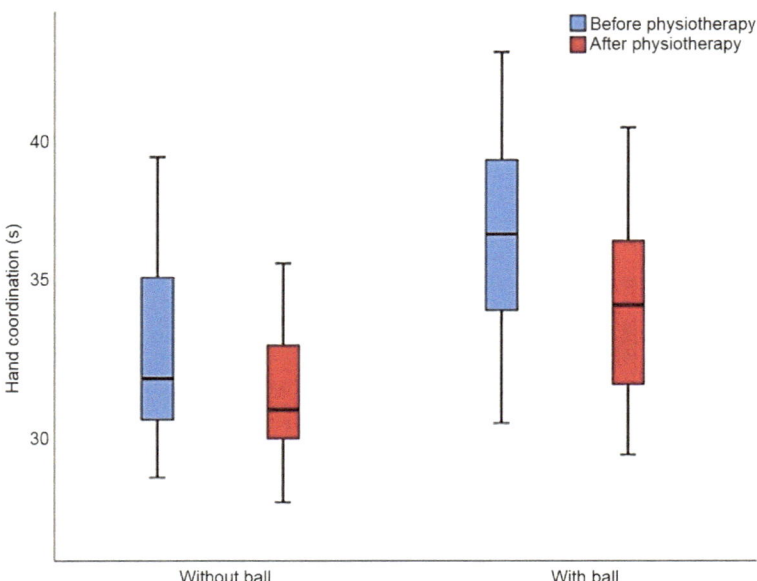

Fig. 3.69 Left hand coordination at baseline and after physiotherapy with or without the vibrational medical device "Vilim ball": *statistically significant difference in comparing the left arm index in the group of physiotherapy without the use of a vibrating ball before and after the procedure ($p < 0.05$). ** statistically significant difference in comparing left hand index of physiotherapy with vibratory ball use before and after the procedure in the group ($p < 0.05$)

significant difference between the groups before ($U = 63.00$, $p = 0.603$) or after interventions ($U = 49.00$, $p = 0.184$). However, it was observed that the tremor power increased by 3.89 % after the "physiotherapy only" and decreased by 30.23 % after the physiotherapy plus "Vilim ball" (see Table 3.14 and Fig. 3.71).

In the physiotherapy group that did not use the vibrational medical device the right-hand grip strength did not change after intervention: at baseline 27.00 kg (min 20.60; max 38.60; arithmetic mean 27.69) versus 26.65 kg (min 19.9; 37.6; 27.65) kg. We also observed no change in right-hand grip strength in the physiotherapy with vibrational medical device group after the intervention: at baseline 27.10 kg (min 18.20, max 38.10, arithmetic mean 27.50) kg versus 28.90 kg (min 19.10, max 37.40, arithmetic mean 28.12) post-intervention. There were no statistically significant differences between the groups before or post-intervention: $U = 71.50$, $p = 0.999$ vs. $U = 67.50$, $p=0.795$, respectively. The median change in right arm muscle strength is shown in Table 3.15 and Fig. 3.72.

Resting tremor remains a significant condition that impairs the quality of life in most Parkinson's disease patients even with symptomatic medical treatment (e.g. levodopa-dopamine replacement agent). Conventional physiotherapy improves motor symptoms, gait, and quality of life in Parkinson's disease, but has little effect on tremors [49]. Research on tremor pathophysiology shows that electrical stimulation of the peripheral

Table 3.13 Right hand tremor intensity data

Group	Baseline Tremor Power (Md (m/s²)²)	Baseline Tremor Power (Md (Min. (m/s²)²)	Baseline Tremor Power (Md (Max. (m/s²)²)	Baseline Tremor Power (Md (A. M. (m/s²)²)	Post Intervention Tremor (Md (m/s²)²)	Post Intervention Tremor (Min. (m/s²)²)	Post Intervention Tremor (Max. (m/s²)²)	Post Intervention Tremor Power (A. M. (m/s²)²)	Z-score	p-value
Physiotherapy	1.135	0.519	2.317	1.195	1.051	0.438	1.941	1.071	−2.040	0.041
Physiotherapy + vibrational medical device	1.372	0.610	3.665	1.527	0.712	0.431	1.028	0.739	−3.06	0.002

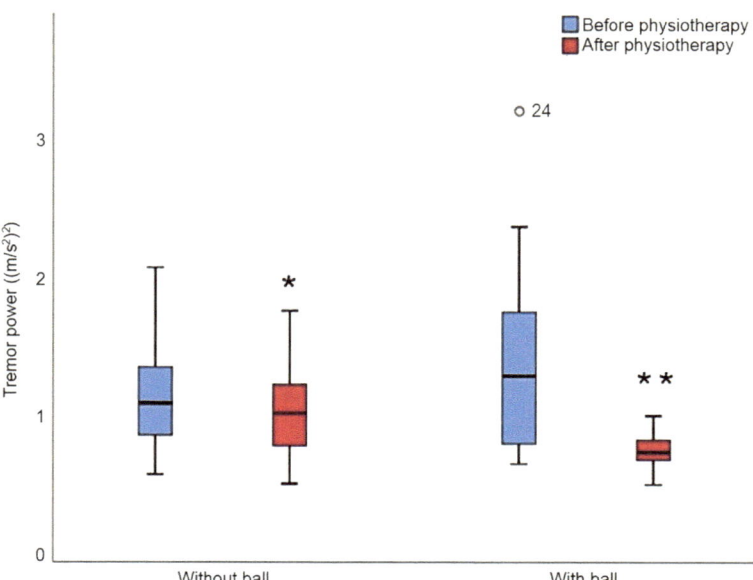

Fig. 3.70 Right-hand tremor intensity changes before vs. after physiotherapy. *Statistically significant difference in comparing the index of the right arm in the group of physiotherapy without the use of a vibrating ball before and after the procedure ($p < 0.05$) ** statistically significant difference when comparing the right-hand index of physiotherapy with the use of a vibratory ball before and after the procedure ($p < 0.05$)

nerves, mechanical perturbation of the limb, or transcranial magnetic stimulation of the motor cortex can alleviate tremor symptoms [50]. Deep brain stimulation remains the most effective intervention to reduce severe tremors [51], while electrical stimulation of muscles has been proposed for patients with less severe forms of Parkinson's disease tremor [52]. Transcutaneous afferent patterned stimulation of the median and radial nerves at the wrist, is the only peripheral electrical stimulation therapy currently approved by the USA Food and Drug Administration for the clinical management of the Essential tremor and Parkinson's disease symptoms. Such therapy involves tens of minutes of noninvasive electrical stimulation that alternates between the median and radial nerves at the wrist at a patient's tremor frequency.

In one related study, 40 Parkinson's disease patients with postural tremor were enrolled in a remote, prospective, single-arm, open-label study with 4 weeks of transcutaneous afferent patterned stimulation. Improvements among other variables were also calculated in a change in postural tremor power using accelerometer data. It was concluded that transcutaneous afferent patterned stimulation reduced postural tremor power by a median of 66% ($p < 0.01$, $N = 35$). This is a better result compared to the results of this study (a decrease of 48.11 % for the right hand and 30.23% for the left hand). However, both studies contained relatively small sample sizes. It must be noted that the transcutaneous

Table 3.14 Left hand tremor intensity data

Group	Baseline Tremor Power (Md (Md (m/s^2)^2)	Baseline Tremor Power (Md (Min (m/s^2)^2)	Baseline Tremor Power (Md (Max (m/s^2)^2)	Baseline Tremor Power (A.M. (m/s^2)^2)	Post Intervention Tremor Power (Md (m/s^2)^2)	Post Intervention Tremor Power (Min (m/s^2)^2)	Post Intervention Tremor Power (Max (m/s^2)^2)	Post Intervention Tremor Power (A.M. (m/s^2)^2)	Z-score	p-value
Physiotherapy	0.612	0.392	1.193	0.714	0.635	0.438	1.941	1.071	−2.04	0.041
Physiotherapy + vibrational medical device	0.821	0.418	1.520	0.840	0.573	0.345	0.968	0.571	−3.06	0.002

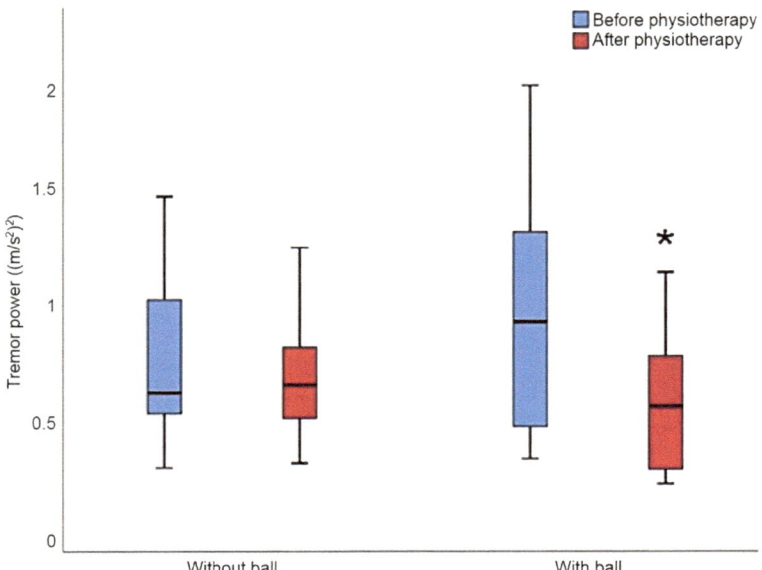

Fig. 3.71 Left hand tremor intensity before and after physiotherapy* statistically significant difference when comparing left hand index of physiotherapy with vibratory ball use before and after the procedure in the group ($p < 0.05$)

afferent patterned stimulation study did not involve physiotherapy. This study authors chose a different frequency range for tremor power calculation compared to this study. However, it is unlikely to cause any issues in comparing the results of the studies as both approaches measure the change in tremor power and not absolute values. Furthermore, both approaches involve the main tremor frequency range. Power in leftover frequency bands is unlikely to be associated with tremor movements.

This study showed that local hand-arm mechanical vibrations generated by the Vilim ball device can be safely and effectively used in Parkinson's disease patients in conjunction with conventional physiotherapy. Such an approach can improve right-hand coordination and decrease tremor power. This result can be explained as an outcome of reduced tremor due to "Vilim ball" therapy.

Quality of life for patients with Parkinson's disease may be affected due to multiple reasons, which include the impact of tremor on activities of daily living, embarrassment due to tremor and its impact on emotional wellbeing, depression and anxiety [53]. Better coordination of hand movements can be beneficial in daily tasks of Parkinson's patients as they face a lot of issues regarding it. Even though the tremor reduction is temporary, in some certain cases it may help to improve quality of life. In addition to the current application of "Vilim ball", the lower limb tremor reduction investigational study may also be conducted but it may require design adjustments as the current shape of the

Table 3.15 Right hand muscle strength data

	Baseline Grip Strength (Md kg)	Baseline (Min kg)	Baseline (Max kg)	Baseline (A.M. kg)	Post Intervention Grip Strength (Md kg)	Post Intervention (Min kg)	Post Intervention (Max kg)	Post Intervention (A.M. kg)	U-value	p-value
Physiotherapy	27.00	20.60	38.60	27.69	26.65	19.90	37.60	27.65	71.50	0.999
Physiotherapy + vibrational medical device	27.10	18.20	38.10	27.50	28.90	19.10	37.40	28.12	67.50	0.795

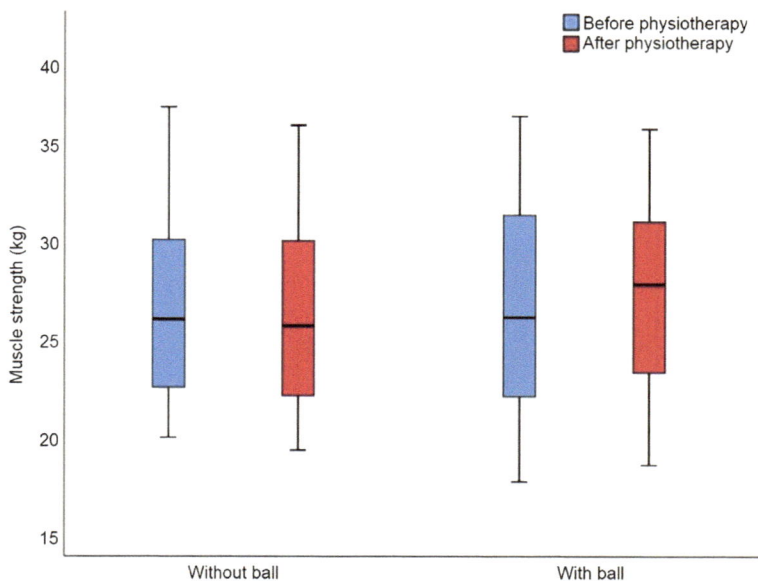

Fig. 3.72 Muscle strength in the right hand before and after physiotherapy

device is not convenient enough for this application. The application of "Vilim ball" to reduce rigidity may also be considered as this symptom is even more frequent than tremor and most of Parkinson's patients face it. Despite the positive findings, the sample size of this study was relatively small. This limitation can affect the generalizability; therefore, results may not be the same on a scale of a larger population.

3.5.3 Essential Tremor Reduction Results

We conducted a prospective, single-center, pragmatic clinical study [54], like routine medical care. In this study, the patients acted as their own controls. We assumed that a single-arm design (without sham control) is appropriate because the primary endpoint is objective, and it is unlikely that patients with essential tremor could achieve spontaneous remission [55]. We recorded the tremor data for 1 min before the intervention and 1 min after the intervention with an accelerometer and transformed the data with Fourier-transformation for power spectrum analysis [56]. The change in power spectrum analysis was the primary efficacy endpoint.

We presented data as the mean (standard deviation) or as the median and interquartile range if the data were asymmetrically distributed. We assessed the data symmetricity with the Normal Q-Q plots. We chose the significance level of $p < 0.05$. We compared the differences between the repeated measures of the primary endpoint with the Wilcoxon signed-rank test. We performed the statistical analysis with R version 3.5.0. All analyzed patients were included in the Efficacy and Safety analysis set. The efficacy and safety analysis sets were equivalent to the Intent-to-Treat Analysis Set.

The clinical investigation plan was developed in line with the EN ISO 14155-1:2009 Clinical Investigation of Medical Devices for Human Subjects—General Requirements, which details the general requirements for the conduct of clinical investigations and EN ISO 14155-2:2009 Clinical Investigation of Medical Devices for Human Subjects. Research with human subjects was performed in line with the Helsinki Declaration adopted by the 18th World Medical Assembly in Helsinki, Finland, in 1964, as last amended by the World Medical Assembly. All measures relating to the protection of human subjects were taken with the core principles of the Helsinki Declaration in mind. A general principle was held, "the rights, safety, and wellbeing of clinical investigation subjects shall be protected consistent with the ethical principles laid down in the Declaration of Helsinki" (EN ISO 14155-1:2009). Bioethics permission (BE-2-90) from the regional research ethics committee was received.

The subjects were asked to hold a smartphone in the dominant hand before vibrational therapy and after it. Tremor data were captured by using a mobile application that was designed to collect raw data (signal frequency 100 Hz) provided by the accelerometer. The primary endpoint was the decrease in the power spectrum (m^2/s^3 Hz) [57] after use of the investigated medical device. The baseline tremor power spectrum was evaluated. After that, vibrational therapy was performed for 5 min for each patient, and the postinterventional tremor power spectrum was evaluated. The difference between baseline and postinterventional tremor power spectrum was determined (as defined in the statistical analysis paragraph). Collected data were filtered to evaluate the range of 4–12 Hz, which is hand tremor frequency with diagnosed essential tremor.

The secondary efficacy endpoint was the patient's assessment of the vibrational therapy effectiveness in a Likert scale. Additionally, the patient's assessment of the tremor intensity before the intervention was assessed (Fig. 3.73).

A Tetras questionnaire was used to evaluate the tremor intensity before intervention [58] to establish a relationship between the accelerometry data and the Tetras estimate. The sample size was estimated during the conduct of the pilot part of the study after the evaluation of 5 patients before and after the use of the investigated medical device. This study was designed to have an α error probability = 0.05; power (1-β error probability) = 0.8; the expected size of difference was at least 0.01, and the effect size was at least 1. The total estimated sample size was 17 patients. The sample size was assessed with G*Power 3.1 [59]. The study population included subjects diagnosed with Essential tremors (Table 3.16).

A retrospective cross-sectional study was planned during the clinical development of the investigated medical device. The study population consisted of adult subjects with neurological diseases that cause movement disorders of hands, who signed informed patient consent during the meeting with the investigator. The primary efficacy outcome was the

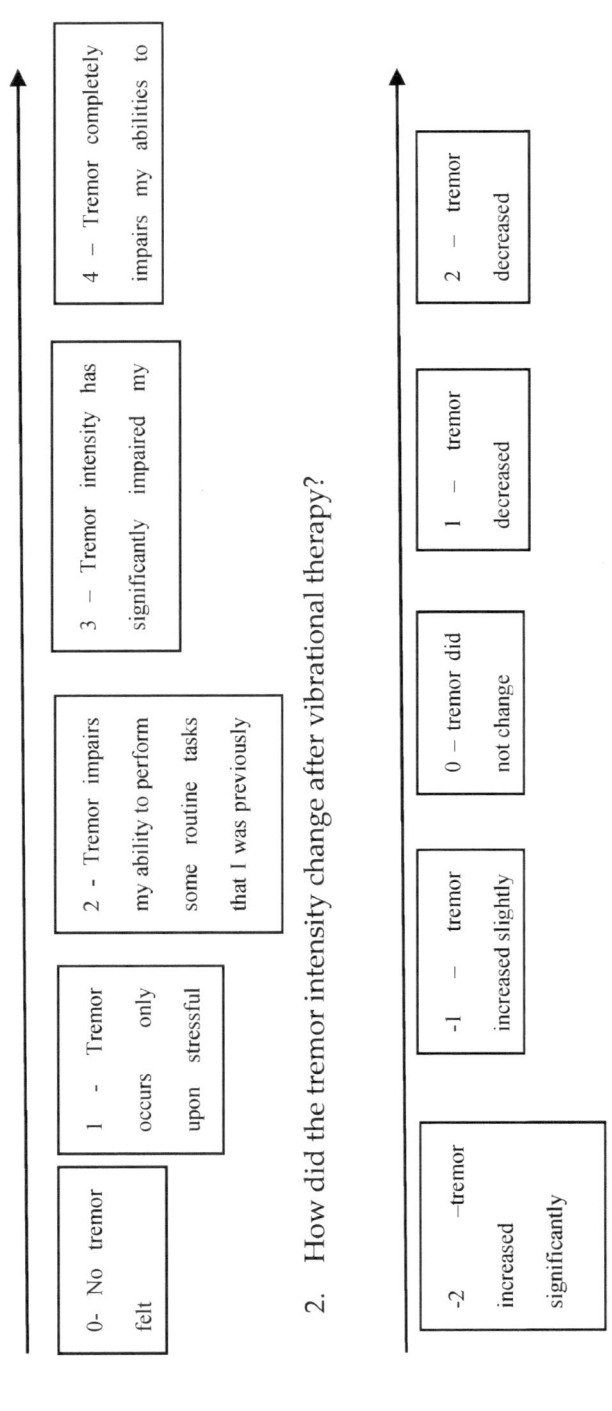

1. Please place a mark at a point on the scale that most accurately defines Your condition:

0- No tremor felt

1 - Tremor occurs only upon stressful

2 - Tremor impairs my ability to perform some routine tasks that I was previously

3 - Tremor intensity has significantly impaired my

4 - Tremor completely impairs my abilities to

2. How did the tremor intensity change after vibrational therapy?

-2 –tremor increased significantly

-1 – tremor increased slightly

0 – tremor did not change

1 – tremor decreased

2 – tremor decreased

Fig. 3.73 Secondary efficacy endpoint

Table 3.16 Inclusion and exclusion criteria

Inclusion criteria

1. Male and female subjects 18–65 years of age at the time of consent
2. Written informed consent provided by the patient
3. Patients are diagnosed with essential tremor

Exclusion criteria

1. Non-compliance
2. Substance-dependence
3. Uncontrolled medical illness (arterial hypertension, diabetes, severe liver or kidney failure)
4. Subjects with following abnormal laboratory values at screening visit:
   a. Hemoglobin <11.0 g/dL (<110.0 g/L) or hematocrit <30% (<0.30 v/v),
   b. White blood cell count <3.0 × 109/L (<3000/mm^3),
   c. Absolute neutrophil count of <1.5 × 109/L (<1500/mm^3),
   d. Absolute lymphocytes count of <0.5 × 109/L (<500/mm^3),
   e. Platelet count <100 × 109/L,
   f. Estimated creatinine clearance <40 mL/min based on the Cockcroft–Gault calculation or serum creatinine value greater than 1.5 times the upper limit of normal,
   g. Aspartate aminotransferase or alanine aminotransferase values greater than 2 times the upper limit of normal,
   h. Subject has positive results for hepatitis B surface antigens, antibodies to hepatitis B core antigens, hepatitis C virus, or human immunodeficiency virus,
   i. Other subjects who, in the opinion of the investigator, have any acute or chronic medical or psychiatric condition or laboratory abnormality at the screening that would impair the subject's capability to follow the study protocol

patient-reported outcome based on a non-validated patient telephone questionnaire [60]. Safety assessments were descriptive and included a summary of adverse events if they were observed. The safety assessment was conducted by the attending physician. The treating physician determined the need for physical examinations, vital signs, electrocardiography, and laboratory measurements (hematology, chemistry, and urinalysis) to assess safety.

In total, 6 men and 11 caucasian women with essential tremor were included in this study from 2017/05/01 and 2017/12/31. The mean age was 70.82 (8.03) years. Seven people reported the use of drugs for essential tremor. Five people reported alcohol consumption. Seven people had family members that had essential tremors. The primary endpoint was the tremor power spectrum. The distributions of the primary endpoint before the intervention and primary endpoint after the intervention were highly asymmetric: primary endpoint before the intervention mean 0.106 ± 0.221 median 0.009 (interquartile range 0.087) and primary endpoint after the intervention mean $= 0.042 \pm 0.078$; median $= 0.009$ (interquartile range 0.012); Wilcoxon signed-rank test V $= 123$; $p = 0.027$ (Table 3.17). Four cases were identified as investigated medical device inefficacy. Seven patients reported that vibrational therapy was not effective. Two patients reported an

Table 3.17 Investigated medical device effectiveness and baseline tremor intensity as reported by patients

	Tremor increased slightly	Tremor did not change	Tremor decreased slightly
Tremor occurs only upon stressful situation	0	0	1
Tremor impairs my ability to perform some routine tasks that I was previously capable of performing	0	4	3
Tremor intensity has significantly impaired my ability to perform daily tasks	2	3	3

increase in tremors after using the device. No other adverse events were reported by the patients included in this study. No serious adverse events were identified by the study investigators.

The primary endpoint before the intervention tremor power spectrum was correlated with the Tetras score. Spearman's rank correlation: rho 0.765, $p < 0.001$. A cross-sectional study was performed in patients with Essential and Parkinsonian tremor that used the "Vilim ball" prototype to assess the safety and efficacy of the "Vilim Ball". The investigation was held by scientists of interested party MB "Fidens" company, which invented the "Vilim ball". Bioethics permission (BE-2-90) from the regional research ethics committees was received. In total, 51 patients with the mean (standard deviation) age of 66.9 (16.28) were included (31 in the essential and 20 Parkinsonian tremors) in the study. The primary efficacy outcome was the Patient-Reported Outcome based on a non-validated patient telephone questionnaire. The secondary outcome was the occurrence of adverse events. Forty-eight patients reported improvement in tremor symptoms, and 49 reported an improvement in function. The patients used the "Vilim ball" for 7.63 (5.41) months. Thirty-eight patients were able to report the duration of improved function, which was 90.79 (68.83) minutes. Two patients reported a lack of efficacy of the proposed medical device during the study. No other serious adverse events were reported.

In the study [61], we found that local vibrational therapy is an effective treatment option in some patients. Our device has novel technological characteristics. However, previous attempts were made to develop medical devices for the treatment of essential tremors. Theoretical (conceptual) articles have been published by several authors regarding the use of the self-balancing device [62] and exoskeleton power-assist robot to treat essential tremors [63]. However, these concepts were not clinically developed.

Other devices went beyond the conceptual phase, and their efficacy was assessed in clinical trials. A pilot randomized sham-controlled pilot trial was conducted to see if local vibration is effective in patients with essential tremors. The pilot study revealed promising results, as the motor performance evaluated with the Archimedes spiral drawing task, improved after stimulation, when compared against baseline [64]. This research (with the same device) was followed with a pivotal study, where it was shown that subjects who received peripheral nerve stimulation did not show a significantly larger improvement in the Archimedes spiral task compared to sham but did show a significantly greater improvement in upper limb Tetras tremor scores ($p = 0.017$) compared to sham. No significant adverse events were reported; 3% of subjects experienced mild adverse events [65]. Vibrating Gaussian noise emitting manipulandum has been shown to improve motor performance. A pilot study showed that the application of Gaussian noise (3–35 Hz) reduces tremor (measured with accelerometric amplitude and electromyography activity) and improves the motor performance in individuals with enhanced physiological tremor [66]. It was also shown that Stochastic resonance of 0–15 Hz (a phenomenon in nonlinear systems characterized by a response increase in the system induced by a particular level of input noise) improves the motor task in healthy individuals and that the higher degree SR is more pleasant with 0–300 Hz and 250–300 Hz noise bandwidths than for 0–15 Hz. The principle of action of the manipulandum used in these studies resembles that of the "Vilim ball" [67]. Wrist tendon vibration (TV, 70 Hz) was applied to the forearm wrist musculature improved arm stability, as evidenced by the decreased magnitude of hand tangential velocity at the target. Improved stability was accompanied by a decrease in muscle activity throughout the arm, as well as a mean decrease in grip pressure in 10 hemiparetic stroke patients [68].

We did not identify major safety risks during the clinical study; however, the local hand arm vibration is associated with the development of certain conditions: Raynaud's phenomenon, carpal tunnel syndrome [69], vibration-induced white finger disease [70], finger pain, back pain, muscular pain or fatigue [71], chronic subdural hematoma (local application to the head) [72], skin irritation, finger blood flow reduction [73], and neck and upper limb musculoskeletal disorders. Vibration can increase the postural and rest tremor [74], exacerbate Dupuytren's contracture, and have various osteoarticular effects (hand and carpal bone vacuoles and cysts, Kienbock's disease, navicular pseudoarthrosis, olecranon spurs, and osteoarthrosis of the wrist and elbow joints). People with the known HTR1B gene may be more susceptible to the development of secondary Raynauds' phenomenon due to vibration exposure [75]. Prolonged vibration may reduce the manual dexterity [76]. Systemic adverse effects that result from local hand-arm vibration may include a cardiovascular response (echocardiographic changes (an increase in ejection fraction and stroke volume, enlarged left ventricular diastolic dimension, and reduction in heart rate) and lower blood pressure) [77], immunological changes (e.g., an increase in T cell lymphocytes of CD4 and CD8), and suppression of serum total cholesterol and triglyceride levels [78]. Vibration may promote vascular injury, endothelial injury, microvasculature changes [79], defects in vascular repair, and intravascular abnormalities (release of vasoactive mediators) [80].

3.6   Alternative Therapeutic Devices

3.6.1   Effect of Electromagnetic Stimulation on Heart Rate Variability

The relationship between solar and geomagnetic factors and the response of the autonomic nervous system to changes in solar and geomagnetic activity in time courses and delays has been established [81]. Autonomic nervous system activity responds to changes in geomagnetic and solar activity during periods of normal undisturbed activity, and it is initiated at different times after the changes in various environmental factors and persists for varying periods of time. Increases in solar wind intensity have been correlated with increases in heart rate, which we interpret as a biological stress response. It has been shown that the increase in solar activity reduces the intensity of the geomagnetic field, which can aggravate heart disease. To address this deficit in the Earth's magnetic field, we proposed the use of an electromagnetic heart pacemaker. Figure 3.74 shows both the analog and digital prototypes of this device.

   Tests conducted on a group of vulnerable individuals have demonstrated that even a very weak electromagnetic field, with a strength equivalent to the geomagnetic field (up to 70 µT), applied either to the whole body or locally for 8–12 min, 1–2 times per day over a period of 10–20 days, provides clinical benefits in most patients (Fig. 3.75). Sensitive

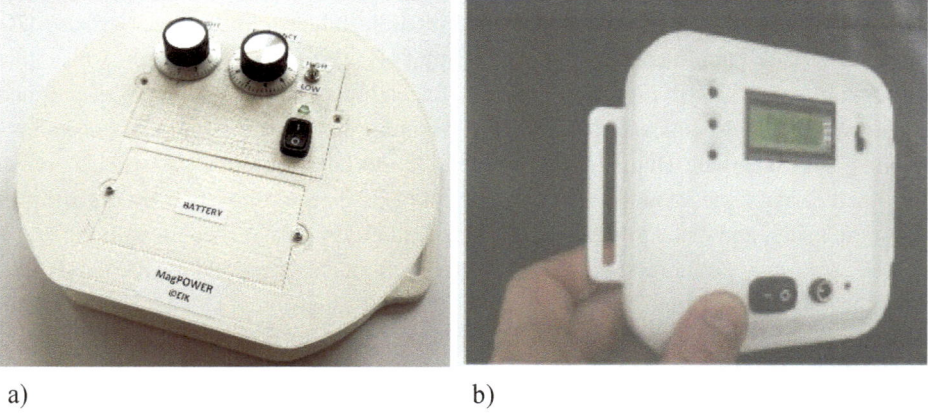

a)   b)

Fig. 3.74 Analog (**a**) and digital (**b**) prototypes of earth's magnetic field compensators for heart stimulation

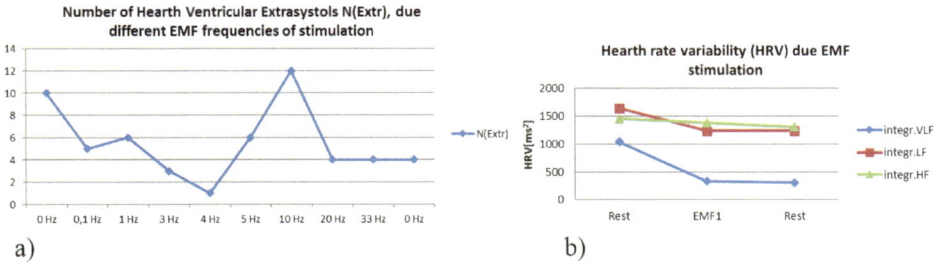

Fig. 3.75 Number of heart ventricular extrasystoles, due different electromagnetic frequencies of stimulation (**a**) and heart rate variability due electromagnetic stimulation (**b**)

patients show improvement within one to two days, while the majority of others require 5–10 days to experience benefits.

Figure 3.75 shows that heart rate variability under the influence of 4 Hz electromagnetic pulses is minimal, suggesting the potential to delay the onset of infarction [82].

3.6.2 Acoustically Compatible Chamber for Whole Body Therapy

Until now, the main attention in the study of the biodynamic characteristics of the human body and the effect of vibrations on the internal organs has been directed to the maintenance of health indicators of vehicle drivers [82, 83]. With the aim of systematically studying how different physiological systems of the human body dynamically interact and collectively behave to influence different physiological states and functions, we created an acoustically compatible chamber (Fig. 3.76). Four powerful loudspeakers installed in this device change the frequency of the sound they produce into a wide spectrum of acoustic vibrations, the specific frequencies of which are excited by the natural vibration modes of human organs. As a result, the vibrations of these individual organs switch to resonance modes with increased amplitudes that accelerate blood circulation and, at the same time, healing processes. This chamber can be used to study physiological, neurological, and biochemical processes under the influence of sound vibrations. Restricting sound to vibration focuses on low-frequency sound (up to 250 Hz), including infrasound (1–16 Hz). The mechanisms of vibration response can be categorized into hemodynamic, neurological, and musculoskeletal effects. Basic mechanisms of hemodynamic effects include endothelial cell stimulation and vibropercussion; neurological effects include protein kinase activation, nerve stimulation with a focus on vibratory analgesia, and oscillatory coherence; musculoskeletal effects include the muscle stretch reflex, bone cell progenitor fate, the influence of vibration on bone ossification and resorption, and anabolic effects on the spine and intervertebral discs. The complexity of the field of vibrational medicine

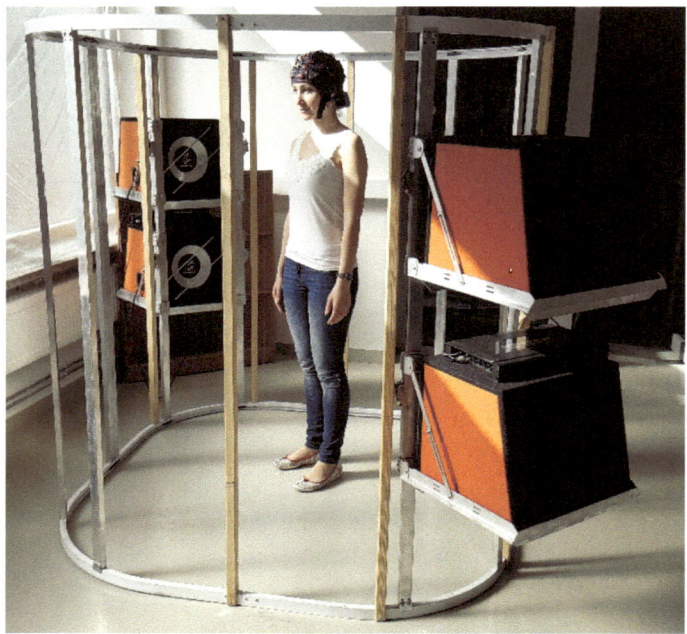

Fig. 3.76 Acoustically compatible chamber for therapy

necessitates specific comparative research on the methods of vibration delivery, the area of the body or surface stimulated, and the effects of specific frequencies and intensities on particular mechanisms, along with greater interdisciplinary cooperation and focus. When conducting such experiments, the complexity of the field of vibrational medicine should be accounted for in specific comparative studies that examine the type of vibration transmission, the area of the body or surface stimulated, the effects of specific frequencies and intensities on particular mechanisms, and the need for greater interdisciplinary cooperation and focus.

3.6.3 Osteopathic Therapy Device

Osteopathy is a type of health care system of diagnosis and therapy that emphasizes the relationship between structure and function in the body, and the ways it can be affected through manipulative therapy and other treatment modalities. Five components should be considered: motility of the central nervous system, fluctuation of the reciprocal tension membranes, mobility of the cranial bones, involuntary movement of the sacrum between the ilia, and fluctuation of the cerebrospinal fluid [84, 85]. A chair (Fig. 3.77) has been designed with a vertical up-down actuator in the back, which activates the cerebrospinal fluid, causing it to pulsate around the spinal cord at a frequency of 6–12 cycles per minute (0.1–0.5 Hz).

Thanks to a sensor around the patient's chest that registers changes in chest volume (Fig. 3.78a), the vertical up-down actuator in the back chair is activated by the respiratory rate, called the cranial rhythmic pulse, which is independent of the heart rate.

The developed sensor is ideal for laboratory testing due to its good measurement repeatability and ability to accurately measure chest volumes. For convenience, respiratory rhythm information can be sent wirelessly to the controller of the therapeutic device

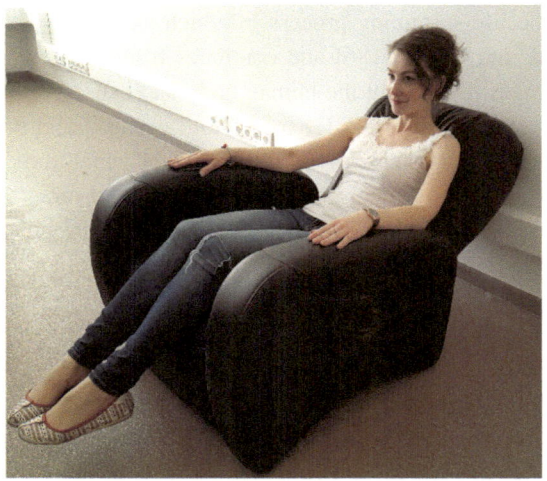

Fig. 3.77   Spinal cord activation chair

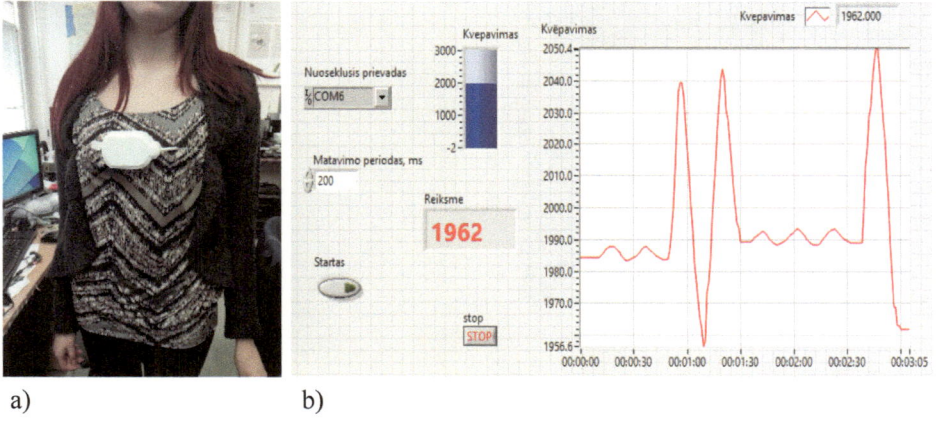

a)   b)

Fig. 3.78   A chest-mounted breath recording device (**a**) and its graphical interface (**b**)

(Fig. 3.78b), and the sensor itself can be used in other cases of remote monitoring of the patient's condition. The graphical user interface is designed to be user-friendly and informative enough to monitor the required parameters. This graphical interface is generated as a standalone executable that can be installed on another computer without the full Lab-View software package. It helps to perform in-depth analysis of breathing by measuring respiratory cycle, amplitude, phase difference and other parameters. The developed sensor has a unique design due to the encoder used in it, which records changes in breathing. This design made it easier to place it on the subject. For data transmission, 2.4 GHz radio modules are used, which are integrated into both the data transmitter and receiver devices.

The respiratory rate, also called the primary respiratory movement, also known as the Breath of Life, is the life-sustaining process in which gases are exchanged between the body and the outside atmosphere [86] and continues from the newborn's first breath. It is a process that spreads throughout the human body and causes various harmonic movements, such as the "Long Tide", 0.05 Hz (of "2 to 3 cycles") and the Cranial Rhythmic Pulse. The "Long Tide" is the basic rhythm, the pace of which directly correlates to the breath of life, oscillating at a frequency of 6 cycles every 10 min. "2 to 3" (also known as 2.5 cycles/minute). 2.5 cycles/minute is a "Long Tide" harmonica that is not modulated by the central or autonomic nervous systems and has a stable rhythm. The Breath of Life flows through the patient's body, activating the patient's healing powers. Activating the spine according to the frequency of breathing can be effective in treating the following ailments: arthritis and back pain, blood circulation and digestive problems, elbow and headaches, accelerating relaxation, neutralizing migraines, alleviating sports injuries and strains, reducing muscle spasms, rheumatic and neck pain, neuralgia. Temperature changes of the massaged back are shown in Fig. 3.79.

During the massage, not only the temperature drops, but also the heart rate (Fig. 3.80).

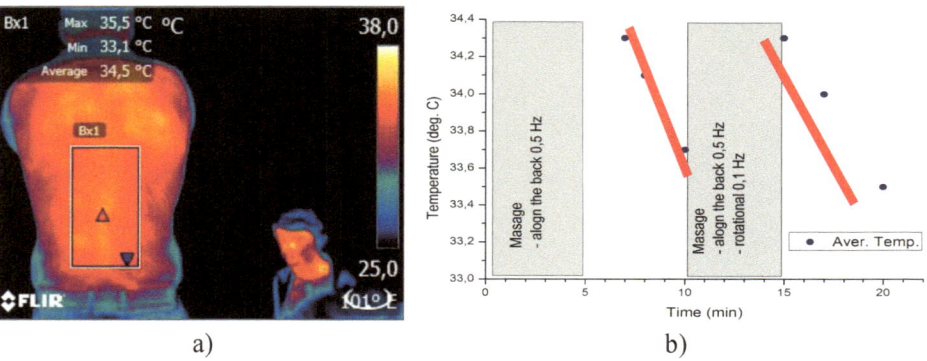

a)   b)

Fig. 3.79 Temperature changes of the massaged back: **a** in the thermal imager, **b** after longitudinal and complex massage

Fig. 3.80 Heart rate variability depending on the intensity and duration of massage movements

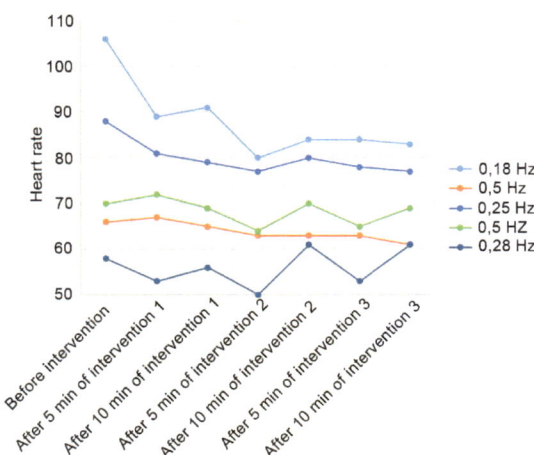

The developed data receiving sensor (Fig. 3.78a) is versatile and can be used in various other projects that require low-power wireless data transmission. It is most convenient to use the currently very popular Bluetooth low energy devices for data registration and storage. Bluetooth low energy is wireless communication that has low power consumption, so it can be powered by small batteries and work for a long time without an external power source. Thanks to a smaller battery, the Bluetooth low energy standard allows the dimensions of wireless devices to be reduced. The main advantages of Bluetooth low energy are durability, simplicity, low power consumption, and price. The Bluetooth low energy connection enables wireless data transfer 8 times faster than the previous version of Bluetooth. The speed of 24 Mb/s allows much faster data transfer. In addition, Bluetooth has a long wireless range. This version provides a reliable wireless connection up to 50 m, but using low power settings reduces the wireless range. The communication distance is also affected by the environment in which communication takes place, e.g. the signal can be suppressed if the communication devices are in different rooms. The system consists of several Bluetooth low energy transmitters and a Bluetooth low energy Wi-Fi transmitter and receiver in one. Each Bluetooth low energy transmitter has its own unique address, which is known to the receiver. The transmitters send data about temperature, pulse, respiration intensity, etc. at every set moment and the receiver registers them. The collected data array is sent via Wi-Fi connection and placed in the "cloud" (server). According to the user's needs, the data (Fig. 3.81) can be displayed in the form of graphs or tables both on a computer and on a smartphone—anywhere there is an Internet connection.

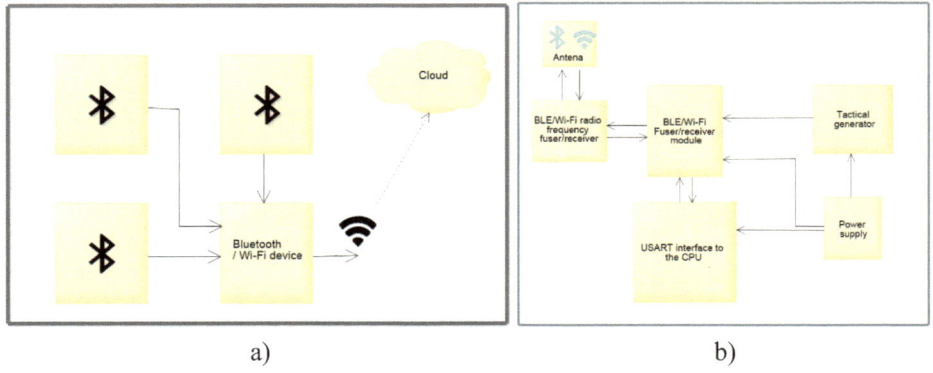

a)   b)

Fig. 3.81 Data collection and transmission system (**a**) and structure of the control device (**b**)

3.6.4 Positioning of the Therapy Device

Gamma Knife can target intracranial lesions with a high degree of accuracy. A headframe is rigidly attached to the patient's skull to establish a stereotactic coordinate system and provide a means to precisely position the patient in stereotactic space. Following stereotactic target localization and radiosurgical treatment planning, the skull and headframe are then moved with sub-millimeter precision to bring a target volume into the radiological focus of the Gamma Knife unit. However, for Gamma Knife models 4C and earlier, the treatable intracranial volume may be limited by collisions between the skull/headframe and the Gamma Knife collimator helmet, or by mechanical travel limitations of the skull/headframe within the collimator helmet. Both of these treatment-limiting conditions can only be identified after the headframe is placed on the patient. If the volume of interest cannot be treated with the initial headframe placement, additional headframe placements or a different treatment approach is required. We have developed and patented [87] a stereotactic pneumatic headframe positioning device for the Gamma Knife system (Fig. 3.82).

In clinical practice, this positioning system has been tested in real conditions by applying the frame to 5 patients. The procedure was performed in the Brain Surgery Department of the LSMU. A shorter procedure time, a smaller number of participating personnel and a smaller need for adjustments made it easier to achieve the desired frame position of the neurosurgeon.

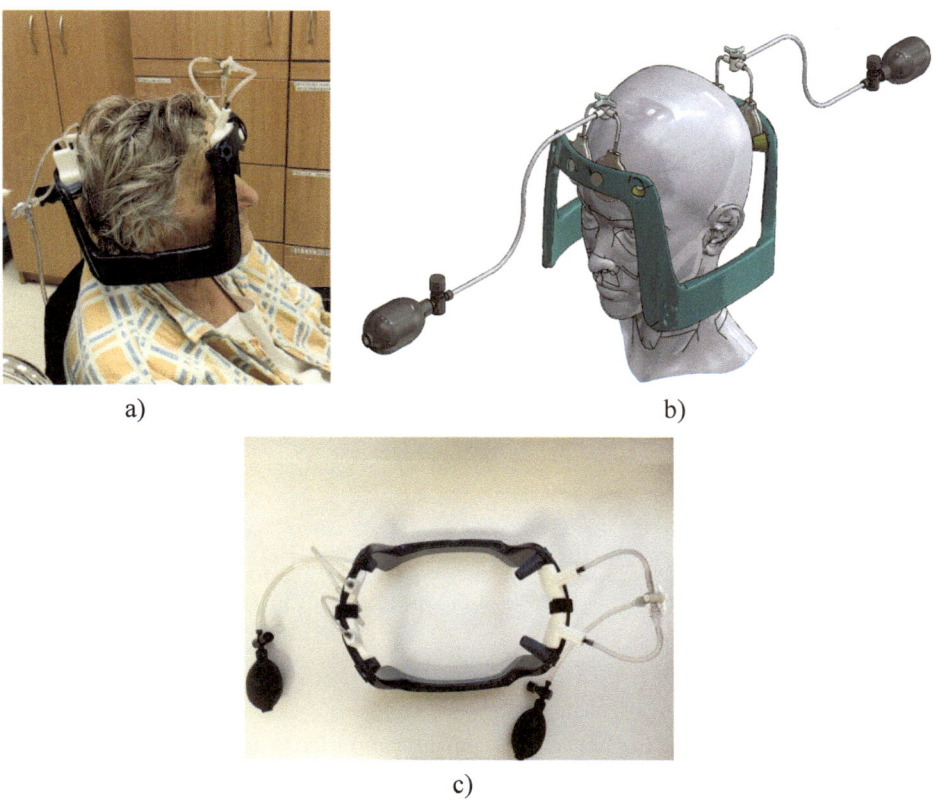

a)   b)

c)

Fig. 3.82 Stereotaxic radiosurgery planning using a stereotaxic frame: **a**—on the patient's head, **b**—shema and **c**—expanded view

3.6.5   Device for Human Vestibular Research

A device has been developed (Fig. 3.83) that allows to evaluate the mechanisms causing dizziness and specific symptoms: dizziness due to peripheral vestibular disorder or dizziness of central origin.

One of the possible methods is measuring the inclination of the head angle in relation to the vertical axis. The essence of this method is based on the assumption that in the presence of vestibular dysfunction, not only the vestibuloocular reflex is damaged, but also parts of other reflexes, due to which the activity of the middle vestibular nuclei of the contralateral side is relatively strengthened, the elevation and intorsion of the eye of the contralateral side is formed, and the damaged extortion of half an eye. Due to an intact vestibulospinal tract, in the presence of a disturbed assessment of gravity, the muscles of the neck on the same side become more spastic (due to erroneously intense

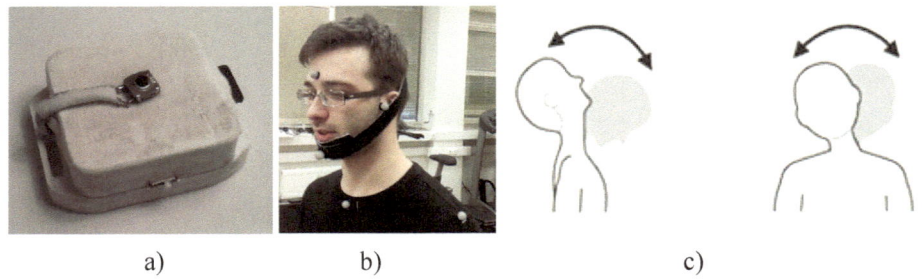

a)   b)   c)

Fig. 3.83 Device for vestibular research: **a** picture, **b** device on the patient's head, **c** head movements

Fig. 3.84 Angular changes in
head position

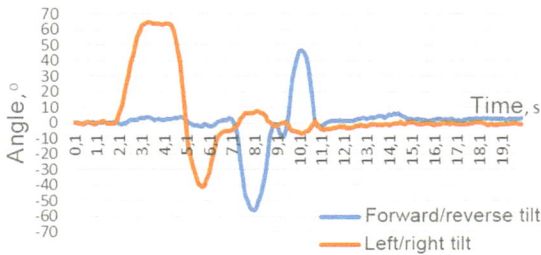

impulse sending), and the corrective neck position in order to maintain proper vision—therefore, over time, the tilt of the head in relation to the vertical axis should become more pronounced. Recorded angular changes in head position are shown in Fig. 3.84.

The accuracy of the device is $\pm 0.2°$. It was tested using a Qualisys 3D motion analysis system with a measurement frequency of 100 Hz and a mechanical goniometer. Data was recorded on a microSD card, transmitted via Bluetooth, and stored in the cloud.

3.7   Personalization of Cardiovascular Flow Reconstruction

3.7.1   Stent-Graft Adaptation

The very first step associated with aortic personalization processes begins with the scanning of this organ affected by *abdominal* aortic aneurysm in the body of the patient for which implantation of the implant of the stent-graft will be made. A computerized tomography scan (Fig. 3.85) shows patient-specific geometry parameters of *abdominal* aortic aneurysm.

Since the modern design process usually starts with simulation, the computational model of the personalized implant is necessary to build from the design scheme which reflects the constructive features of a scanned aortic shape (Fig. 3.86).

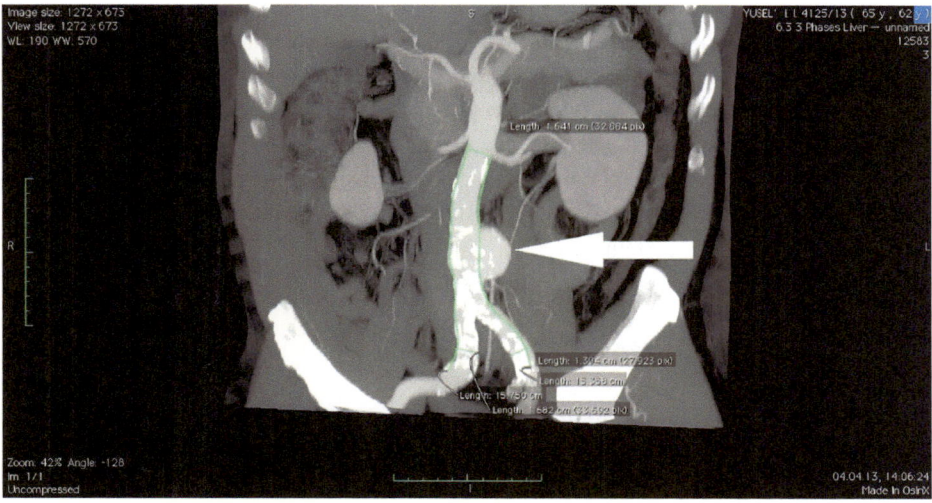

Fig. 3.85 A computerized tomography scan of *abdominal* aortic aneurysm

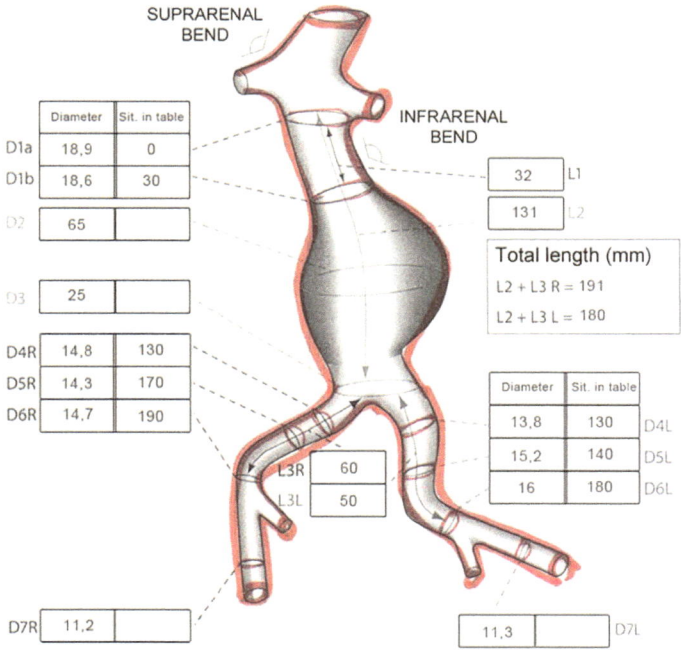

Fig. 3.86 The computational model of *abdominal* aortic aneurysm

The main parameter for the initial computational model according to Fig. 3.86 is the interior diameter of scanned aorta. In our case it is equal to 25 mm. Other initial data are related to the blood pressure, velocity, and the shape of the stent-graft. In the COMSOL Multiphysics interface, the input parameters of fluid, pressure and velocity are necessary to define. The aortic pressures were derived from non-invasive measurement of brachial blood pressure and suprasystolic waveform. Noninvasive magnetic resonance velocity mapping, to determine the hemodynamic significance of blood flow in aorta was used for a certain patient in a certain condition.

3.7.2   Mathematical Model of Blood Flow

The main objective of this study is to create a model of blood flow in COMSOL Multiphysics software for future design and manufacturing of personalized endovascular prostheses [88, 89]. The model should be adequate to the real conditions of fluid flow and comply with the laws of hydrodynamics. Therefore, to achieve this, the initial parameters were taken from the results of patient diagnosis. Verifying the adequacy of the simulation results in the mathematical model to those in the physical one, the liquid flow parameters should correlate with the experimental data.

The computational model is presented in the form of the Navier–Stokes equations that describe the motion of fluids and can be considered as Newton's second law imposed on the fluid flow [90]. In the case of a compressible Newtonian fluid, we have

$$\rho\left(\frac{\partial u}{\partial t} + u \cdot \nabla u\right) = -\nabla p + \nabla \cdot \left(\mu\left(\nabla u + (\nabla u)^{\mathrm{T}}\right) - \frac{2}{3}\mu(\nabla \cdot u)\mathrm{I}\right) + F, \qquad (3.34)$$

where ρ is the density, $u = (u, v)$ is the fluid velocity, p is the pressure, I is the unit diagonal matrix, η is the dynamic viscosity, and F is the volume force.

The equations are always solved as a system using the following equality:

$$\frac{\partial \rho}{\partial t} + \nabla \cdot (\rho u) = 0. \qquad (3.35)$$

The Navier–Stokes equations define the conservation of momentum, while the previous equation represents the conservation of mass.

In the case of high Reynolds numbers, the initial forces are much higher than the viscous forces. These turbulent flow problems are temporary in nature. The simulations using Navier–Stokes equations are often beyond the computational power under such conditions. Therefore, Reynolds-Averaged Navier–Stokes formulation of the Navier–Stokes equations could be used, which averages the velocity and pressure fields in time [91]:

$$\rho(U \cdot \nabla U) + \nabla \cdot \mu_\tau \left(\nabla U + (\nabla U)^T - \frac{2}{3} \mu_\tau (\nabla \cdot U) I \right)$$

$$= -\nabla P + \nabla \cdot \left(\mu (\nabla U + (\nabla U)^T) - \frac{2}{3} \mu (\nabla \cdot U) I \right) + F \tag{3.36}$$

$$\nabla \cdot (\rho U) = 0, \tag{3.37}$$

where U is the time-averaged velocity and P is the time-averaged pressure. μT defines the turbulent viscosity.

First, a mathematical 2D model (Fig. 3.87) of straight channel was designed according to the dimensions of scanned aorta and was idealized by passing the liquid through a direct channel.

According to the requirements of the housing and fixing points of the experimental setup, a stent-graft model was designed. The measurement area of 80 mm in length was considered because in the experimental setup the stent-graft had to be inserted on the input and output channels. This shortens the measurement area yet does not affect the experimental or simulation results. The mirror diameters and lengths on the left and right sides of the stent-graft model were designed in compliance with the experimental setup. These irregularities of the channel surface affect fluid flow and output parameters, therefore it is necessary to imitate a model that is as like such conditions as possible. The main output parameter is expressed by the Δp (pressure differential). Therefore, the pressure distribution on the entire plot in the COMSOL graphical extent was selected when

Fig. 3.87 Mathematical 2D model of straight channel imitating aorta

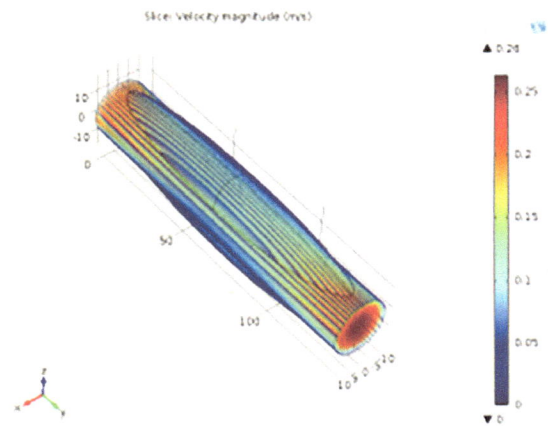

analyzing the results of blood flow simulation. The steady and unsteady 3D blood flows via stent-implant models were proposed. In the steady case, an aortic aneurysm model of 10.0 cm in length was simulated using the Reynolds numbers of 350 and 700; whereas in the unsteady case an aortic aneurysm model was simulated using the Reynolds numbers of 350, 700 and 1400 [92].

3.7.3 Modeling and Manufacturing of Stent-Graft Prostheses

The next step was to build a COMSOL Multiphysics model of fluid flow passing through the endovascular prosthetic stent-graft. The scheme was carried out according to the patient aorta scan. Pressure was considered as the main input parameter ($p = 24\text{kPa}$). A similar study of a stent-graft model was conducted to compare results and find out how the channel roughness affects the pressure gradient.

The result obtained from the analysis during flow simulation inside implant (inlet $V = 0.226$ m/s, outlet $P = 22$ kPa) is represented in Fig. 3.88. As we can see, the pressure mean increases and drops before and after the mounting rings of the implant. These alterations indicate how these rings influence curves' inconsistency to the theoretical one in the ideal conditions of the straight channel.

Further, the blood stream flow rates for various parameters (Q-flow rate) taken from patient diagnosis results, namely $Q = 400$, 480 550, 680, 760, 838 and 900 L/h, were

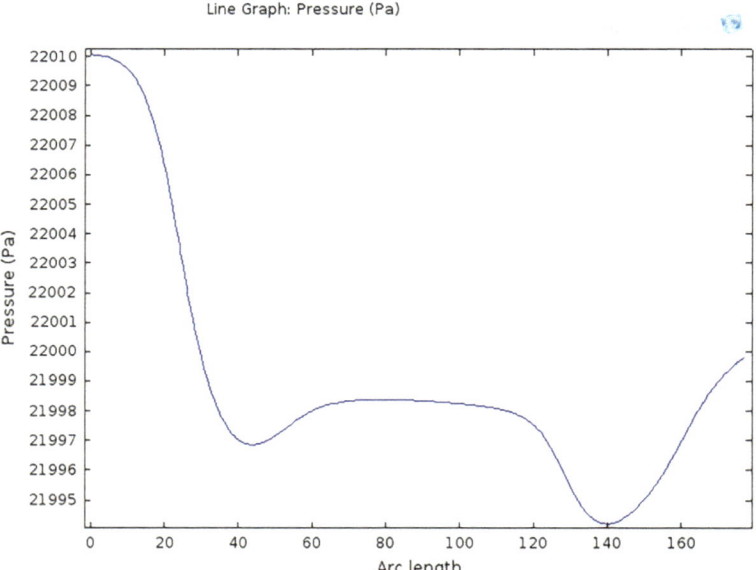

Fig. 3.88 The blood pressure changes in aorta

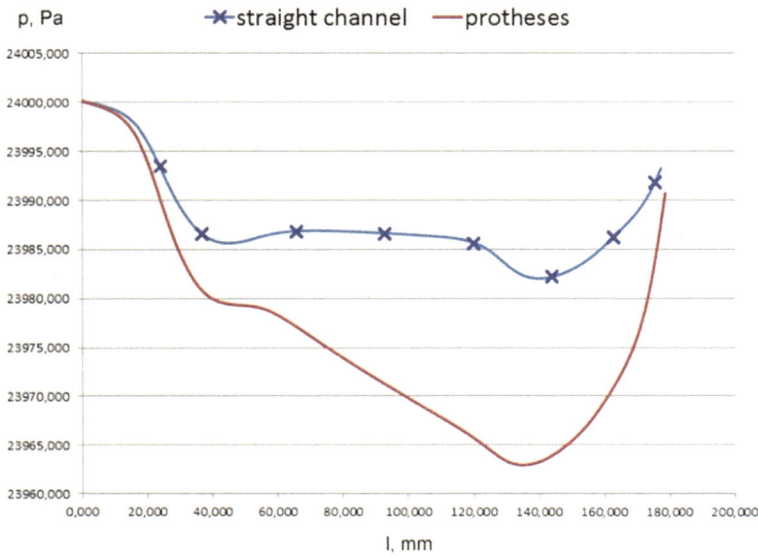

Fig. 3.89 The characteristic curves of the pressure in aorta and prosthesis at different Δp

identified. Comparing the pressure distribution graphs in the cases of fluid passing through the direct channel and the endovascular prosthesis, the characteristic curves of the pressure at different Δp could be illustrated by Fig. 3.89. As we can see, the pressure gradient in stent-graft type of the channel is sharper comparing to a straight channel. Pressure means becomes lower during the length of measurement area.

As in the case with the passage of liquid through the straight channel, it is necessary to analyze the behavior of pressure in the case of an incoming velocity parameter. The result of the simulation under conditions (inlet $V = 0.232$ m/s, outlet $P = 19$ kPa) showed the same behavior patterns. The maximum difference in pressure Δp_{max} for both cases could be determined. During the simulation, for the inlet P it was $\Delta p_{max} = 28$ Pa, while for the inlet V it was $\Delta p_{max} = 25$ Pa.

Next, the calculations were repeated considering human blood perfusion parameters. For the initial study, velocity and pressure values were assumed: $V = 150, 170, 190, 210, 230$ and 250 mm/s; $P = 13,333$ Pa. The blood consistency has distinct characteristics of water, which was used previously; therefore, set the following values: density $\rho = 1060$ kg / m^3, dynamic viscosity $\mu = 0.005$ Pa s.

A 2D endovascular prosthesis model (with the dimensions $L = 80$ mm, $D = 25$ mm) like a physical one was used in the experiment. The height of corrugations was 1 mm. The obtained simulation results are presented in Table 3.11. On closer examination it is possible to conclude similarities between the behavior patterns and relationship of linearity. The relation between the velocity, the Reynolds number, and the output pressure difference is shown in Table 3.18.

Table 3.18 The simulation results

v, mm/sec	Reynolds number	Δp, Pa
150	7950	15
170	9010	18
190	10,070	21
210	11,130	25
230	12,190	29
250	13,250	33

Furthermore, the analysis of the shape of the resulting curve, namely, comparing the cases of inlet V and outlet P, enables us to speak of a homogeneous nature of the fluid flow. It is also necessary to consider the maximum value of the pressure difference. Thus, for the first case, in which the incoming flow parameter is pressure, we have $\Delta p_{max} = 18$ Pa. For the second one, where the incoming flow parameter is speed, we get $\Delta p_{max} = 16$ Pa. The parameters are different, yet very close in value. Furthermore, the results where non-disruptive flow was observed, permits to start the manufacturing process of the aorta stent-graft.

Only when the ideal blood flow at the site of the abdominal aorta is reached, derived parameters are passed to the manufacture, where high-precision equipment (Fig. 3.90) creates a personalized stent-graft. The special machines can produce as many as three branches from the main channel of the aorta, which is sufficient for a successful application in practice.

The implant was designed for a particular patient, considering the basic calculations of these parameters with the maximum coverage of the iliac arteries. A unique design of the aortic stent-graft enabled surgical treatment of aneurysms of the thoracic aorta during operations with artificial circulation. A blood vessel prosthesis of the original

Fig. 3.90 Stent-graft manufacturing unit

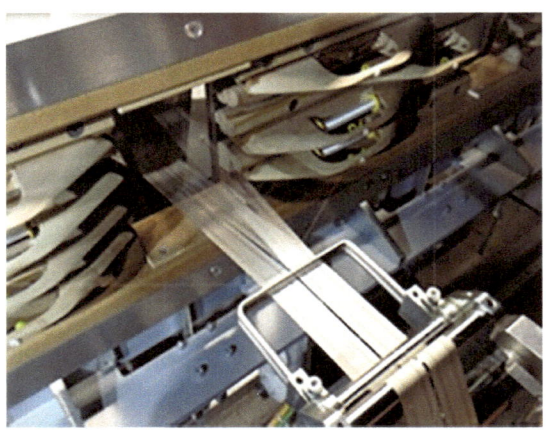

multi-layered weave seamless design was manufactured using ultra-high-strength threads that provide zero permeability of blood. The competitive advantage gained is the availability of transverse fluting, which allows the blood vessel prosthesis to restore its original shape after stretching, and inner-outer gelatin coating which, after implantation into the body, provides neointima formation on the inner surface and germination of the connective tissue.

A device for occlusion of the left atrial appendage with a special weave technology ensuring minimal risk of blood clots and high fixation process was developed. It assures the following: reliability of installation in the cavity (left atrial appendage); minimum risk of blood clots; high likelihood of complete occlusion of the left atrial appendage; low probability of residual blood flow, which contributes to the rapid shutdown of the cavity from circulation and thrombosis of the distal part of the left atrial appendage (blood clots prevent migration of the left atrial appendage into the general circulation); and high flexibility and control structure that helps to prevent dislocation of the occlusions during implantation. The available manufacturing equipment enable to develop such stent-implants manufacturing issues:

- Spiral blood flow in aorta. Since the heart is twisted on its axis and the aortic arch is curved, tapered, and twisted, it is normal that blood circulation acquires spiral motion. Blood flowing in a spiral pattern helps to reduce damage to the arterial wall as it diminishes forces acting laterally and reduces energy needed to move blood around the arterial system. Angioscopy has revealed a rifled endoluminal arterial surface characteristic of most of the arteries. This internal structure of the vessel may be considered to generate the spiral torque in the blood flow passing through the vessel and could be realized in the stent-graft during manufacturing. The main task of the stent-graft design prepared for manufacturing is related to the simulation results that the structural parameters of the internal helical surface of stent-graft depends on the patient cardiovascular system physiological peculiarities. Therefore, developed mathematical and experimental models confirm the opportunity to generate flow patterns like that in blood vessels with the aim to maintain spiral blood flow and thus improve patency rates.
- Glass-like coatings for cardiovascular implant application. Cardiovascular implants might be improved by using glass in their manufacturing, i.e. nitinol alloys used as a stent material may be coated with thick layers of glass. To tackle the issue of chronic inflammation as a response to a foreign body and to meet the needs for patient comfort, the surface material should possess the features of biocompatibility, i.e. ability to properly respond in a particular situation, and immunogenicity, i.e. ability to trigger an immune reaction (for example, inflammation). This method ensures a range of attractive properties which make them adequate in many applications such as drug delivery, bone tissue regeneration, and implant manufacturing.

• Restenosis and thrombosis reduction with stent lining. Research and development
  activities carried out on alternative stenting therapies and such devices as polymer
  and metal bio absorbable implants and drug eluting stents were tested to make them
  adequate for use. Naturally occurring vascular endothelial cells are attracted by electrical field acting on a stent. These cells are inherently present in the arterial system and,
  if planted on the stent's lumen, they would accept the stent as body part. The cell lipid
  membrane covers all human cells, and its outer surface carries a polarized electrical
  charge. In the human body, most cells contain a net negative going potential. It is also
  important that a unique electrical signature characterizes each cell type.

After the production stage of a stent-graft, the manufactured prototype of stent-graft needs
to be tested experimentally. Therefore, the experimental set-up (Fig. 3.91) was assembled
to ensure precise measurements of flow parameters.

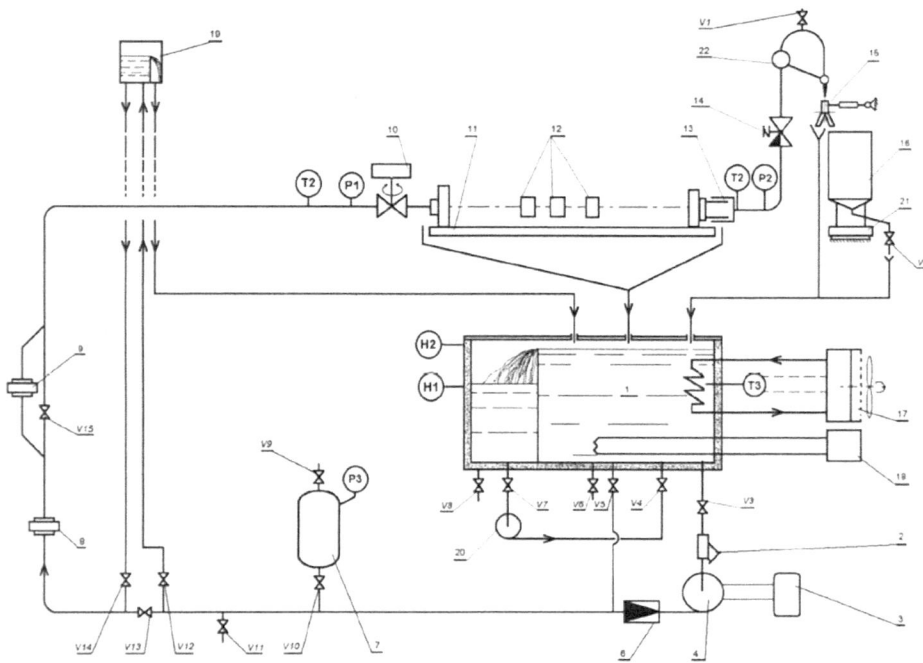

Fig. 3.91 Experimental set-up for flow measurement

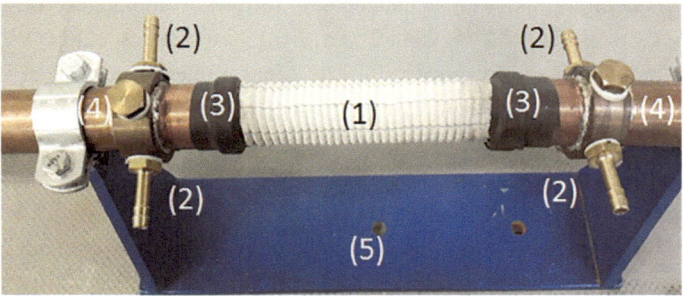

Fig. 3.92 Stent anchoring bracket: 1-stent, 2- supports, 3- nozzles, 4- outlet tubes

3.7.4 Validation of the Mathematical Model Adequacy

Fluid from the main tank 1 goes through the mechanical cleaning filter 2 and with a centrifugal pump 4, consisting of a frequency converter 3, is fed to the pressure line equipped with a non-return valve 6, which prevents leakage of fluid into the vessel 7 when the main pump is suspended. Fluid is supplied to the reference flow meters 8 and 9 knot through the pressure line, after which it enters a working Sect. 11 where pilot flow meters are mounted 12. Between these flow meters, a manufactured stent-graft was integrated (Fig. 3.3.91, 10). Fluid flowing by a longitudinal compensation node 13 and a control valve 14 is routed by a flow directing device 15 to the balance tank 16 or to the main container 1. A refrigerating machine 17 evaporator is mounted on the main tank for fluid cooling, which was not used in our experiment. An electric heater 18 with adjustable temperature is equipped for raising the temperature. Depending on the flow rate, one of two flowmeters 8 and 9 could be selected.

The fabricated stent was fixed in the flow measurement stand in a special holder 5 (Fig. 3.92), where stent 1 was fixed in supports 2 through special nozzles 3 at the fluid inlet and outlet tubes 4.

The experiment was conducted with three types of different stent-grafts. First, a straight plastic stent-graft was used to compare experimental results with theoretical calculations. After the identification of adequacy between theoretical and experimental models of three types of stent-grafts (straight, corrugated and involuted) were integrated in the measurement part of the hydraulic scheme. The experiment was conducted with low-stream equipment, where the stable flow rate from 0.01 to 3 m^3/h was ensured with an accuracy of $\pm 0.2\%$.

Measurement conditions were changed as follows: temperature T from 18 to 40 °C, ±0.07 °C, working pressure from 2 kPa, ±0.1%, when flow rate Q was 100 L/h, to 80 kPa, when water flow rate reaches 1200 L/h. Measurements were taken in 1.2 m-long section of the working channel, comprising pressure measurement gauges installed before and after the integrated stent-graft. Pressure difference was measured using FKCW (Fuji Electronics) transmitter, the accuracy of which is ±0.3 Pa.

First, pressure difference was measured in the straight plastic stent-graft which was 100 mm long, 25 mm diameter and the distance between pressure measurement slots was 190 mm. The pressure means were compared to the recalculated ones according to theoretical formulas. Pressure alteration depends on channel roughness, resistance coefficient, and flow type, which is turbulent.

Pressure calculations [93] for the round channel are as follows:

$$\Delta p = \xi \frac{l}{d} \cdot \frac{\rho \bar{v}^2}{2} \tag{3.38}$$

where ξ is the resistance coefficient, l is the specific length, m; d is the channel diameter, m; ρ is the density kg/m^3, and v is the stream velocity, m/s.

Velocity is calculated from flow rate Q:

$$Q = v \cdot A = v\pi r^2 \tag{3.39}$$

where r is the channel radius, m.

Resistance coefficient is calculated using the following:

$$\xi = 0.31464 \cdot (\text{Re})^{-1/4}, \tag{3.40}$$

where the Reynolds number defining a flow type is calculated [94] as follows:

$$\text{Re} = \frac{\rho v d}{\mu} \tag{3.41}$$

where μ is the dynamic viscosity, kg/(ms).

Experimental results of all three different stent-grafts are plotted in Fig. 3.93. The shapes of the curves are alike and correlate between each other. From these curves, we can see how the shape of the channel wall affects pressure difference comparing Reynolds numbers. The pressure difference is much higher in the corrugated stent-graft.

The experimental results of a straight plastic stent-graft and the corrugated stent-graft with water were compared with simulation results (Fig. 3.94). In the graph we can see that simulation results of the corrugated stent-graft with water and blood correlate between each other.

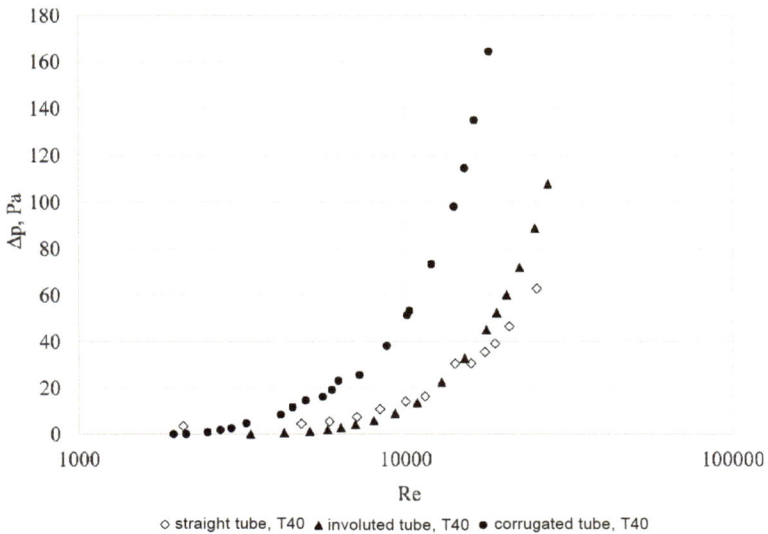

Fig. 3.93 Experimental results of all three different stent-grafts

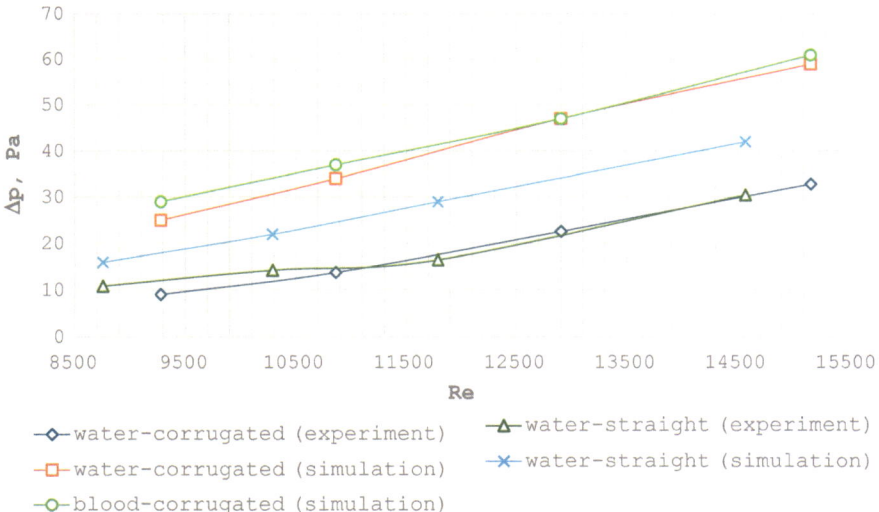

Fig. 3.94 The experimental results of a straight plastic stent-graft and the corrugated stent-graft

Pressure differences in the experimental model are lower compared to that in the simulation one because of the connections in the experimental setup. The correlation between these curves proves that a stent-graft could be designed and tested with numerical simulation software, and the experimental testing phase could be eliminated further from the personalization process. Thus, by comparing the diagnostics and simulation results, the homogeneous nature of the dependence of Δp on Q is confirmed. In turn, this means that the model built in software COMSOL Multiphysics is adequate to the actual flow of the fluid. In this case, the entire process is very fast and effective giving the possibility in a short time to design, produce and implant the personalized stent-graft.

Since each person is unique from birth, and even more so according to their style of life, the blood flow in the cardiovascular system also has its own peculiarities which must be considered in case of avoiding unpleasant consequences for the human body. It is well known that the specific anatomic need of each individual patient is an exciting possibility that may reduce complications [95]. Therefore, it is especially important, based on data obtained in the diagnosis of the patient, to create such an endoprosthesis that considers all the factors and characteristics of the cardiovascular system leading to minimal or no negative effects of its implantation surgery. The situation is complicated in the case of the formation of an abdominal aortic aneurysm due to trauma.

The personalization process necessary steps have been started by the scanning of the aorta affected by abdominal aortic aneurysm in the body of the patient for whom the implant stent- graft will be implanted. From the computerized tomography scan, the design scheme allowed to identify the interior diameter of scanned aorta. As initial data for numerical model the aortic pressure of the individualized specific patients was measured using non-invasive measurement technique of brachial blood pressure and suprasystolic waveform as well as magnetic resonance velocity mapping, let (enabled) to determine the hemodynamic significance of blood flow. The usability of computational methods for the purpose of improved function of implants the cardiovascular system is the future of the medicine [96], thus COMSOL Multiphysics software was used to simulate the blood flow. The computational model was presented in the form of the Navier–Stokes equations. A graphical interface allowed the user to predict stent-graft deformation under different pressures and positions simulating the blood flow. It was found, that in the case of high Reynolds numbers, the inertial forces were much higher than the viscous forces. For the first approach the virtual blood stream has been passed through a direct channel and stent-graft was designed according to the requirements of the housing and fixing points of the experimental set-up. The steady and unsteady 3D blood flows via stent-graft implant models were proposed. The mathematical model of fluid flow passing through the endovascular prosthesis stent-graft was created and the influence of channel roughness evaluated. The simulation results have shown the homogeneous nature of the fluid flow. The blood pressure distribution graphs in the cases of fluid passing through the direct channel and the endovascular prosthesis have showed that the pressure difference in stent-graft was bigger comparing to a straight channel mainly due to the roughness effect. Therefore, it was created the mathematical model in the form of endovascular graft inside the human body.

As the size and shape of the cardiovascular implant determines the fluid flow type, the avoidance of the turbulent flow regime should be ensured in the implant integrated into the cardiovascular system. Furthermore, according to previous studies, the high stress in the aortic wall could be a risk factor in aortic dissections [97]. Therefore, our method enables the validation process of the stent-graft. The simulation results have showed different pressure gradients in every model and any undesirable augmentation in pressure value could be noticed and eliminated by modifying the shape of the implant. These simulation results became the base for the implant prototype design.

Shape optimization in the design of Nitinol self-expandable stent-grafts with the aim to achieve better fatigue safety factor and higher radial stiffness is clearly described [98]. Even after decades of implantation, most prosthetic vascular grafts implanted in humans have no endothelium [99]. This is a minor defect for large bore prostheses in aortic or iliac position that has no impact on their clinical performance; however, in the case of small- to medium-sized grafts, this becomes a serious fault resulting in high failure rate. Therefore, there has been a substantial amount of research devoted to solving this problem recently, with no success yet. Furthermore, the vascular implants used currently in clinics lack the ability to revive lost biomechanical function of the diseased artery [100]. Therefore, our available implant manufacturing equipment involves not only the specialized loom for endovascular prosthesis manufacturing, but also the equipment for testing samples for implants radial stiffness and inner-outer gelatin coating which, after implantation into the body, provides neointima formation on the inner surface and germination of the connective tissue. A device for occlusion of the left atrial appendage with a special weave technology ensuring minimal risk of blood clots and high fixation process was developed. During manufacturing, the blood vessel prosthesis of the original multi-layer weave seamless design with the use of ultra-high-strength threads that provide zero permeability of blood was produced. It is related to the availability of transverse fluting, which allows the blood vessel prosthesis to restore its original shape after stretching.

References

1. Venslauskas M, Ostasevicius V, Vilkinis P (2017) Influence of low-frequency vibrations on blood flow improvement in human's limbs. Bio-Med Mat Eng: IOS Press 28(2):117–130
2. Hou G, Wang J, Layton A (2012) Numerical methods for fluid-structure interaction—a review. Com Comp Phys 12:337–377
3. Moore B, Jaglinski T, Stone DS, Lakes RS (2007) On the bulk modulus of open cell foams. Cell Polym 26(1):1–10
4. Lythgo N, Eser P, de Groot P, Galea M (2008) Whole-body vibration dosage alters leg blood flow. Scand Soc Clin Physiol Nucl Med 29(1):53–59
5. Benevicius V, Gaidys R, Ostasevicius V, Marozas V (2014) Identification of rheological properties of human body surface tissue. J Biomech 47(6):1368–1372
6. Huang J-Y, Li L-T, Wang H, Liu S-S, Lu Y-M, Liao M-H, Tao R-R, Hong L-J, Fukunaga K, Chen Z, Wilcox CS, Lai EY, Han F (2013) In vivo two-photon fluorescence microscopy

reveals disturbed cerebral capillary blood flow and increased susceptibility to ischemic insults in diabetic mice. Hypert 62:A93

7. Lensink AV, Van Rooy M-J, Soma P, van Papendorp D, Lipinski B, Pretorius E (2013) Changes in red blood cell membrane structure in type 2 diabetes: a scanning electron and atomic force microscopy study. Card Diabet 12(1):25
8. Mester J, Kleinoder H, Yue Z (2006) Vibration training: benefits and risks. J Biomech 39(6):1056–1065
9. Martinez-Pardo E, Romero-Arenas S, Alcaraz PE (2013) Effects of different amplitudes (high vs. low) of whole-body vibration training in active adults. J Streng Cond Rese 27(7):1798–806
10. Mauroy B (2007) Following red blood cells in a pulmonary capillary. ESAIM Proc 23:48–65
11. Yu L, Sheng Y, Chiou A (2013) Three-dimensional light-scattering and deformation of individual biconcave human blood cells in optical tweezers. Opt Exp 21(10):12174–12184
12. Wang T, Xing Z (2010) Characterization of blood flow in capillaries by numerical simulation. J Modern Phys 1:349–356
13. Park YK, Best CA, Kuriabova T, Henle ML, Feld MS, Levine AJ, Popescu G (2011) Measurement of the nonlinear elasticity of red blood cell membranes. Phys Rev E Stat Nonlinear Soft Matter Phys 83(5 Pt 1):051925
14. Rahman M, Islam R, Rana SM, Halder MR, Hassan T, Ahmed S (2014) Design, construction and performance test of a rotational digital viscometer. Int Conf Mech, Ind Ener Engin, Khulna, Bangladesh
15. Dulinska-Molak I, Targosz M, Strojny W, Lekka M, Czuba P, Balwierz W, Szymonski M (2006) Stiffness of normal and pathological erythrocytes studied by means of atomic force microscopy. J Bioch Bioph Meth 66(1–3):1–11
16. Fung Y (1993) Biomechanics: mechanical properties of living tissues, 2nd edn. Springer-Verlag, NY
17. Minamitani H, Tsukada K, Kawamura T, Sekizuka E, Oshio C (2000) Analysis of elasticity and deformability of erythrocytes using micro-channel flow system and atomic force microscope. Microtech Med Biol, 1st Ann Int Conf 68–71
18. Fornal M, Lekka M, Pyka-Fościak G, Lebed K, Grodzicki T, Wizner B, Styczeń J (2006) Erythrocyte stiffness in diabetes mellitus studied with atomic force microscope. Clin Hemorheol Microcirc 35(1–2):273–276
19. Gregersen MI, Bryant CA, Hammerle WE, Usami S, Chien S (1967) Flow characteristics of human erythrocytes through polycarbonate sieves. Science 157(3786):825–827
20. Pennec F, Achkar H, Peyrou D, Plana R, Pons P, Courtade F (2007). Verification of contact modelling with COMSOL multiphysics software. Rapport LAAS: 07604
21. Yalla SK, Kareem A (2000) On the beat phenomenon in coupled systems. In: Proceedings of the 8th ASCE Joint Spec Conference on Probabilistic Mechanics and Structural Reliability, Notre Dame, Indiana
22. Yalla SK, Kareem A, Kantor JC (1998) Semi-active control strategies for tuned liquid column dampers to reduce wind and seismic response of structures. In: Proceedings of the second world conference on structural control, Kyoto, John Wiley
23. Meriam JL, Kraige LG (1987) Engineering mechanics 2, dynamics, 2nd edn. ISBN 0-471-84912-X (620.104 MER)
24. Lutron electronic enterprise co., Ltd, [Cited: 2014/11/22]. Available at: http://www.lutron.com.tw

25. Cardinale M, Wakeling J (2005) Whole body vibration exercise: are vibrations good for you? Br J Sports Med 39(9):585–589

26. Kunz RW, Pitcher GK (1986) Vibrator massager using beat frequency. US patent 4570616 A, Available at: https://www.google.co.cr/patents/US4570616

27. Venslauskas M, Ostasevicius V, Marozas V (2013) Limb's vibrations exercise monitoring with MEMS accelerometer to identify influence of cardiovascular system. Vibroengineering procedia: international conference on "Vibroengineering- 2013", vol 1, pp 48–52

28. Venslauskas M, Ostasevicius V, Jurenas V (2014) Development of vibrating bracelet for the actuation of the blood circulation at capillaries. J Vibroeng 16(3):1535–1542

29. Venslauskas M, Ostasevicius V, Jurenas V, Stankevicius E (2018) A device for stimulating blood circulation in the limbs and a method of inducing low-frequency vibrations LT 6527 B

30. Plagenhoef S, Evans FG, Abdelnour T (1983) Anatomical data for analyzing human motion. Res Quart Exerc Sport 54:169–178

31. Venslauskas M, Ostasevicius V, Jurenas V (2015) Novel training machine for stimulation of blood circulation in feet. Mechanika 21(3):201206

32. Gore WL and Associates (2015) AP2400-EN124Gore hybrid vascular graft Available at http://www.goremedical.com/hybrid/technical/

33. Palevicius A, Ragulskis K, Bubulis A, Ostasevicius V, Ragulskis M (2004) Development and operational optimization of micro spray system. Proc SPIE 5390:429–438

34. Pust O (2000) PIV: Direct cross-correlation compared with FFT-based cross-correlation. In: Proceedings of the 10th international symposium on applications of laser techniques of fluid mechanics, Lisbon, Portugal

35. Hagsater MS (2008) Development of micro-PIV techniques for aplication in micrfluidic systems. Lyngby: DTU Nanotech Dep Micro-Nanotech

36. Wikipedia. Katsuzo Nishi – Wikipedia, [Online] [Cited: 30 March 2013]. Available at http://en.wikipedia.org/wiki/Katsuzō_Nishi

37. Microlife (2013) Available at http://www.microlife.com/products/hypertension/automatic/bp-a100/

38. Reeve A, Simcox E, Turnbull D (2014) Ageing and Parkinson's disease: why is advancing age the biggest risk factor? Ageing Res Rev 14(100):19–30

39. Tröster AI, Pahwa R, Fields JA, Tanner CM, Lyons KE (2005) Quality of life in essential tremor questionnaire (QUEST): Development and initial validation. Parkinsonism Relat Disord 11(6):367–373

40. Brillman S, Khemani P, Isaacson S, Pahwa R., Deshpande R, Zraick V, Rajagopal A, Rosenbluth K, Khosla D (2022) Transcutaneous afferent patterned stimulation provides upper limb motor symptom relief in patients with Parkinson's disease. Neurology 98(18)

41. Bloem BR, de Vries NM, Ebersbach G (2015) Nonpharmacological treatments for patients with Parkinson's disease. Mov Disord 30(11):1504–1520

42. Pascual-Valdunciel A, Rajagopal A, Pons JL, Delp SL (2022). Non-invasive electrical stimulation of peripheral nerves for the management of tremor. J Neurol Sci 435:120195

43. Stegemöller EL, Vallabhajosula S, Haq I, Hwynn N, Hass CJ, Okun MS (2013) Selective use of low frequency stimulation in Parkinson's disease based on absence of tremor. NeuroRehab 33(2):305–312

44. Bubulis A, Juknevicius AR, Litvinas E, Stankevicius E, Venslauskas M (2019) Vibration therapy device. Patent A61H 23/00

45. Lendraitiene E, Rekus E, Volkeviciute A, Tunaityte A, Venslauskas M, Abramavicius S, Stankevicius E (2024) Research of upper limb tremor reduction with a vibrational medical device for parkinson's disease. Technol Disability 36(1–2):29–38
46. Nine-Hole Peg Test, Nine-Hole Peg Test - Physiopedia (physio-pedia.com)
47. Steady hands Steady Hand: Definition, Meaning, and Origin (usdictionary.com)
48. Heinzel G, Rüdiger A, Schilling R (2002) Spectrum and spectral density estimation by the Discrete Fourier transform (DFT), including a comprehensive list of window functions and some new at-top windows. Max Plank Institute
49. Haas CT, Turbanski S, Kessler K, Schmidtbleicher D (2006) The effects of random whole-body-vibration on motor symptoms in Parkinson's disease. NeuroRehabil 21(1):29–36
50. Jöbges EM, Elek J, Rollnik JD, Dengler R, Wolf W (2002) Vibratory proprioceptive stimulation affects Parkinsonian tremor. Parkinsonism Relat Disord 8(3):171–176
51. Kremer NI, Pauwels RWJ, Pozzi NG, Lange F, Roothans J, Volkmann J, Reich MM (2021) Deep brain stimulation for tremor: update on long-term outcomes, target considerations and future directions. J Clin Med 10(16):3468
52. Meng L, Jin M, Zhu X, Ming D (2022) Peripherical electrical stimulation for Parkinsonian tremor: a systematic review. Front Aging Neurosci 14:795454
53. Greenland JC, Barker RA (2018) The differential diagnosis of Parkinson's disease. In: Stoker TB, Greenland JC (eds) Parkinson's disease: Pathog Clin Asp [Internet]. Codon Publications, Brisbane (AU). Chapter 6
54. Ford I, Norrie J (2016) Pragmatic trials. N Engl J Med 375:454–463
55. Morant AV, Jagalski V, Vestergaard HT (2019) Characteristics of single pivotal trials supporting regulatory approvals of novel non-orphan, non-oncology drugs in the European Union and United States from 2012–2016. Clin Transl Sci 12:361–370
56. Grimaldi G, Manto M (2010) Neurological tremor: sensors, signal processing and emerging applications. Sensors 10:1399–1422
57. Daneault JF, Carignan B, Codère CÉ, Sadikot AF, Duval C (2012) Using a smart phone as a standalone platform for detection and monitoring of pathological tremors. Front Hum Neurosci 6:1–31
58. Elble R, Comella C, Fahn S, Hallett M, Jankovic J, Juncos JL, Lewitt P, Lyons K, Ondo WG, Pahwa R, Sethi K, Stover N, Tarsy D, Testa C, Tintner R, Watts R, Zesiewicz T (2012) Reliability of a new scale for essential tremor. Mov Disord 27:1567–1569
59. Faul F, Erdfelder E, Lang AG, Buchner A (2007) G*Power 3: a flexible statistical power analysis program for the social, behavioral, and biomedical sciences. Behav Res Meth Psychon Soc Inc 175–191
60. Bahgat D, Raslan AM, McCartney S, Burchiel KJ (2012) Lesioning and stimulation in tremor-predominant movement disorder patients: an nstitutional case series and patient-reported outcome. Stereot Funct Neurosurg 90:181–187
61. Abramavicius S, Venslauskas M, Vaitkus A, Gudziunas V, Laucius O, Stankevicius E (2020) Local vibrational therapy for essential tremor reduction: a clinical study. Medicina 56:552
62. Chuanasa J, Songschon S (2015) Essential tremor suppression by a novel self-balancing device. Prosthet Orthot Int 39:219–225
63. Kiguchi K, Hayashi Y (2013) Upper-limb tremor suppression with a 7DOF exoskeleton power-assist robot. In: Proceedings of the annual international conference on IEEE engineering in medicine and biology society (EMBS), pp 6679–6682
64. Lin PT, Ross EK, Chidester P, Rosenbluth KH, Hamner SR, Wong SH, Sanger TD, Hallett M, Delp SL (2018) Noninvasive neuromodulation in essential tremor demonstrates relief in a sham-controlled pilot trial. Mov Disord 33:1182–1183

65. Pahwa R, Dhall R, Ostrem J, Gwinn R, Lyons K, Ro S, Dietiker C, Luthra N, Chidester P, Hamner S, Ross E, Delp S (2019) An acute randomized controlled trial of noninvasive peripheral nerve stimulation in essential tremor. Neuromod Techn Neural Interf 22:537–545

66. Trenado C, Amtage F, Huethe F, Schulte-Mönting J, Mendez-Balbuena I, Baker SN, Baker M, Hepp-Reymond M-C, Manjarrez E, Kristeva R (2014) Suppression of enhanced physiological tremor via stochastic noise: Initial observations. PLoS ONE 9:e112782

67. Trenado C, Mikulić A, Manjarrez E, Mendez-Balbuena I, Schulte-Mönting J, Huethe F, Hepp-Reymond M-C, Kristeva R (2014) Broad-band Gaussian noise is most effective in improving motor performance and is most pleasant. Front Hum Neurosci 8:22

68. Conrad MO, Scheidt RA, Schmit BD (2011) Effects of wrist tendon vibration on targeted upper-arm movements in poststroke hemiparesis. Neurorehabil Neural Repair 25:61–70

69. Nilsson T, Wahlström J, Burström L (2017) Hand-arm vibration and the risk of vascular and neurological diseases—a systematic review and meta-analysis. PLoS ONE 12(7):e0180795

70. Sauni R, Toivio P, Pääkkönen R, Malmström J, Uitti J (2015) Work disability after diagnosis of hand-arm vibration syndrome. Int Arch Occup Environ Health 88:1061–1068

71. Kluger N (2017) National survey of health in the tattoo industry: observational study of 448 French tattooists. Int J Occup Med Environ Health 30:111–120

72. Park H-R, Lee K-S, Bae H-G (2013) Chronic subdural hematoma after eccentric exercise using a vibrating belt machine. J Korean Neurosurg Soc 54:265–267

73. Ye Y, Mauro M, Bovenzi M, Griffin MJ (2015) Reduction in finger blood flow induced by hand-transmitted vibration: effect of hand elevation. Int Arch Occup Environ Health 88:981–992

74. Bovenzi M, Prodi A, Mauro M (2016) A longitudinal study of neck and upper limb musculoskeletal disorders and alternative measures of vibration exposure. Int Arch Occup Environ Health 89:923–933

75. Palmer KT, Bovenzi M (2015) Rheumatic effects of vibration at work. Best Pract Res Clin Rheumatol 29:424–439

76. Popević MB, Janković SM, Borjanović SS, Jovičić SR, Tenjović LR, Milovanović APS, Bulat P (2014) Assessment of coarse and fine hand motor performance in asymptomatic subjects exposed to hand-arm vibration. Arh Hig Rada Toksikol 65:29–36

77. Abramavičius S, Volkevičiūtė A, Tunaitytė A, Venslauskas M, Bubulis A, Bajoriūnas V, Stankevičius E (2020) Low-frequency (20 kHz) ultrasonic modulation of drug action. Ultras Med Biol 46:3017–3031

78. Gudas R, Siupsinskas L, Gudaite A, Vansevicius V, Stankevicius E, Smailys A, Vilkytė A, Simonaitytė R (2018) The Patello-femoral joint degeneration and the shape of the patella in the population needing an arthroscopic procedure. Medicina 54:21

79. Krajnak K (2018) Health effects associated with occupational exposure to hand-arm or whole-body vibration. J Toxicol Environ Heal Part B Crit Rev 21:320–334

80. Wang YJ, Huang XL, Yan JW, Wan YN, Wang BX, Tao JH, Chen B, Li BZ, Yang GJ, Wang J (2015) The association between vibration and vascular injury in rheumatic diseases: a review of the literature. Autoimmunity 48:61–68

81. Alabdulgader A, McCraty R, Atkinson M, Dobyns Y, Vainoras A, Ragulskis M, Stolc V (2018) Long-term study of heart rate variability responses to changes in the solar and geomagnetic environment. Sci Rep 8(1)

82. Ostasevicius V, Markevicius V, Venslauskas M, Mikuckyte S, Domeika A, Grigaliunas V, Aleknaite-Dambrauskiene I (2019) Conceptual solutions for driver-vehicle interfaces and interaction. Transport Means 2019:1485–1490

83. Bubulis A, Jurenas V, Mikuckyte S, Ostasevicius V, Minchenya V (2020) Device for the effect of acoustic waves on the organs of the human body LT 6759 B

84. Mikuckyte S, Ostasevicius V (2020) Investigation of fluid flow velocity within the lumbar intervertebral disc. Mechanika 26(6):497–502

85. Ostasevicius V, Venslauskas M, Jurenas V, Mikuckyte S (2019) Device for improving the nutrition of the intervertebral discs and strengthening the deep muscles of the back LT 6585 B

86. Bordoni B, Escher AR (2023) Rethinking the origin of the primary respiratory mechanism. Cureus 15(10):e46527

87. Ostasevicius V, Bubulis A, Jurenas V, Eidukynas D, Radziunas A, Tamasauskas A, Tamasauskas S (2024) Positioning system of a stereotactic frame EP4385451A1

88. Ostasevicius V, Tretsyakou-Savich Y, Venslauskas M, Bertasiene A, Minchenya V, Chernoglaz P (2018) Adaptation of cardiovascular system stent implants. Biomed Eng Biomediz Techn Berlin: Walter de Gruyter 63(3):279–290

89. Ostasevicius V, Minchenya V, Tretsyakou-Savich Y (2015) Blood flow simulation and material choice for individualized human cardiovascular prostheses. Mechatronic systems and materials: abstracts of the 11th international conference. MSM 2015:120–121

90. Wendt JF (2009) Computational fluid dynamics, 3rd edn. 15c Springer-Verlag Berlin

91. Heidelberg Tennekes H, Lumley JL (1992) A first course in turbulence. Mass MIT Press, Cambridge. ISBN 978-0-262-20019-6

92. Taylor TW, Yamaguchi T (1994) Three-dimensional simulation of blood flow in an abdominal aortic aneurysm-steady and unsteady flow cases. J Biomech 116(1):89–97

93. Crane CO (1988) Flow of fluids through valves, fittings, and pipe, 25th edn. Crane Conf

94. Cohn R, Russell J (2012) Reynolds number. VSD

95. Rousseau H, Elaassar O, Marcheix B, Cron C, Chabbert V, Combelles S, Dambrin C, Leoban B, Moreno R, Otal P, Auriol J (2012) The role of stent-grafts in the management of aortic trauma. Card Vasc Interv Radiol 35(1):2–14

96. Zarins CK, Taylor CA (2009) Endovascular device design in the future: transformation from trial and error to computational design. J Endovasc Ther 16:I12-21

97. Gao F, Watanabe M, Matsuzawa T (2006) Stress analysis in a layered aortic arch model under pulsatile blood flow. BioMed Engin 5:25

98. Abad EMK, Pasini D, Cecere R (2012) Shape optimization of stress concentration-free lattice for self-expandable Nitinol stent-grafts. J Biomech 45(6):1028–1035

99. Zilla P, Bezuidenhout D, Human P (2007) Prosthetic vascular grafts: wrong models, wrong questions and no healing. Biomat 28(34):5009–5027

100. Singh C, Wong CS, Wang X (2015) Medical textiles as vascular implants and their success to mimic natural arteries. J Funct Biomat 6(3):500–525

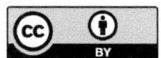

Separation of Bioparticles Using Acoustofluidics

4

4.1 Introduction

Preserving erythrocytes can facilitate blood transfusion in harsh environments, such as rural clinics, long-distance military operations and long-distance travel. Currently, the storage of erythrocytes is limited by the short storage time of 42 days at 4 °C. There is a clear need for low-cost and energy-efficient bioparticle separation devices that can be easily transported and quickly prepared for use in extreme conditions. Sound frequency and ultrasound separation technologies for bioparticles are proposed. Using digital twins of both of these separation technologies, portable devices have been designed, manufactured and patented to rapidly separate bioparticles from larger volumes of spilled blood for further use.

4.2 Simulation of Bioparticles Separation Process

Based on the findings of literature review and the formulated objectives, the possibilities of blood particles separation from larger volumes should be theoretically investigated before proceeding to the next steps. This chapter presents the information regarding the design and operation principles of the object under consideration. Numerically it is demonstrated that the low-level pressure field nodal circles of acoustic radiation waves, separate blood particles at different velocities. Using COMSOL Multiphysics software it was found that the distribution of blood particles in biological suspension or water in the acoustic pressure field is the same, yet the velocity of particle convergence to the low-level pressure field excited in piezoelectric cylinder differs few times [1].

The aim is to investigate the presence of a steady-state ultrasonic wave for fluids and particles in an acoustic field. To this end, the COMSOL Multiphysics software platform

V. Ostasevicius et al., *Noninvasive Therapeutic Technologies*, Synthesis Lectures on Biomedical Engineering, https://doi.org/10.1007/978-3-031-79025-6_4

(COMSOL, Inc., Burlington, Mass., USA) was used to model the effects of acoustic pressure on sonic and ultrasonic frequencies. The forces acting on the particles while they are in the acoustic field, which allows them to separate, or concentrate are related to:

1. Radiation power—of the most important forces which affect the body in an acoustic field. Action force leads to particle movement in the acoustic standing wave field.
2. Stokes strength moving particles in an acoustic standing wave field [2], which acts due to resistance or friction forces.
3. The strength of the Bjerknes [3]. When particles reach the pressure node, they are sub-jected to the force of interaction, called Bjerknes force. The strength of the interaction is a radiation force experienced by the particle due to the acoustic wave from the other particle.
4. The strength of gravity. At any particle in the earth's gravitational field, the force of gravity, or the force of attraction of the earth's surface exist. The particles that are already in the field of acoustic pressure node, the force of gravity, which causes the particles to settle, if they are in a stationary state, or deviate from a straight course to the nearest node of pressure.
5. The strength of Bernoulli [4]. When the particles are in the field of acoustic pressure node in the fluid, which moves with a velocity v, the force of attraction Bernoulli arises due to the reduced pressure between the particles.

The standing acoustic wave generates a force of acoustic radiation which acts on the particles. This force arises from the pressure and the acoustic field interaction with the particles. In the initial time the elastic particles are evenly distributed in a constant acoustic field then due to emerged acoustic radiation force and drag force, they begin their movement.

Acoustic radiation force is an important nonlinear force exerted by acoustic fields on particles. The acoustic radiation force F_{rad} on the particle can be calculated as the time averaged second-order forces acting on a fixed surface $\partial\Omega$ in the inviscid bulk, encompassing the particle. For inviscid fluids, vector F_{rad} is the sum of the time-averaged second-order nonlinear acoustic pressure field $\langle p_2 \rangle$ and momentum flux tensor $\rho_0 \langle v_1 v_1 \rangle$ [5],

$$
\begin{aligned}
F_{rad} &= -\int_{\partial\Omega} dr \{ \langle p_2 \rangle n + \rho_0 \langle (n \cdot v_1) v_1 \rangle \} \\
&= -\int_{\partial\Omega} dr \left\{ \left[\frac{\kappa_0}{2} \langle p_1^2 \rangle - \frac{\rho_0}{2} \langle v_1^2 \rangle \right] n + \rho_0 \langle (n \cdot v_1) v_1 \rangle \right\}
\end{aligned}
\tag{4.1}
$$

where: ρ_0—fluid density, v_1—the first-order acoustic velocity field, $\langle p_1 \rangle$—the first order linear pressure field, κ_0—explicit expression for the compressibility, n—normal vector.

The radiation force acting on a small particle placed in a standing wave is a gradient force of the potential function U_{rad} [6]:

$$F_{rad} = -\nabla U_{rad} \tag{4.2}$$

$$U_{rad} = V_p\left[f_1\frac{1}{2\rho_0 c^2}\langle p^2\rangle - f_2\frac{3}{4}\rho_0\langle v_1^2\rangle\right] \tag{4.3}$$

$$f_1 = 1 - \frac{K}{K_p}, \quad f_2 = \frac{2(\rho_p - \rho_0)}{2\rho_p + \rho_0} \tag{4.4}$$

where ρ_p—particle density, c—speed of sound, f_1 is really valued and depends only on the compressibility ratio between the particle and the fluid.

The dipole scattering coefficient f_2 is related to the translational motion of the particle, it depends on the viscosity of the fluid, K—bulk modulus of the fluid (blood), K_p—bulk modulus of the particle (erythrocyte), V_p—volume of the particle.

4.3   Sonic Frequency Manipulation of Bioparticles

4.3.1   Simulation of Sonic Frequency Acoustic Wave Manipulation of Bioparticles

The aim is to investigate the blood particles separation possibility using sonic frequency acoustic waves in fluids. For this purpose, a conical plastic container with a rigid bottomed disc-shaped bimorph type piezoelectric transducer was chosen (Fig. 4.1).

The equations of direct and inverse piezoeffects in the disc-shaped bimorph type piezoelectric transducer take the form [7]:

$$\begin{aligned} D &= E\varepsilon + eS \\ \sigma &= -eE + c_0 S \end{aligned} \tag{4.5}$$

where D denotes electric induction in the piezoelectric transducer; E—the tension of the electric field; ε dielectric constant; e piezoelectric coefficient; S transverse deformation; σ elastic stress; c_0 the velocity of acoustic deformation waves in the container with biofluid.

If the piezo transducer operates at resonant frequency, Eq. (4.5) is transformed to

$$\begin{aligned} D\exp(-j\omega t) &= E\varepsilon + e\frac{\partial U_0}{\partial x} \\ \sigma &= -eE + \frac{\lambda_0\omega}{2\pi}\cdot\frac{\partial U_0}{\partial x} \end{aligned} \tag{4.6}$$

where j denotes imaginary unit; ω the resonant frequency; Uo—the displacement; t—time; $\lambda_0 = 2\pi c_0/\omega$.

Then the elastic stress in the piezoelectric transducer can be expressed like:

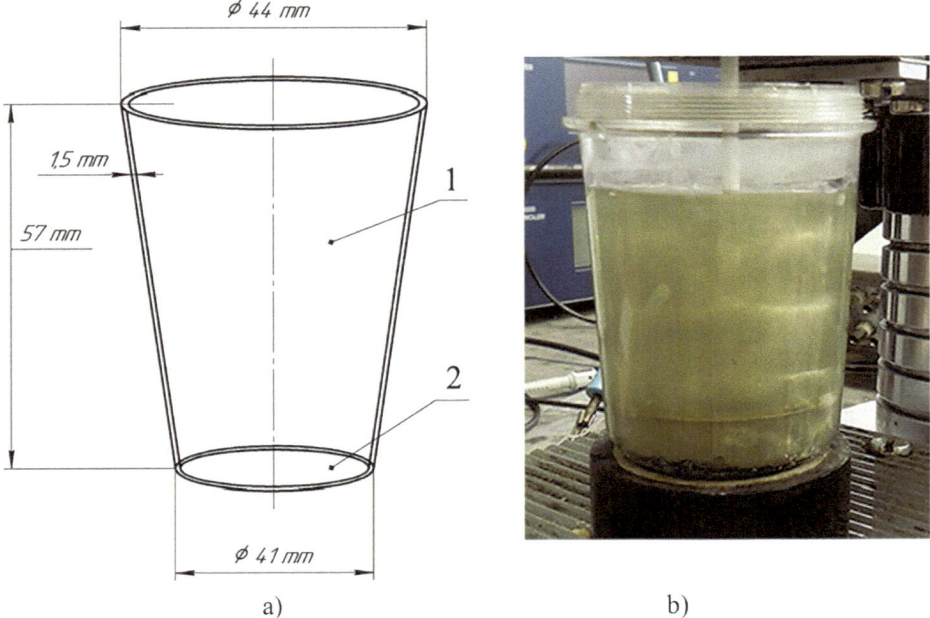

Fig. 4.1 **a**—scheme of conical plastic container with a rigid bottomed disc-shaped bimorph type piezoelectric transducer: 1—container, 2—disc-shaped bimorph type piezoelectric transducer; **b**—practical model of conical plastic container with a rigid bottomed disc-shaped bimorph type piezo-electric transducer

$$\sigma = \frac{\lambda\omega}{2\pi} \cdot \frac{\partial U_0}{\partial x} - \frac{e}{\varepsilon}\left(D\exp(-j\omega t) - e\frac{\partial U_0}{\partial x}\right) \tag{4.7}$$

The oscillatory motion of the piezoelectric exciter is described by the following system of equations:

$$\begin{array}{l}\frac{\partial^2 U_0}{\partial t^2} = c_0^2 \frac{\partial^2 U_0}{\partial x^2} \\ \frac{\partial^2 U_1}{\partial t^2} = c_1^2 \frac{\partial^2 U_1}{\partial x^2}\end{array} \tag{4.8}$$

with the following boundary conditions:

$$U_0 = U_1$$
$$\frac{\lambda_1\omega}{2\pi} \cdot \frac{\partial U_1}{\partial x} = \frac{\lambda_0\omega}{2\pi} \cdot \frac{\partial U_0}{\partial x} - \frac{e}{\varepsilon}D\exp(j\omega t) + \frac{e^2}{\varepsilon} \cdot \frac{\partial U_0}{\partial x} \tag{4.9}$$

where U_1 denotes the displacement; c_1 the velocity of acoustic deformation waves in the container; $\lambda_1 = 2\pi c_1/\omega$.

When the piezoelectric transducer performs the harmonic oscillations, the solution of Eq. (4.8) with conditions Eq. (4.9) can be approximated by the following relationships:

$$-V_1 \sin \frac{\omega l}{c_1} = V_0 \sin \frac{\omega a}{c_0}$$

$$\rho_1 c_1 \omega V_1 \cos \frac{\omega l}{c_1} = V_0 \omega \cos \frac{\omega a}{c_0} \left(\rho_0 c_0 + \frac{e}{\varepsilon c_0} \right) - \frac{e}{\varepsilon} D \tag{4.10}$$

where V_0 and V_1 the amplitudes of harmonic vibrations of the piezoelectric transducer and the container (waveguide); a—height of the piezo transducer; l—height of the container; ρ_0 and ρ_1 material densities of the piezoelectric transducer and the container.

The force transferred from piezoelectric transducer to the container can be calculated from the following relationship:

$$F_1 = Q \frac{\lambda_1 \omega}{2\pi} \cdot \frac{\partial U_1}{\partial x} \tag{4.11}$$

where Q denotes the contact area between the piezo transducer and the container. Finally, the expression of contacting force takes the form:

$$F_1 = \frac{-\rho_1 c_1 \frac{e}{\varepsilon} DQ \exp(-j\omega t)}{\rho_1 c_1 \cos \frac{\omega l}{c_1} + \sin \frac{\omega l}{c_1} ctg \frac{\omega a}{c_0} \left(\rho_0 c_0 + \frac{e^2}{\varepsilon c_0} \right)} \tag{4.12}$$

The optimal height of the container can be selected from the condition of maximization of the transferred force [8]:

$$l = \frac{c_1}{\omega} arctg \left(\frac{\rho_0 c_0 + \frac{e^2}{\varepsilon c_0}}{\rho_1 c_1} ctg \frac{\omega a}{c_0} \right) \tag{4.13}$$

Equation (4.13) shows that the maximum force of pressing is achieved when the length of the waveguide is integer number and one quarter of the acoustic deformation wavelength in the container.

COMSOL Multiphysics software platform for simulating physics-based pressure acoustics problem in frequency domain was used. Acoustic fluid pressure was applied to the frequency domain. Among all types of free elastic vibrations, it is possible to identify modes of oscillations whose frequency spectrum corresponds well to the experimental results of micro/nanoparticles separation theoretical calculations in the approximation of plane motion. Such modes of oscillations are capable of exciting acoustic standing waves in fluids under consideration.

After carrying out the modeling of a fluid-column and disc-shaped bimorph type piezoelectric transducer, the following results were obtained [9]. Oscillations in the first mode were at 1.40 kHz (Fig. 4.2a), the second mode was 5.39 kHz (Fig. 4.2b), the third at 13.0 kHz (Fig. 4.2c) [9]. The simulation results are presented from two positions—the type of deformation from the side of piezo ceramics in the upper line (I) and from the side of the fluid column surface in the lower line (II) of Fig. 4.2.

Based on the results of the simulation, it is seen how the oscillations of the disc-shaped bimorph type piezoelectric transducer are changed upon contact with the fluid. The

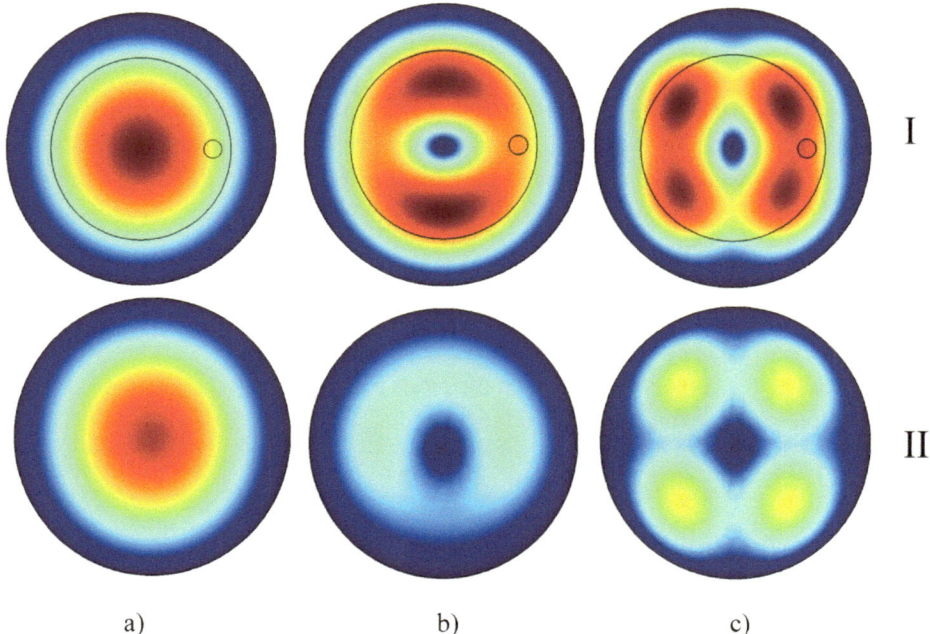

Fig. 4.2 Results of a disc-shaped bimorph type piezoelectric transducer modeling in interaction with a fluid column. I—line, which shows the oscillations modes from the side of piezoceramics; II—line shows the oscillations modes from the side of viscoelastic fluid: **a**—first mode at 1.40 kHz, **b**—second mode at 5.39 kHz and **c**—third mode at 13.0 kHz

value of the deformations decreases, and after passing through the fluid, it significantly weakens. Another interesting fact is that the force of pressure drops when the resonance mode increases. The strength F_z of the radiation pressure in the direction of the acoustic axis of the bimorph type piezoelectric transducer is determined by the flux of the pulse through the surface of the object [5]:

$$F_z = - \int_s \Pi_{zi} n_i ds \qquad (4.14)$$

where Π_{zi} $\bar{p}\delta_{zi} + \rho v_z v_i$ is the acoustical impulse density tensor, n_i is the projection of the normal to the surface of the object in the direction i, $\bar{p} = \frac{\rho}{2c^2}\left(\frac{\partial \Phi}{\partial t}\right)^2 - \frac{\rho v^2}{2}$ is the time-averaged overpressure in the acoustic wave, $v = \text{grad } \Phi$ is the vibrational velocity, Φ is the potential, ρ is the density of the fluid, c is the velocity of sound in the fluid, v_z and v_i are the components of the vibrational velocity.

Since the disc-shaped bimorph type piezoelectric transducer is rigidly mounted on the bottom of the conical container, it also excites the walls of that container. As shown in Fig. 4.3, mechanical vibration of disc-shaped bimorph type piezoelectric transducer activates a deformable container body, triggers a corresponding field of acoustic pressure level, the minimum of which coincides with the minimum point of the amplitude of the radial oscillation of the deformable container body. On the surface of the container five pressure level bands are formed at 13.8 kHz. It is known that during the separation of particles in the field of acoustic wave, they propagate precisely to a low acoustic pressure level zone.

This physical phenomenon can be applied to the separation of bioparticles using low sonic frequency mechanical vibrations. At the initial time t = 0 s, the bioparticles are evenly distributed in volume of the contaminated or shaken fluid (blood) (Fig. 4.4). The axial section of container below shows the distribution of the acoustic pressure level field in the fluids volume: the three upper zones of low pressure level are in the perpendicular fluid flow across the longitudinal axis, and two low levels are not.

In Fig. 4.5, bioparticle positions in the field of sound pressure level at t = 12 s and their trajectories are presented. As can be seen, the bioparticles "cling" to the vessel wall

Fig. 4.3 Vibrating container and acoustic pressure level (dB) on its surface when excitation frequency—13.8 kHz

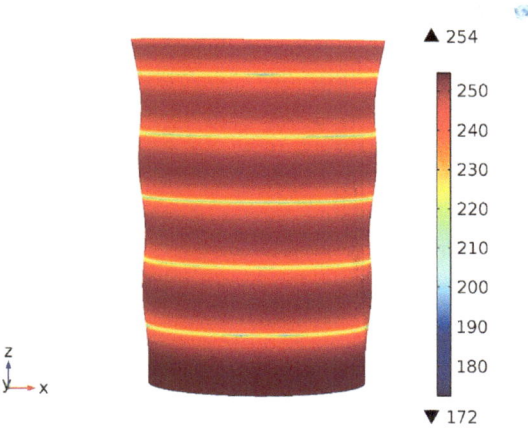

Fig. 4.4 Axial section in yz plane of vibrating container and acoustic pressure level (dB) with distributed bioparticles in suspension at time t = 0 s of disc-shaped bimorph type piezoelectric transducer excitation on 13.8 kHz frequency

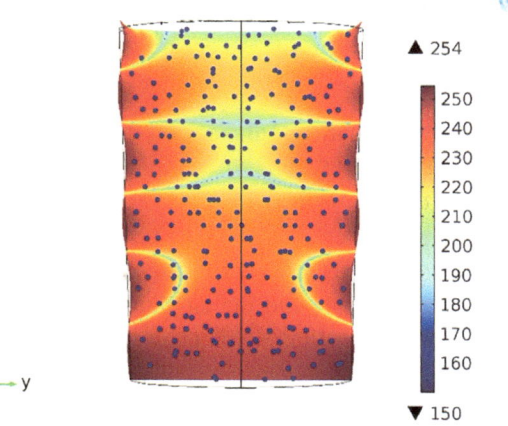

Fig. 4.5 Axial section in yz plane of vibrating container and acoustic pressure level (dB) and positions of the particles at time t = 12 s and their motion trajectories. Excitation frequency—13.8 kHz

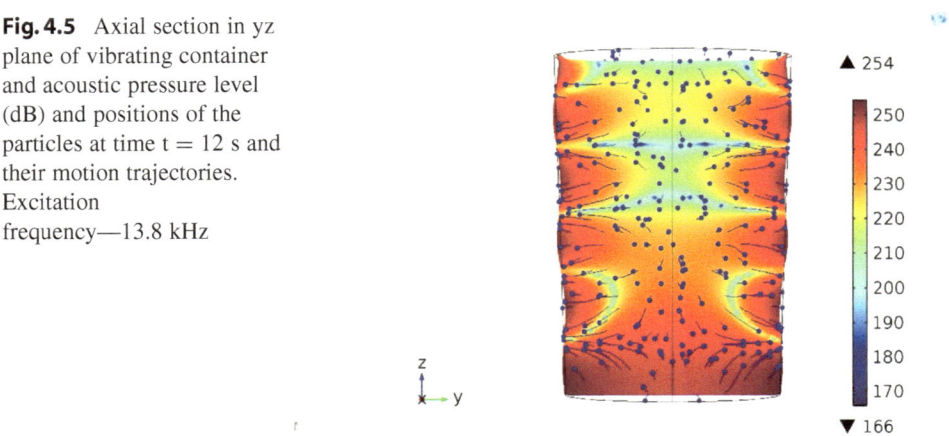

in low acoustic pressure levels zones. When analyzing the effect of acoustic waves on the volume of fluid with microparticles, we notice that the bioparticles accumulate in certain areas of this volume where the zones of acoustic wave nodes or anti-nodes settle down. The microparticle movement is vertical near anti-node, horizontal at the node and inclined in between. Therefore, there is a net force pushing the hydrophobic (heavier) particle to the anti-node and a hydrophilic (lighter) particle towards the node. When applying the acoustic waves on one another, it can be seen resonating fluid, which leads to a distribution of bioparticles in the volume.

Figure 4.6 shows the bioparticles trajectories in the other plane, observing from the top of the container, which corresponds to the xy plane in Fig. 4.5. At the initial time point, the particle positions are shown in Fig. 4.6a, b—after 12 s.

As it can be seen, the bioparticles "drift" towards the surface of the container. This is due to self-vibrations of the wall of the container, which deforms on one of its own forms, depending on the frequency of the excitation. A traveling acoustic wave generates a stream of fluid with bioparticles, and when these bioparticles run off, they fall into the lower pressure nodal sections of the vibrating wall.

4.3.2 Experimental Validation of Bioparticles Separation by Sonic Frequency Acoustic Waves

Several experimental studies are needed to ensure high dynamic accuracy of operation for controlling the flow of bioliquid substances. In most cases the exciting frequencies are quite high, and the amplitudes of the piezoelectric transducer corresponding to them are measured in micrometers. Therefore, the holographic method can be effectively applied for the visual representation of vibrating processes taking place in the disc-shaped bimorph type piezoelectric transducer. The most effective method for studying is the

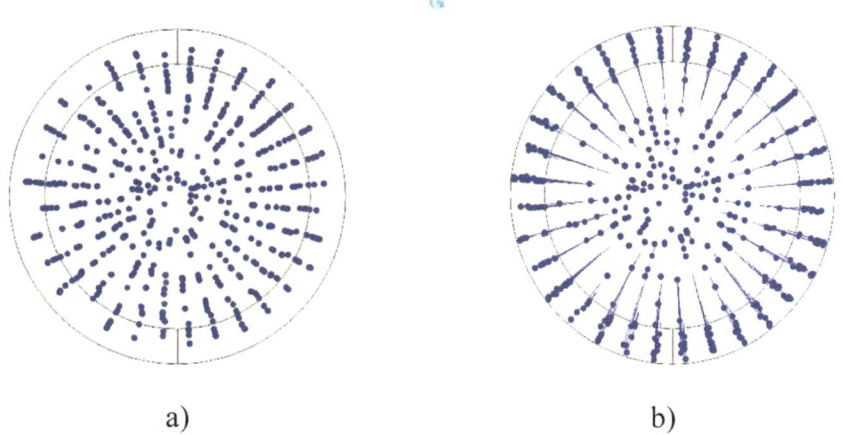

a)   b)

Fig. 4.6 Microparticles positions from the top of vessel: **a**—at the initial time t = 0 s, **b**—after 12 s

method of holographic interferometry with time averaging. It should be noted that the most clearly expressed bands in the holographic interferograms are those recorded at the positions of minimum amplitudes.

To study the proposed theory, a disc-shaped bimorph type piezoelectric transducer was evaluated with steady state vibrations in frequency range from 1.3 to 25 kHz was used. For the validation of simulation results the holographic interferometry set-up was used. Figure 4.7 shows an optical scheme for recording holographic interferograms of a vibrating disc-shaped bimorph type piezoelectric transducer: 1—vibrating disc-shaped bimorph type piezoelectric transducer; 2—high-frequency signal generator; 3—amplifier. Means of signal control: 4—frequency meter, 5—voltage amplitude of the power source is controlled by a voltmeter. The optical scheme includes a holographic table with a helium–neon laser, which serves as a source of coherent radiation. First, the beam from the optical laser 6 decays into two coherent beams, and one of them passes through the beam separator 7. The so-called object beam reflected from mirror 8 and the widely distributed lens 10, illuminates the surface of the vibrating disc-shaped bimorph type piezoelectric transducer 1 and, after reflection from it, illuminates photographic plate 12. The reference beam reflected by mirror 9 and lens 11 illuminates' photographic plate 12 where is recorded interference of these two beams. Block-scheme of experimental set-up with laser holographic interferometry system is presented in Fig. 4.8.

The holographic method was used to analyze the stability of an optical scheme. In the tests, the PRISM system was used (Fig. 4.9).

The characteristic function defining the complex amplitude of the laser beam M_T in the plane of the hologram formed by the time-averaging holography techniques takes the form [10]:

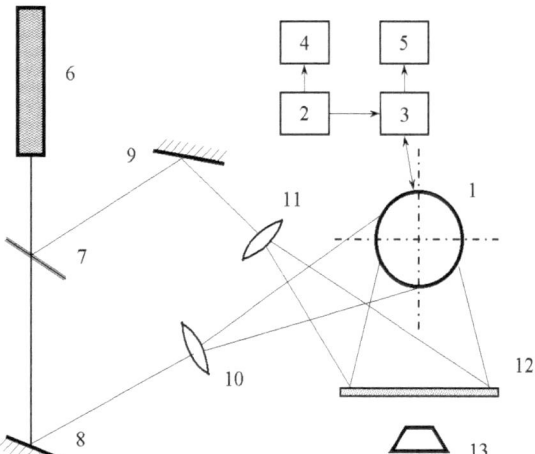

Fig. 4.7 Optical scheme of the laser holographic interferometry system: 1—tubular working tube; 2—high-frequency signal generator; 3—amplifier; 4—frequency meter; 5—voltmeter; 6—laser; 7—beam splitter; 8, 9—mirror; 10, 11—lenses; 12—photographic plate; 13—recorder

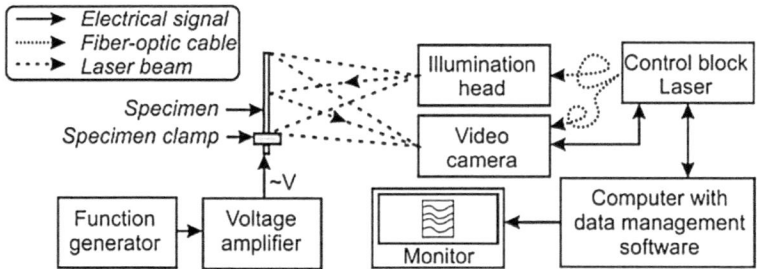

Fig. 4.8 Block-scheme of the experimental set-up with laser holographic interferometry system

$$M_T = \lim_{T \to \infty} \frac{1}{T} \int_0^T \exp\left(i\left(\frac{4\pi}{\lambda}\right)Z(x)\sin\omega t\right)dt = J_0\left(\left(\frac{4\pi}{\lambda}\right)Z(x)\right) \qquad (4.15)$$

where T—the exposure time of the hologram, $(T \gg 1/\omega)$; ω—the frequency of structural vibrations, λ—the laser wavelength; J_0—zero order Bessel function of the first type.

Then, the resulting intensity I of the point (x, y) on the hologram is:

$$I(x, y) = a^2(x, y)|M_T|^2, \qquad (4.16)$$

where a(x,y)—the distribution of the amplitude of the incident laser beam.

Fig. 4.9 Holographic interferometry set-up used in the experiment

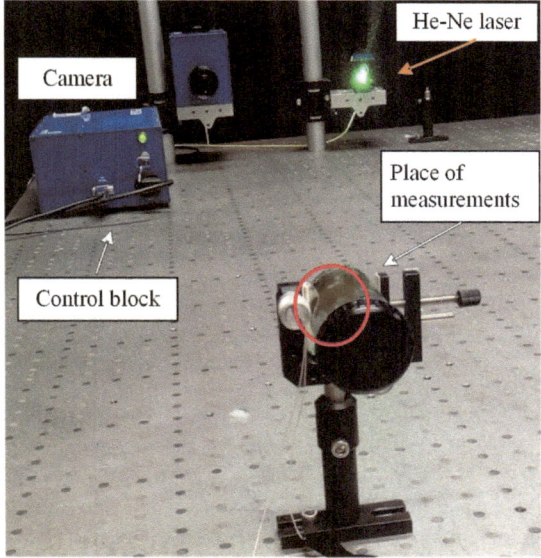

It can be noted that the centers of dark interference bands in the holographic inter-ferogram coincide with such values of Z(x) which turn the Bessel function to zero. The structure of the distribution of the interference bands does not depend on the static deformations of the structure, nor from the distance between the structure and the hologram.

The practical problem using the time-averaging holographic interferometry is related to the fact that the surface of an analyzed object must perform steady state vibration, otherwise the interference band pattern can be hardly interpretable. As the construction elements of the analyzed system oscillate but do not perform translational motion, the application of this convenient holographic analysis turned out to be not very effective.

Quantitative 3D reconstruction of velocity vector fields from the pattern of fringes requires construction of holographic images of the same vibrating surface with different angles of illumination between the incident laser beam and the vector of displacement (Fig. 4.10). The generated pattern of interference bands in the hologram reveals the motion of the analyzed surface in the direction of the incident laser beam. Therefore the direction of illumination plays a key role in the procedures of interpretation of holographic images. Further, the angle between the incident laser beam and the tangent to the analyzed surface will be specified. The methodology of interpretation 3-D vibration is presented in [11].

The problem of determination of the amplitude–frequency response characteristics of a vibrating surface, which vibrates in three dimensions in the majority of cases, is encoun-tered in the analysis of vibrations of mechanical system. The development of methods for calculating the characteristics of three-dimensional (3D) vibrations contributes to the solution of vital problems in the investigation, design, testing, and diagnostics of systems.

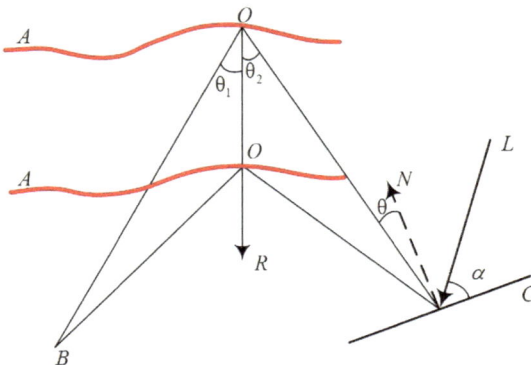

Fig. 4.10 The scheme of holographic experiment: A—oscillating object; B—laser light source; C—hologram plate; O—point on the surface of the body; R—vector of displacement; L—reference laser beam; N—normal vector of the hologram plate; α—angle between the reference laser beam and the tangent of the hologram plate; θ—angle between the reflected laser beam and the normal to the hologram plate; θ_1—angle between the incident laser beam and the vector of displacement

In the present section a method of calculating the amplitudes of the normal and tangential components of the displacement vector of 3D vibrations of the surface of deformable elements on the basis of experimental holographic-interferometry data and the theory of vibrations of mechanical systems is described. The proposed method permits a several fold reductions in the quantity of input data for analysis of vibrations from holographic interferograms. The wave phase changes as the laser light beam travels from the source up to the point O on the surface of the analyzed body, and back to the hologram, will be:

$$\Omega = \frac{2\pi}{\lambda}\vec{R}\cdot\vec{K}, \tag{4.17}$$

where λ—laser wave length $\vec{R}$—vibration vector, $\vec{K}$—sensitivity vector, Ω distances between the centers of appropriate interference bands.

The vibration vector $\vec{R}$ can be expressed as follows:

$$\begin{aligned}
\vec{R}(\tau) &= U_i(\tau)\cdot\vec{t} + W_i(\tau)\cdot\vec{z}, \\
U_i(\tau) &= U_0^i\cos(\omega\tau + \alpha_i), \\
V_i(\tau) &= V_0^i\cos(\omega\tau + \beta_i), \\
W_i(\tau) &= W_0^i\cos(\omega\tau + \gamma_i),
\end{aligned} \tag{4.18}$$

where U_i, V_i, W_i—coordinates of the solid point under forced vibrations, ω—frequency of forced vibrations, α_i, β_i, γ_i—appropriate phase shifts, τ—time. Further on, the corresponding amplitudes may be expressed exploiting the fact that the steady state regime of motion may be decomposed into a mixture of natural oscillations:

$$U_0^i = \sum_{j=1}^{k} A_j^U F_{ij}^U,$$

$$V_0^i = \sum_{j=1}^{k} A_j^V F_{ij}^V, \qquad (4.19)$$

$$W_0^i = \sum_{j=1}^{k} A_j^W F_{ij}^W,$$

where F_{ij} is the value of the j-th mode for the i-th point, A_j is the coefficient of influence of the j-th mode, and k is the number of modes analyzed. Consequently, to calculate the component of the 3D vibration vector, it is necessary to determine the values of $F_{ij}^U, F_{ij}^V, F_{ij}^W, A_j^U, A_j^V, A_j^W, \alpha_i, \beta_i, \gamma_i$. The amplitudes of the first k modes can be calculated according to Comsol Multiphysics model of vibration, with respect for the geometry of investigated links and their boundary conditions. Parameters of are $A_j^U, A_j^V, A_j^W, \alpha_i, \beta_i, \gamma_i$ determined from the solution (4.20) using results of analysis of holographic interferometry.

$$\frac{\Omega^i \lambda^2}{4\pi} = \left[\left(\sum_{j=1}^{k} A_j^W F_{ij}^W \right) \cos \gamma_i K_r^i + \left(\sum_{j=1}^{k} A_j^V F_{ij}^V \right) \cos \beta_i K_t^i + \left(\sum_{j=1}^{k} A_j^U F_{ij}^U \right) \cos \alpha_i K_z^i \right]^2$$
$$+ \left[\left(\sum_{j=1}^{k} A_j^W F_{ij}^W \right) \sin \gamma_i K_r^i + \left(\sum_{j=1}^{k} A_j^V F_{ij}^V \right) \sin \beta_i K_t^i + \left(\sum_{j=1}^{k} A_j^U F_{ij}^U \right) \sin \alpha_i K_z^i \right]^2,$$
$$(4.20)$$

Solution of the nonlinear Eq. (4.20) requires several holographic interferograms which must be obtained for different angles of illumination and observation of the investigated transducer. Methodology of solution of this equation is presented in paper [11]. The coefficients $F_{ij}^U, F_{ij}^V, F_{ij}^W$ are calculated using FEM model of the investigated mechanical system. The components of the vector sensitivity are determined from the scheme of the optical set-up knowing the values of the angle of the observation and illumination of the object.

To determine the working and resonant frequencies of the disc-shaped bimorph type piezoelectric transducer, a study of a loaded actuator on a holographic installation was initially carried out (Fig. 4.11). The results showed that the first three modes of the disc-shaped bimorph type piezoelectric transducer excited with harmonic signal of 200 Mv voltage are: first mode is 4.4 kHz (Fig. 4.11a), the second is 9.4 kHz (Fig. 4.11b), and third is 13.9 kHz (Fig. 4.11c).

The next step in the study of the disc-shaped bimorph type piezoelectric transducer was to verify theoretical results and identify its deformations using the Polytec PSV-500-D-HV device (Fig. 4.12). The studies were carried out in steady state vibration mode with different input signal frequencies. Each of the forms of deformation were determined from the peak values of the deformation.

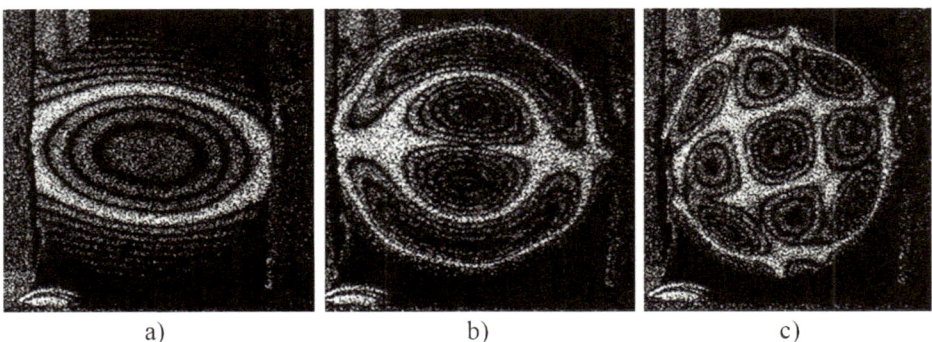

a)   b)   c)

Fig. 4.11 Holographic pattern of the change in the surface of bimorph type piezoelectric transducer, depending on the resonance mode: **a**—1.4 kHz, **b**—5.4 kHz, **c**—13.9 kHz

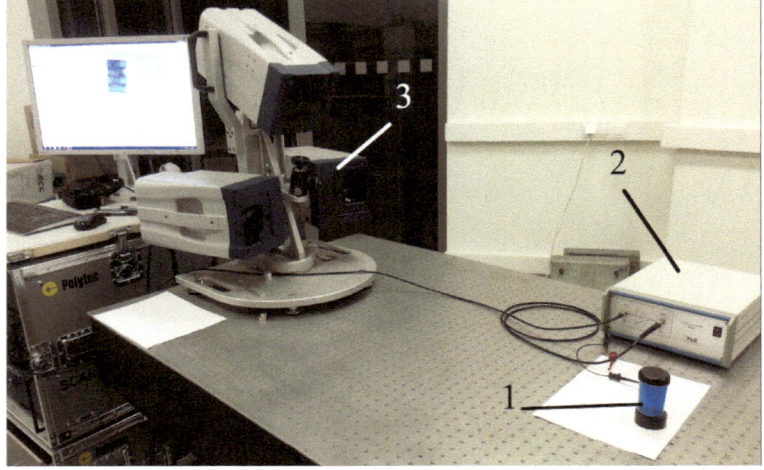

Fig. 4.12 Experimental set-up: 1—an experimental object; 2—liner amplifier P200 (FLC Electronics AB, Sweden), 3—3D scanning vibrometer PSV-500-3D-HV (Polytec GmbH, Germany)

Each of the following shapes of deformation has its own peculiarities in the zonal distribution. The higher the disc-shaped bimorph type piezoelectric transducer mode, the smaller the deformation region each of the peak points has, but the number of points increases (Fig. 4.13).

Since the disc-shaped bimorph type piezoelectric transducer is rigidly mounted on the bottom of the conical container, it also excites the wall of that container (Fig. 4.14).

The five vibration modes of the disc-shaped bimorph type piezoelectric transducer can be distinguished in the frequency response diagram (Fig. 4.15). The frequencies of the

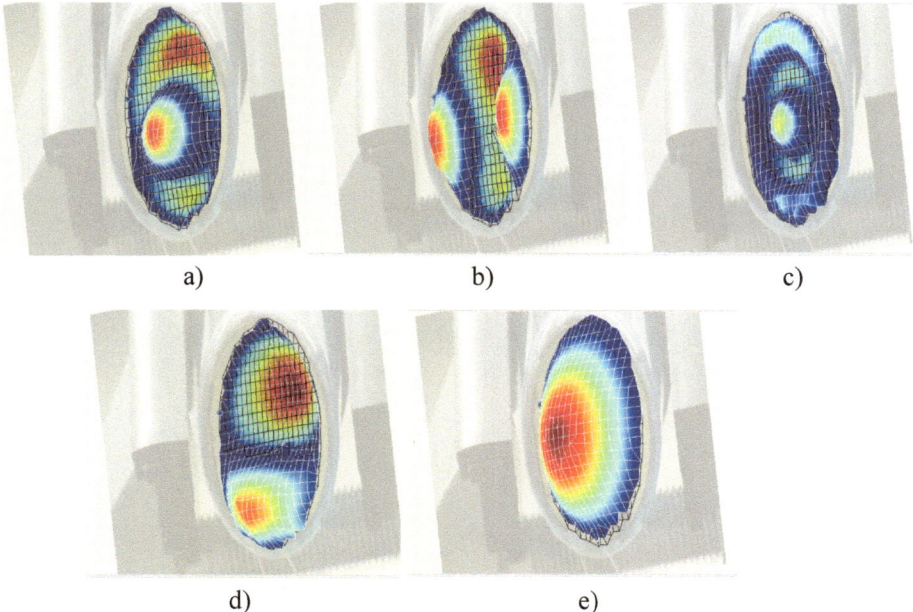

a)   b)   c)

d)   e)

Fig. 4.13 Investigation of deformation of the disc-shaped bimorph type piezoelectric transducer and the vibration modes of the frequencies: **a** 13.81 kHz; **b** 5.01 kHz; **c** 3.95 kHz; **d** 2.48 kHz; **e** 1.03 kHz

modes are: first mode—1.03 kHz; second mode—2.48 kHz; third mode—3.95 kHz; fourth mode—5.01 kHz; fifth mode—13.81 kHz.

Considering the amplitude–frequency characteristic given in Fig. 4.15 we see that it is possible to obtain stable results [12]. The obtained results are a prerequisite for the development of an experimental prototype for blood bioparticle purification. The proposed purification method could be used in different emergency situations to keep spilled blood ready for further use.

The experimental set-up of blood particles separation in suspensions is presented in Fig. 4.16a. During the experiment, it was found that after 5–8 s from the excitation signal applied to the resonator bioparticles begin to accumulate around the acoustic nodal circles of conical container wall thus stratifying in the test container sections disposed at same distances from each other. The third and most stable resonance result is at 12.2 kHz. For the clarity of the experiment, observations were made regarding the effect of the amount of fluid in the test container on the result. As a result, a proportional number of concentrated clusters of particles fractions of the suspension is obtained, depending on the height of the fluid column (Fig. 4.16b and c).

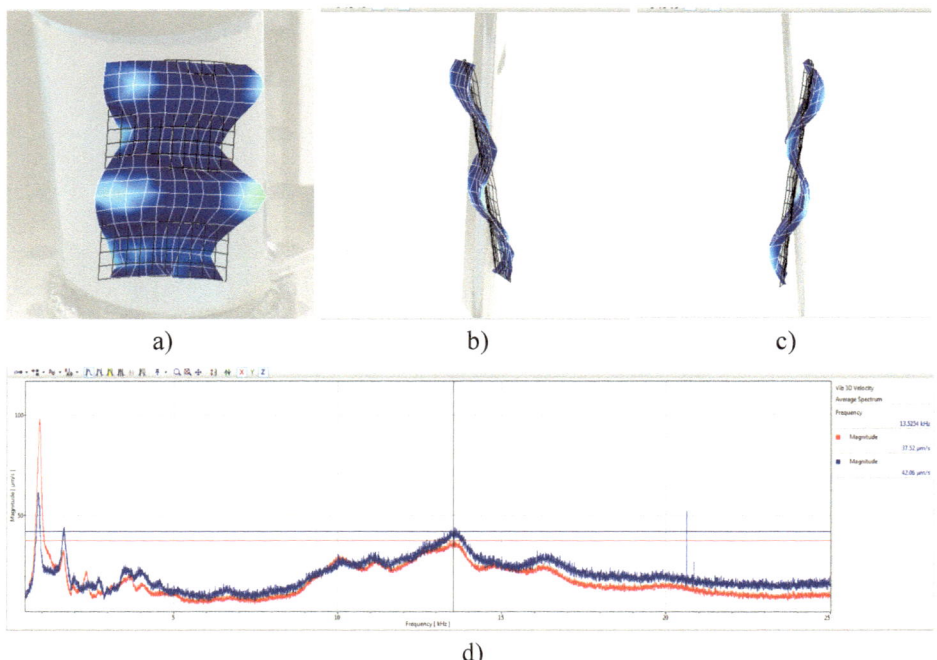

Fig. 4.14 Deformations of the wall (**a–c**) of the conical container at 13.52 kHz and its peak strain plot (**d**)

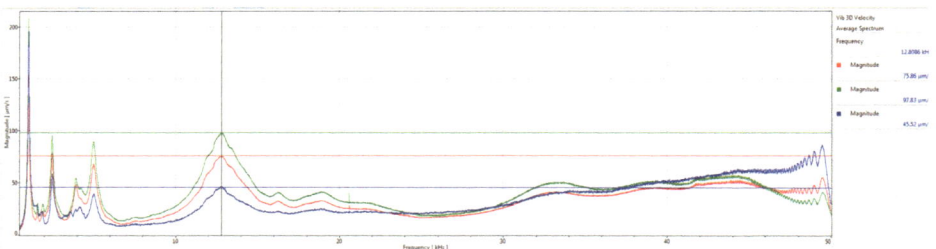

Fig. 4.15 Frequency response of the disc-shaped bimorph type piezoelectric transducer at 13.81 kHz

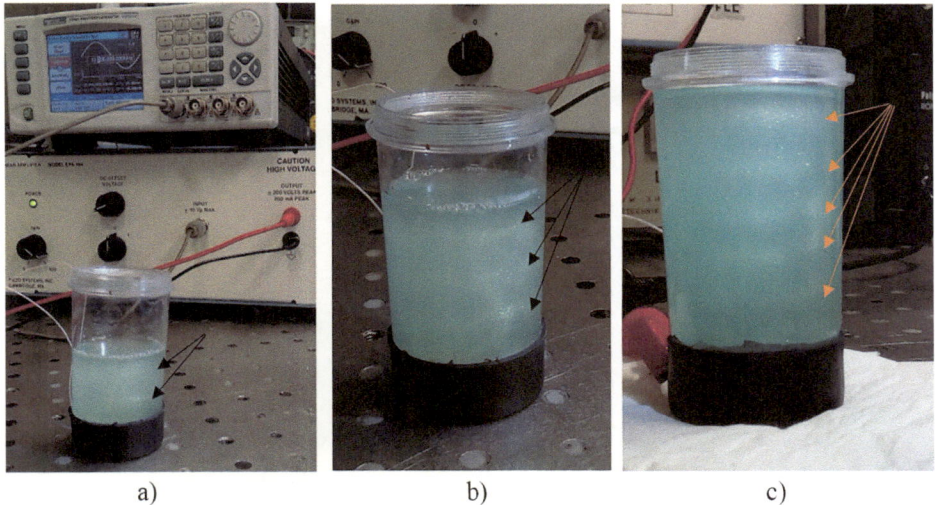

Fig. 4.16 Experimental set-up (**a**) and bioparticle concentration circles (**b**, **c**), depending on the height of the fluid column at a frequency of 12.2 kHz

4.4   Simulation of Ultrasonic Manipulation of Bioparticles

4.4.1   Ultrasonic Bioparticle Manipulation

The aim is to investigate the bioparticles separation possibility using ultrasonic frequency acoustic waves in fluid. For this purpose, a tube-shaped piezoceramic transducer was chosen (Fig. 4.17). For modeling a piezo-driven tube-shaped piezoceramic transducer for biofluid sonication has been used (with dimensions of $\varnothing15 \times \varnothing11 \times 27$mm). The piezo-ceramic material type PZT-4 [13] was used for the transducer. This material is ideally suited for ultrasonic, high-power acoustic radiation applications and can produce large mechanical drive amplitudes while maintaining low mechanical and dielectric losses. PZT-4 material properties are given in Table 4.1.

A tube-shaped piezoelectric cylinder element was filled with a fluid and excited at resonant frequency of $f_0 = 350$ kHz and the standing waves were simulated in it. The pressure field of the acoustic standing wave is shown in Fig. 4.18 as well as the acoustic pressure level in Fig. 4.19.

The acoustic radiation force on a compressible, spherical, micrometer-sized particle of radius $r = 5 \cdot 10^{-6}$ m suspended in a viscous fluid in an ultrasound field of wavelength $\lambda = 4.5 \cdot 10^{-3}$ m at room temperature was analyzed, thus $r \ll \lambda$. The numerical model contained a piezoelectric actuator cylinder with an internal radius of $R = 5.5 \cdot 10^{-3}$ m and a direct piezoelectric effect, which was electrically excited by harmonic law at frequencies $f_0 = 350$ kHz. The cylinder was filled with a fluid, and by exciting the piezoelectric cylinder at

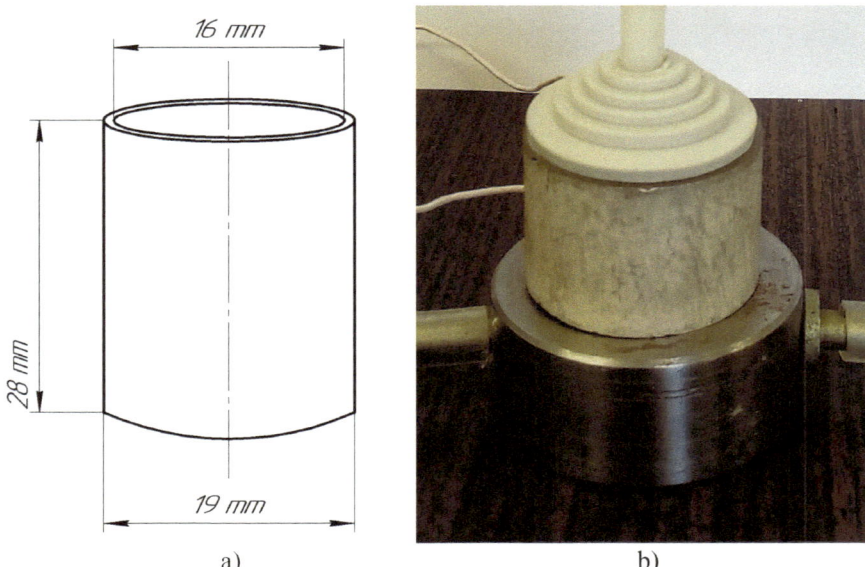

Fig. 4.17 **a**—Scheme of tube-shaped piezoceramic transducer for blood particles separation; **b**—photo of the tube-shaped piezoceramic transducer

Table 4.1 Physical properties of piezoceramic material type PZT-4

Density (10^3 kg/m^3)	7.7
Young's modulus (10^{10} N/m)	7.3
Curie point (°C)	350
Mechanical Q	1000
Relative dielectric constant $\varepsilon_{33}^T/\varepsilon_0$	1725
Dielectric loss (1 kHz)	0.4
k_{31}	0.32
k_p	0.54
d_{31} (10^{-12} m/V)	-130

a certain frequency, the standing waves were exposed in it. The modeling procedure was composed of two stages: in the first stage, the particles in a water suspension were simulated; in the second stage, blood properties were attributed to the biological suspension. Particle parameters were the same in both cases. A 2D model of the system was studied (Fig. 4.19). The model uses the following physical quantities: speed of sound in water: $c = 1.57 \cdot 10^3$ m/s; the speed of sound in biological suspension: $c = 1.48 \cdot 10^3$ m/s; $\rho_p = 4 \cdot 10^3$ kg/m^3 is the particle density; $K_p = 2.2$ GPa is a bulk modulus of the particle; and the amplitude of the excited acceleration of the transducer is $a_0 = 7.5 \cdot 10^6$ m/s^2.

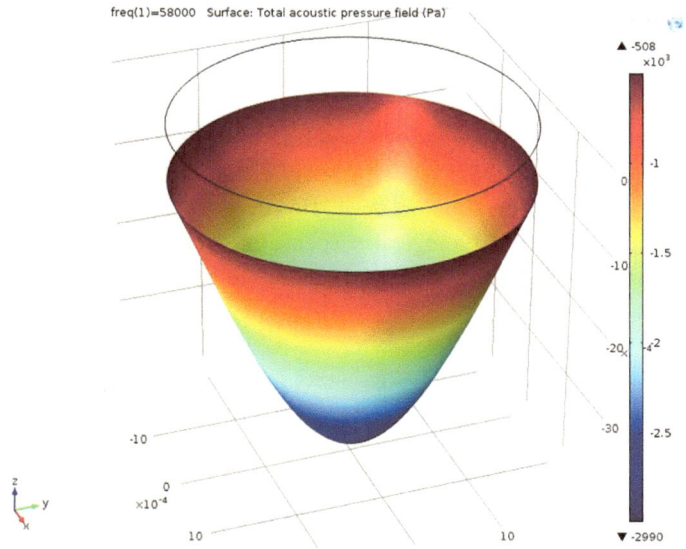

Fig. 4.18   Sound pressure field of the acoustic standing wave

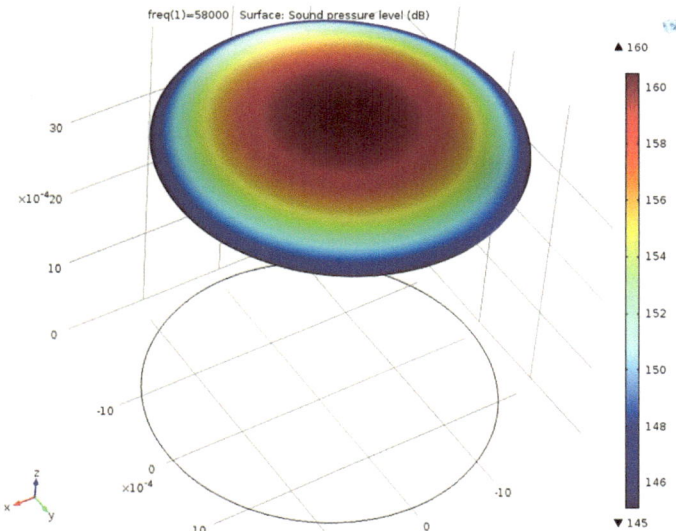

Fig. 4.19   Sound pressure level of acoustic standing wave

For the effective separation of bioparticles the frequency of excitation of the acoustic waves was chosen that concentrates the microparticles in two rings and equal to 350 kHz. The pressure fields of the standing waves in biological and in water suspension are shown in Fig. 4.20.

The acoustic pressure levels for these two substances are presented in Fig. 4.21.

The acoustic pressure field is analogous in both fluids, i.e., there are three high-pressure areas and two low-pressure areas in between. However, the low-pressure areas differ in different fluids: in the case of biological suspension, they are wider in comparison to those of water suspension. Consequently, this is caused by different parameter values of

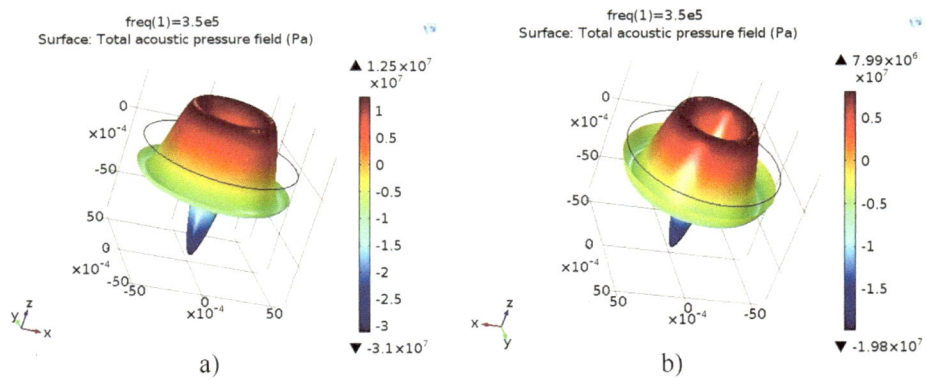

Fig. 4.20 Pressure field (Pa) of the standing wave in biological (**a**) and water suspension (**b**). Excitation frequency 350 kHz. The high-pressure area is represented in red and blue areas of low pressure. The values of the high and low pressure reach several kPa but in opposite directions

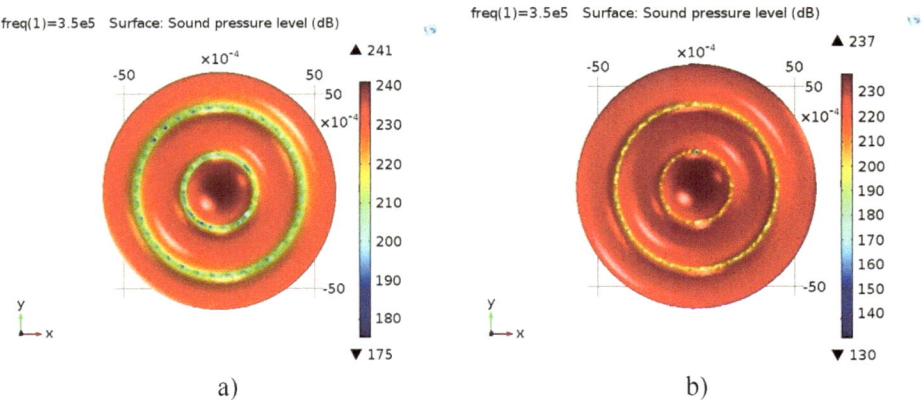

Fig. 4.21 Acoustic pressure level (dB) in biological (**a**) and water suspension (**b**). Excitation frequency 350 kHz

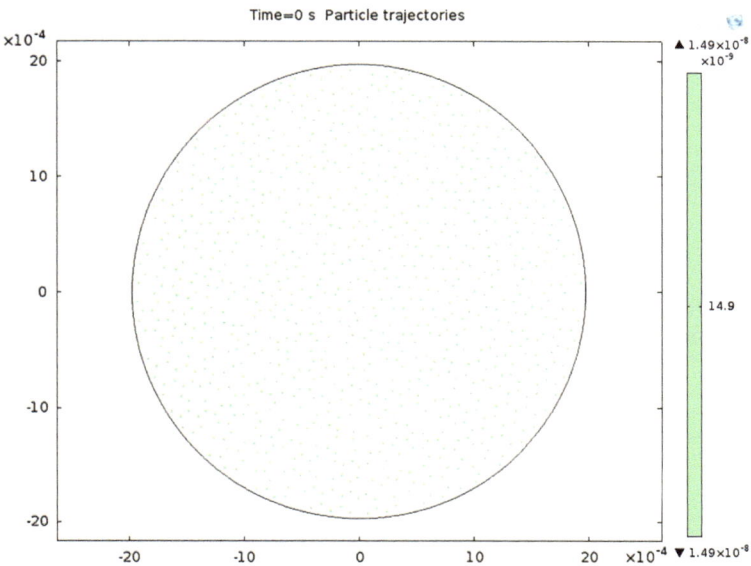

Fig. 4.22 The distribution of microparticles in the acoustic pressure field in the biological suspension at the initial moment of time t_0

the fluids (biological and water suspensions in this case). Due to standing acoustic waves, an acoustic radiation force arises which acts on microparticles. This force occurs due to pressure and acoustic field interaction with the microparticles. At the initial moment of time t_0, the microparticles are uniformly distributed in the acoustic field (Fig. 4.22), and later, due to the acoustic radiation forces and drag force that are generated, their movement begins.

The distribution of the microparticles in the acoustic field at different points in time is shown in Fig. 4.23 for biological suspension. The color of the microparticles represents the speed at the moment of time t_i which is calculated by integrating the equations of motion.

The distribution of the microparticles in the acoustic field at different points in time is shown in Fig. 4.24 for water suspension.

It was found that the distribution of both biological and water suspension microparticles in the acoustic pressure field is the same, yet the velocity of microparticle convergence to the low-level pressure field is different. When the fluid is water, the microparticles get into the low acoustic pressure field in 4s, whereas in the case of biological suspension, it takes twice the time, i.e., 8 s. Another difference between the fluids under investigation is the microparticle distribution in low acoustic pressure fields. Concentration areas of biological suspension microparticles at the end of the process, i.e., when the fluid becomes stationary, are broader in comparison to areas obtained using

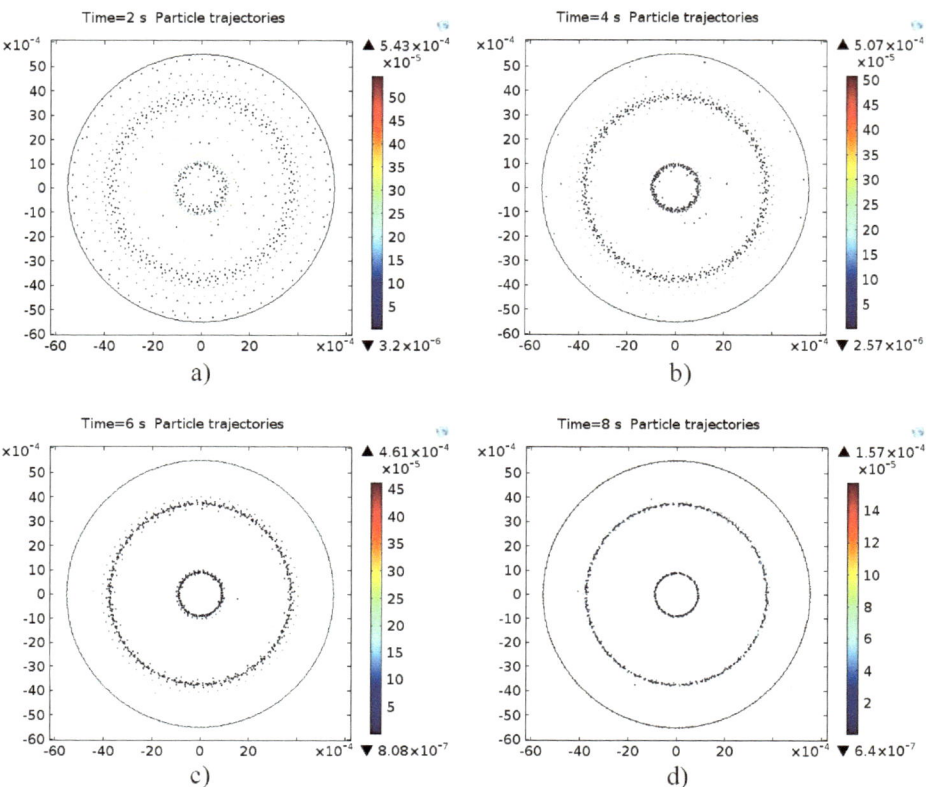

Fig. 4.23 The distribution of blood particles in the acoustic pressure field in the biological suspension at different times t_i: **a**—2 s; **b**—4 s; **c**—6 s; **d**—8 s

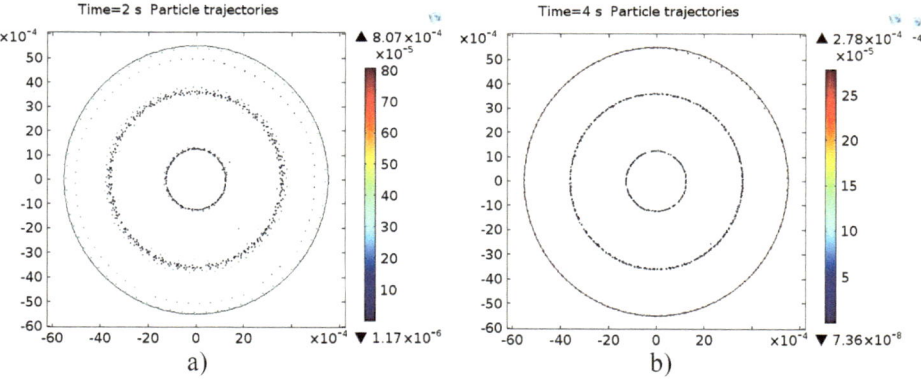

Fig. 4.24 The distribution of bioparticles in the acoustic pressure field for the water suspension at different time t_i: **a**—2 s; **b**—4 s

water as a fluid (see Fig. 4.24). Both peculiarities may be explained by different values of analyzed fluid properties. Finally, the third difference lies in the geometrical discrepancy of the small radius low acoustic pressure level areas: in the case of biological suspension as a fluid, the area radius is smaller by 30% in comparison to that of water suspension. This fact should be taken into consideration when separating biological suspensions of various viscosity. Considering this effect enables us to control the microparticles distribution in the desired areas of the acoustic field. This entails a quick and reliable microparticle concentration in the desired acoustic field areas (by changing the characteristics of vibrations generated by the transducer). This is a technological approach for the removal of microparticles from suspensions.

The simulation results have shown that bioparticle density does not affect the acoustic pressure, because it is created by an external effect, in this case it is the reverse piezo effect. But the density of the microparticles influences the separation time interval. This time interval is particularly increased when the fluid and the microparticle density ratio is approaching unity. As the fluid and the microparticle density ratio is very important, from the engineering point of view this ratio directly affects the tube-shaped piezoceramic transducer length. In our case the length of tube-shaped piezoceramic transducer and the flow rate of fluid were sufficient for the microparticles separation time interval equal to 8 s. In theory, if the fluid and the microparticle density are close the process of purification time increases considerably, thus requiring a larger length of a separator.

4.4.2   Experimental Validation of Bioparticles Separation by Ultrasonic Waves

To validate the results of modeling, experiments with a piezo-driven ultrasonic tube-shaped piezoceramic actuator for fluid sonication have been conducted [14, 15]. To assess the separation process of microparticles suspended in a suspension using ultrasonication and to determine vibrating deflection shapes and eigenmodes of the piezoceramic tube-shaped actuator, an experimental set-up with a Polytec 3D scanning vibrometer (Type PSV-500-3D-HV, Polytec GmbH, Waldron, Germany) was developed and is shown in Fig. 4.25a.

The experimental set-up consists of the scanning vibrometer 10, the piezoelectric tube-shaped actuator 6 driven by an ultrasonic frequency signal generator 1 (Agilent Technologies, Inc., Loveland, Colorado 80537, USA) and voltage amplifier 2 (P200— FLC Electronics AB, Sweden). For the fluid flow rate control and transfer to the actuator, a peristaltic pump 4 (model NP-1M, LOIP Ltd.) is used. Container 3 with the fluid is connected to the inlet tubing of the peristaltic pump, and the outlet tubing of the pump is connected to the inlet 5 of the tube-shaped actuator 6. The bottom end surface of a tube-shaped piezo actuator (dimensions $\varnothing 19 \times \varnothing 16 \times 28$ mm) is glued with elastic silicone to the ring-shape surface of outer diameter $\varnothing 17$ mm of the manufactured collector.

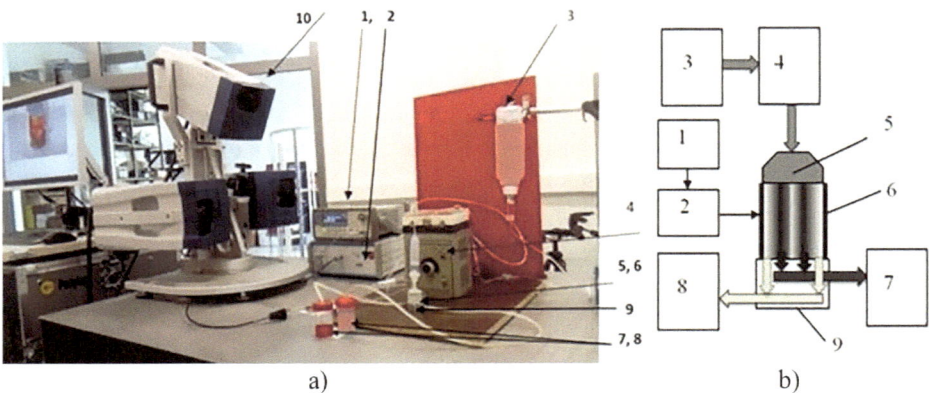

Fig. 4.25 Photo of the experimental set-up a and block diagram b for separation of blood particles: ultrasonic frequency signal generator (Agilent 33220A)—1, voltage amplifier P200 (FLC Electronics)—2, container of the suspension—3, peristaltic pump (model NP-1M)—4, inlet of the actuator—5, piezoelectric tube-shaped actuator—6, containers for the microparticles phase and the fluid phase—7 and 8, collector of the fluid—9 and Polytec 3D scanner-vibrometer—10

Sonication of the fluid is carried out using a tube-shaped actuator; an ultrasound standing wave is applied to separate/distribute microparticles in the researched fluid. The separated particles and liquid phase through the fluid collector 9 are collected in containers 7 and 8. The deformation of the piezoelectric tube-shaped actuator and its frequency response are measured by using Polytec 3D scanning vibrometer PSV-500-3D-HV (Polytec GmbH, Germany) 10.

A block diagram of the experimental set-up is presented in Fig. 4.25b. It explains the direction of fluid movement in the system for separation of blood particles suspended in a fluid. In the suspension container 3, fluid with bioparticles is stirred and transferred to the peristaltic pump 4, which regulates the flow rate of the fluid before entering the actuator inlet 5 and the separation chamber of the piezoelectric tube-shaped actuator 6. An ultrasonic standing wave sonication of the fluid in the flow was established by the piezoelectric actuator driven by signal generator 1 and the voltage amplifier 2. After sonication, the suspended blood particles were separated into an enriched and a cleared phase, by collector 9, and then they were transported into separate containers 7 and 8. The duration of the sonication process in the separation chamber of the tube-shaped actuator was controlled by the flow rate of the peristaltic pump 4. The stable separation pattern of blood particles was formed after 5–10 s and was monitored by the Nikon microscope Eclipse LV100 (Nikon Corp., Tokyo, Japan) with CMOS camera-INFINITY1-1C (Lumenera Corporation, Capella Court, Ottawa, ON, Canada).

In the experiments, blood particle suspensions of water and artificial blood, which correspond to human blood by their viscosity, density, and acoustic velocity parameters, were used. As a microparticle phase in the suspension, the material of zeolite with color

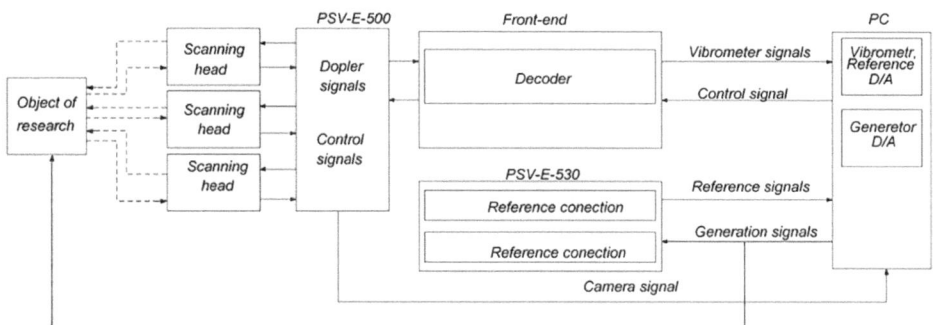

Fig. 4.26 Block-scheme of experimental setup with a Polytec 3D scanning vibrometer

pigments was used (made in SIGMA-ALDRICH 3050 Spruce Street, Saint Louis, MO 63103, USA). Microparticle dimensions were 0.5–15 μm.

To assess the separation process of blood particles suspended in a liquid using ultrasonic sonication and to determine vibrating deflection shapes and eigenmodes of the piezoceramic tube-shaped actuator, an experimental set-up with a Polytech 3D scanning vibrometer (Type PSV-500-3D-HV) was developed and is shown in Fig. 4.26.

The vibrating deflection shapes and eigenmodes of the tube-shaped piezoelectric actuator were determined by a Polytec 3D scanning vibrometer. The outer surface of the tubular actuator was virtually segmented, and each segment was 3D scanned. Figure 4.27a shows the scanned segment and the grid of the measurement points. To minimize the terrestrial gravity influence on a blood particle separation process, the tubular actuator was positioned vertically. To determine the resonance frequency of the researched actuator suitable for the blood particles separation, the frequency spectrum was obtained in an operational frequency range from 100 to 650 kHz.

Figure 4.27b–d show the deformations of the scanned surface of the actuator (a segment of the outer surface) at operational frequency 345 kHz with different fluids. Measurements were taken for the actuator without a suspension (Fig. 4.27b), with a water-based suspension (Fig. 4.31c) and with a biological suspension-synthetic viscous fluid (Fig. 4.27d). As can be seen from the results deformations of the actuator without and with the viscous fluid are similar. This is due to viscous damping and fluid inertia. The frequency spectra of the actuator with the fluid were measured with a 3D scanner (Fig. 4.28) and confirmed the simulation results.

A stable resonance frequency of 345 kHz allowed to obtain a constant fluid flow separation into fractions. At a frequency of 202 kHz, the amplitude of deformation is the greatest, but the practical study showed flow instability that led to suspension mixing rather than its separation. So, we had to give up the greater amplitude to continually collect blood particles and move them to the desired trajectory of the audio signal. Here, (a) denotes the deformation in the fluid without suspension, (b) stands for a signal for a water

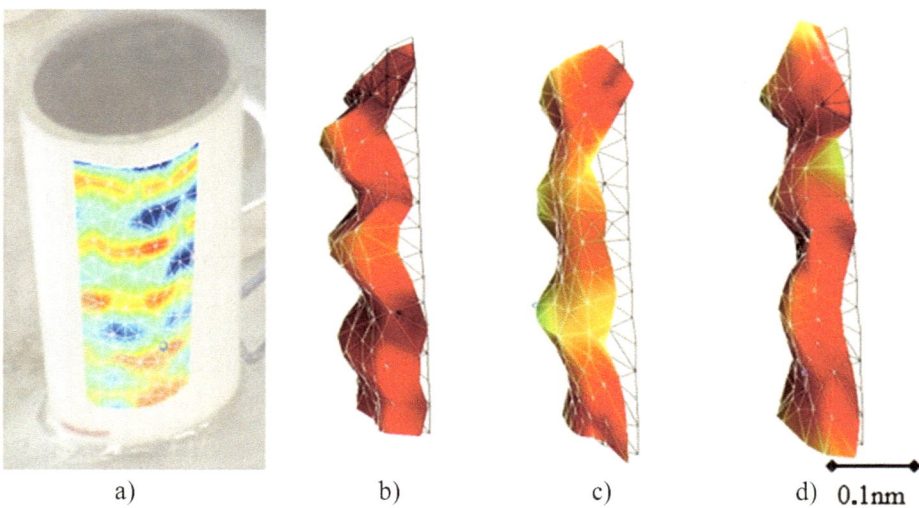

Fig. 4.27 Photo of the tube-shaped prototype actuator and a segment of its surface **a**, which is 3D-scanned to determine vibrating deflection shapes and eigenmodes of the actuator **b–d**

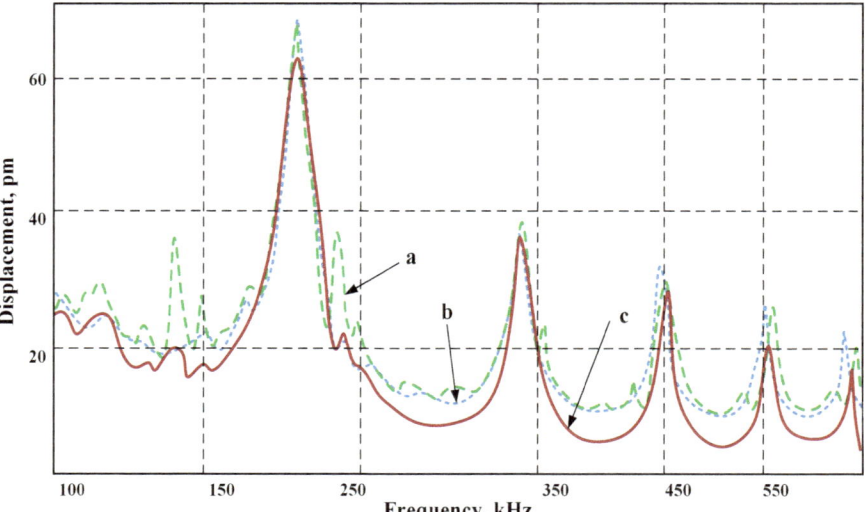

Fig. 4.28 Frequency average spectrum of the actuator scanned surface obtained by measurement via a 3D scanner: **a**—fluid without suspension; **b**—with water suspension; **c**—with biological suspension-viscous fluid

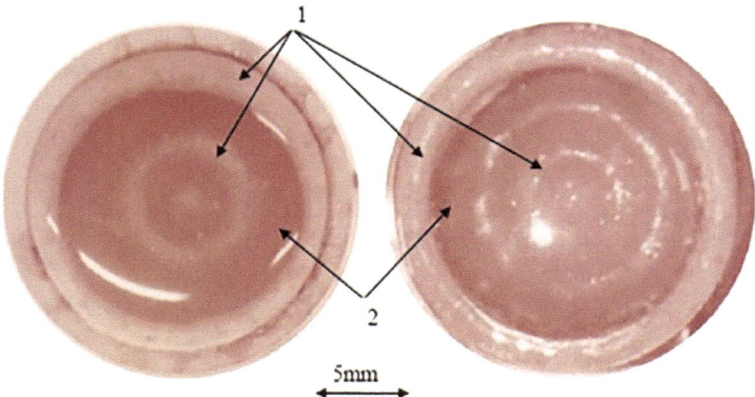

Fig. 4.29 The distribution of the blood particles in the cylinder with suspension under the influence of a standing ultrasonic wave: **a**—excitation frequency of 202 kHz; **b**—excitation frequency of 345 kHz

suspension and (c) describes the operation when using a biological suspension-viscous fluid. As can be seen from the chart, with a viscous flow there is a certain quenching strain on non-resonant frequencies.

The separation of the bioparticles from suspension in the piezoelectric cylinder under the influence of the standing ultrasonic wave is shown in Fig. 4.29. For comparison, data are given for a frequency of 202 kHz (Fig. 4.29a) and for a frequency of 345 kHz (Fig. 4.29b). The time spent on the separation of the suspension flow into fractions was 4 s for a water-based fluid and 8 s for a biological suspension-viscous fluid.

4.4.3 Evaluation of the Effect of High and Low Frequency Ultrasound on Bioparticles

In the first chapter, we revealed the influence of low-frequency ultrasound on the separation of erythrocytes from aggregates, while in this chapter we propose the opposite technology—the application of high-frequency ultrasound in concentrating or aggregating bioparticles. These results confirm that high-frequency ultrasound concentrates bioparticles in the nodal zones of the standing acoustic wave, unlike the traveling acoustic wave of low-frequency ultrasound, which breaks up erythrocyte aggregates. The results of both the simulation (Fig. 4.23) and the experimental study (Fig. 4.29) of this chapter show that the concentration of bioparticles into aggregates takes about 8 s, while the opposite process of separation of erythrocytes from aggregates under the influence of low-frequency ultrasound begins in the second minute of the natural experiment with sheep evaluating variation in oxygen concentration in the blood (Fig. 2.29), variation in sheep pulse rate

(Fig. 2.30) and changes in blood pressure (Fig. 2.31). In addition to the obvious confirmation of the differences between low and high frequency ultrasound, we see that the effect of ultrasound on a living organism is slowed down compared to its direct effect on the blood. This can be explained by the interaction between the living body and many very complex effects of ultrasound on it.

4.5   Bioparticles Separation Devices

4.5.1   Sonic Frequency Acoustic Waves Device for Bioparticles Separation

To carry out the experiment with fluid, a plexiglass flask, a piezoceramic bimorph disk-shape transducer and a suspension of water and glycerin 50/50%, silicate mica with a particle size of 5–15 μm and a water-soluble pigment staining for contrasting results were used. A device was also developed and patented [16] that would allow the separation of concentrated accumulations of microparticles and fluids. Schematic diagram of the device is shown in Fig. 4.30, where 1—is a container of the fluid with microparticles; 2—inlet valve; 3—a chamber of the acoustic separator with fluid; 4—disc-shaped bimorph type piezoelectric transducer; 5—enriched phase of the fluid; 6—cleared phase of the fluid; 7—outlet valve of the enriched phase of the suspension; 8—outlet valve of the cleaned phase of the suspension; 9—an air escape valve. When the control valve is opened on container 1, through the inlet valve 2 the suspension enters the chamber of the acoustic separator composed from conical vessel 3 and piezoelectric disc-shaped bimorph 4, where, under the action of the acoustic standing wave, the microparticles drift in the volume of the fluid and accumulate in the nodal zones of the vessel wall standing wave. Then the enriched phase of the suspension from nodal circles through the outlet valve 7 flows to container 5 and are cleaned from microparticles phase of the suspension, and through the outlet valve 8 flows to the container 6. Valve 9 serves for air escape.

According to this scheme, a device was assembled, which is shown in Fig. 4.31.

When examining the conical container of the acoustic separator after 12 s, it can be seen microparticles accumulated on its wall (Fig. 4.32).

Since the disk-shaped bimorph type piezoelectric transducer vibration modes are different at different frequencies, the following effect occurs in the first and second modes: active mixing of the suspension due to large parasitic forces, such as radiation pressure and streaming has place, and it is not possible to obtain one or two stable circles of particle concentration on the inner surface of container resonator. When switching to a higher mode, the number of concentration circles increases, but the radiation pressure no longer has such a great mixing influence. As a result, a stable process of the distribution of microparticles in a suspension without mixing streaming, which prevented from the formation of concentric zones, was obtained (Fig. 4.33).

Fig. 4.30 Schematics of the blood particle separation system: 1—is a container of the fluid with microparticles; 2—inlet valve; 3—a chamber of the acoustic separator with fluid; 4—disc-shaped bimorph type piezoelectric transducer; 5—enriched phase of the fluid; 6—cleaned phase of the fluid; 7—outlet valve of the enriched phase of the suspension; 8—outlet valve of the cleaned phase of the suspension; 9—air escape valve

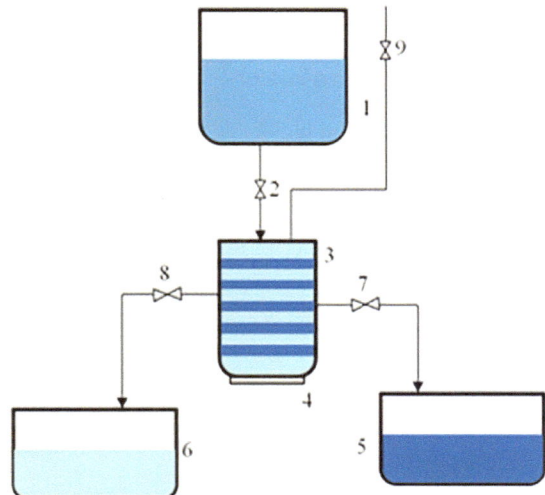

Fig. 4.31 Device for the blood particle separation: 1—is a container of the fluid with microparticles; 2—inlet valve; 3—a conical container of the acoustic separator with fluid; 4—disc-shaped bimorph type piezoelectric transducer; 5—enriched phase of the fluid; 6—cleaned phase of the fluid; 7—outlet valve of the enriched phase of the suspension; 8—outlet valve of the cleaned phase of the suspension; 9—air escape valve

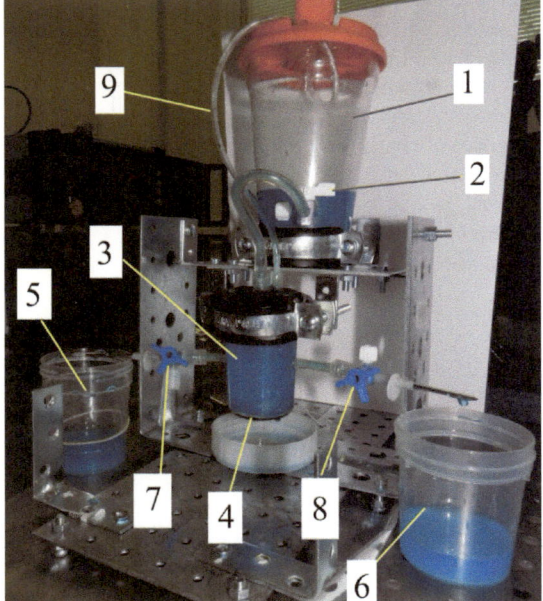

It is known from the classical theory of the propagation of acoustic waves that the wavelength of sound could be found from the equation:

$$\lambda = v/f \tag{4.21}$$

where, λ is the wavelength, v is the wave velocity, and f is the wave frequency.

Fig. 4.32 Arrangement of
concentrated zones with blood
particles in a suspension under
the influence of acoustic
waves, frequency 13.5 kHz

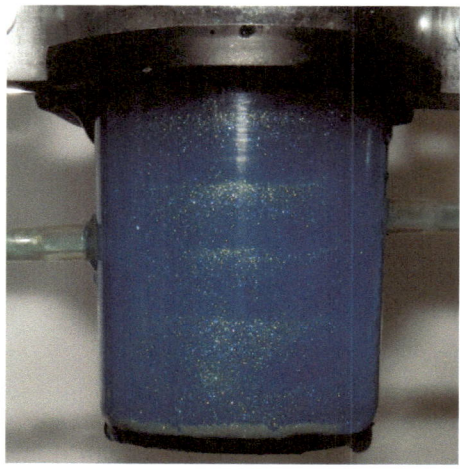

Fig. 4.33 Distribution of
microparticles in a suspension
at piezoelectric transducer
mode of 13.5 kHz frequency:
1—container with
microparticles in a suspension,
2—zones of concentration of
microparticles in a suspension
column, 3—a disk-shaped
bimorph type piezoelectric
transducer

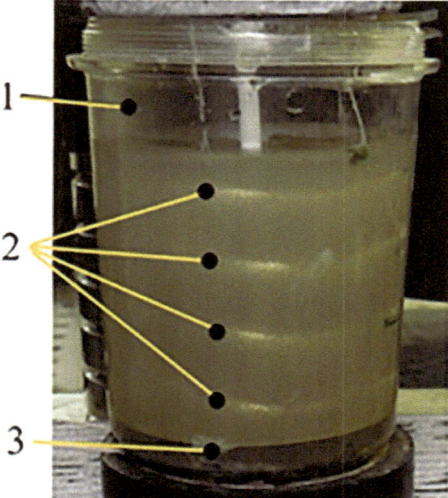

Based on this formula, it's possible to calculate the wavelength in the fluid at $v = 1430$ m/s and $f = 13,500$ Hz is 0.1059 m. It turns out that the height of the container for obtaining at least one concentric circle of bioparticles on the container inside wall should be equal to or greater than 0.11 m. The experimental data showed that the wavelength in the container with to the bottom attached active disc-shaped bimorph type piezoelectric transducer was 0.02 m, which according to the classical formula should be obtained at a frequency $f = v/\lambda = 1430/0.02 = 71.50$ kHz. To confirm the classical theory, a vibration single-component vibrator was used, with a range of operating frequencies from 100 Hz to 80 kHz. The resonant frequency of this vibrator was at 70.5 kHz, the fluid used was the same as for the previous experiments. The wavelength in this case was 0.021 m, which corresponds to the received data. Thus, with the help of disc-shaped bimorph type piezoelectric transducer it was possible with the sonic frequency and low power acoustical excitation to obtain the same results as for the ultrasonic frequency of powerful vibrators.

4.5.2 Ultrasonic Acoustic Waves Device for Bioparticles Separation

For the extraction of bioparticles from biological suspension, the special collector was designed, manufactured and patented [17] (Fig. 4.34). The distribution of channels of this collector are in the circles which diameters coincide with the diameters of acoustic standing wave nodes circles or low-pressure areas in which the bioparticles precipitate (Fig. 4.29). After eight seconds of ultrasonic treatment in the tube-shaped piezoceramic cylinder the enriched by bioparticles mixture was accumulated via collectors' channels.

To determine the effectiveness of the bioparticles separation in suspension, two separate samples were examined under a microscope. The results are shown in Fig. 4.35. The image (a) depicts a sample of microparticles in biological suspension before and (b) after separation procedure.

With these results, it can be concluded that even for suspensions with bioparticles of different shape and density, separation in the suspension is possible.

As only the physical experiment with elaborated purification device could confirm the appropriateness of a mathematical model, the experimental set-up was assembled to ensure precise measurements. Two types of fluid suspension were considered: biological and water that included the microparticles of the diameter of erythrocytes. We choose

Fig. 4.34 Photo of manufactured collector: 1—openings for collection of the blood particles enriched phase; 2—openings for collection of the suspension phase; 3—volume of the suspension phase

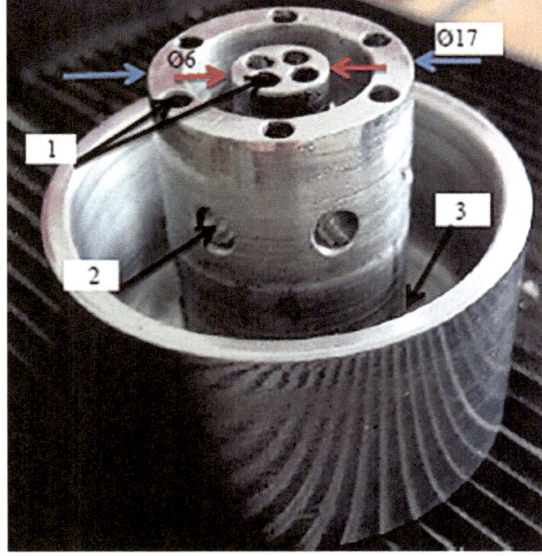

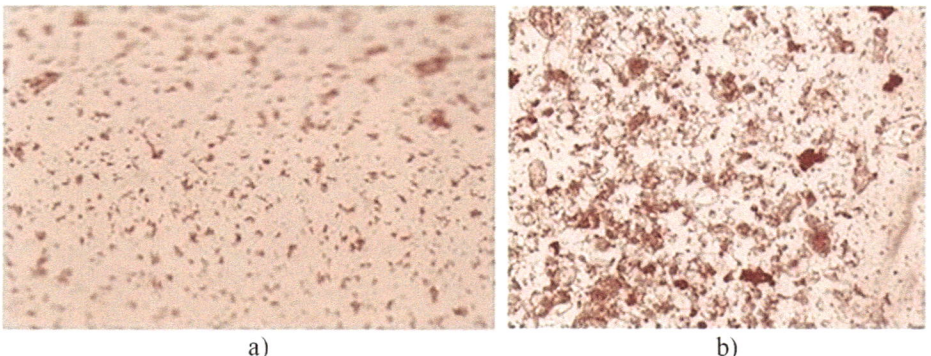

a)   b)

Fig. 4.35 Microscopic view of the biological suspension samples before (**a**) and after (**b**) bioparticles separation procedure

these types of suspensions to demonstrate the universality and validity of the proposed separation technologies by experiment, which would be complicated due to the rapidly changing properties of erythrocytes in the blood. Standard guidelines for blood sample handling state that plasma or serum should be separated (20–30 min) from cells as soon as possible after clot formation is complete to avoid clot-induced changes in the concentration of serum analytes [18]. Agglutination of erythrocytes can occur within a few minutes after finding the blood outside the body. Separately, the same red blood cell mass, when maintained at room temperature for more than 1 h, is not to be used for transfusion; rather, it should be sent for recycling. For experimentation, artificial blood was taken to act as a substitute for erythrocytes [19]. While true blood serves many different functions, artificial blood is designed for the purpose of transporting oxygen and carbon dioxide throughout the body.

Two main parameters of the microparticles that form a nodal circle are related to the fluid acoustical excitation frequency and constructive dimensions of the piezo actuator. Since the number of nodal circles or low-pressure areas in which the solid microparticles precipitate is increased by higher frequencies and was concentrated at frequency of 345 kHz the lower frequency of 202 kHz was abandoned in favor of stable and efficient acoustic forces produced at a frequency of 345 kHz. The diameters of microparticles concentration circles coincide in both simulation and experimentation cases.

As it was shown experimentally and theoretically, the diameters of microparticle aggregation circles for both suspensions were identical, whereas the period of circle formation differed two-fold. This period (from 4 to 8 s) could be considered as very short compared to other known methods of blood purification [20]. Keeping in mind the simplicity of purified particle separation from biological suspensions, this method could be used in different emergency situations to keep spilled blood ready for further use. The results show that by increasing the amount of fluid and moving it away from the microarray, it is possible to get the same results as in the microflow [21]. Even though biological fluid is very suscep-tible to the influence of ultrasonic signals, our experience has shown that the frequency of 345 kHz is safe for cell membranes [22]. Whereas a theory should make predictions, and a good theory's predictions should be supported by the results of the experiment, the matching of simulation (350 kHz) and experimentally obtained (345 kHz) ultrasonic exci-tation frequencies as well as coincidence of the diameters of blood particles concentration circles in both—simulation and experimentation cases testify that the mathematical model imitates the real blood purification process.

Ethical Statement The study of human pulmonary arteries was conducted according to the princi-ples defined in the Declaration of Helsinki [23]. Permission to perform this study was obtained from the local institutional review board of the Kaunas Regional Biomedical Research Ethics Committee (No. 2022-03-10 Nr. BE-2-39).

Permission to perform experimental research with animals was obtained from the Lithuanian experimental animal ethics board by Lithuanian veterinary and food services (Issued date 2022-02-02; Nr. G2-195).

References

1. Ostasevicius V, Jurenas V, Golinka I, Gaidys R, Aleksa A (2018) Separation of microparti-cles from suspension utilizing ultrasonic standing waves in a piezoelectric cylinder actuator. Actuators 7(2–14):1–12
2. Wang S, Allen JS, Ardekani AM (2017) Unsteady particle motion in an acoustic standing wave field. Eur J Comput Mech 26(1–2):115–130
3. Wang J, Dual J (2012) Theoretical and numerical calculation of the acoustic radiation force act-ing on a circular rigid cylinder near a flat wall in a standing wave excitation in an ideal fluid. Ultrasonics 52(2):325–332
4. Saadatmand M (2012) A study on vibration-induced particle motion under microgravity. PhD thesis, University of Toronto, p 259
5. Settnes M, Bruus H (2012) Forces acting on a small particle in an acoustical field in a viscous fluid. Phys Rev E 85(016327):1–12
6. Gor'kov LP (1962) On the forces acting on a small particle in an acoustical field in an ideal fluid. Sov Phys Dokl 6:773
7. Sezer N, Koc M (2021) A comprehensive review on the state-of-the-art of piezoelectric energy harvesting. Nano energy 80, 105567:1–25
8. Palevicius A, Ragulskis K, Bubulis A, Ostasevicius V, Ragulskis M (2004) Development and operational optimization of micro spray system. In: Proceedings of SPIE the international soci-ety for optical engineering, vol 5390, p 0277
9. Ostasevicius V, Jurenas V, Zukauskas M (2014) Investigation of energy harvesting from high frequency cutting tool vibrations. Mexanika 20(5):500–505
10. Lichnov P (1988) Dynamics of a system with cylindrical shell. Mashinostroenije
11. Vasiliauskas R, Palevicius A, Ragulskis K (1988) Analysis of holographic interferograms of ultrasonic piezoelectric transducers in the investigation of three-dimensional vibrations. J Sov Phys Acoust 34(6)

12. Ostasevicius V, Jurenas V, Gaidys R, Golinka I, Kizauskiene L, Mikuckyte S (2020) Development of a piezoelectric actuator for separation and purification of biological microparticles. Actuators 9(3):61:1–13
13. Morgan Advanced Materials (2016) High-density, defect-free PZT components from Morgan
14. Ostasevicius V, Golinka I (2015) Theoretical and experimental investigation to improve particles separation in liquid. In: Mechatronic systems and materials: abstracts of the 11th international conference, MSM 2015, pp 115–116
15. Ostasevicius V, Golinka I, Jurenas V, Gaidys R (2017) High frequency separation of suspended micro/nanoparticles. Mechanika 23(3):408–411
16. Ostasevicius V, Jurenas V, Kizauskiene L, Bubulis A, Gaidys R (2021) Acoustic suspension separation device, Patent LT 6834 B
17. Bubulis A, Jurenas V, Golinka I, Ostasevicius V, Gaidys R (2018) Ultrasonic emulsion separation device. Patent LT 6568 B
18. Turchiano M, Nguyen C, Fierman A, Lifshitz M, Convit A (2013) Impact of blood sample collection and processing methods on glucose levels in community outreach studies. J Environ Public Health (3) 256151:4
19. Otterstedt JE, Brandreth DA (2013) Small particles technology. Springer Science & Business Media, pp 206–208
20. Stegmayr BG (2005) A survey of blood purification techniques. Transfusion Apher Sci 32(2):209–220
21. Devendran C, Gralinski I, Neild A (2014) Separation of particles using acoustic streaming and radiation forces in an open microfluidic channel. Microfluid Nanofluid 17:879–890
22. Wu J, Nyborg WL (2008) Ultrasound, cavitation bubbles and their interaction with cells. Adv Drug Deliv Rev 60:1103–1116
23. Carlson RV, Boyd KM, Webb DJ (2004) The revision of the declaration of Helsinki: past, present and future. Br J Clin Pharm 57(6):695–713

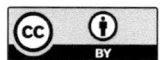